Oxford Medical Publications

Postpsychiatry

International Perspectives in Philosophy and Psychiatry

Series editors

Bill (KWM) Fulford
Katherine Morris
John Z Sadler
Giovanni Staghellini

Other volumes in the series:

Mind, Meaning and Mental Disorder, 2e
Bolton and Hill

Disembodied Spirits and Deanimated Bodies
Giovanni Stanghellini

Nature and Narrative
Fulford, Morris, Sadler and Stanghellini (eds)

The Philosophy of Psychiatry
Radden (ed)

Values and Psychiatric Diagnosis
Sadler

Forthcoming books in the series:

Oxford Textbook of Philosophy and Psychiatry
Fulford, Thornton, and Graham

Postpsychiatry

Patrick Bracken

and

Philip Thomas

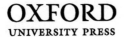

OXFORD
UNIVERSITY PRESS

OXFORD

UNIVERSITY PRESS

Great Clarendon Street, Oxford OX2 6DP

Oxford University Press is a department of the University of Oxford.
It furthers the University's objective of excellence in research, scholarship,
and education by publishing worldwide in

Oxford New York

Auckland Cape Town Dar es Salaam Hong Kong Karachi
Kuala Lumpur Madrid Melbourne Mexico City Nairobi
New Delhi Shanghai Taipei Toronto

With offices in

Argentina Austria Brazil Chile Czech Republic France Greece
Guatemala Hungary Italy Japan Poland Portugal Singapore
South Korea Switzerland Thailand Turkey Ukraine Vietnam

Oxford is a registered trade mark of Oxford University Press
in the UK and in certain other countries

Published in the United States
by Oxford University Press Inc., New York

British Library Cataloguing in Publication Data

Data available

Library of Congress Cataloging in Publication Data

Data available

Typeset by Newgen Imaging Systems (P) Ltd., Chennai, India
Printed in Great Britain
on acid-free paper by
Biddles Ltd., King's Lynn

ISBN 0-19-852609-1   978-0-19-852609-4

Acknowledgements

We are very grateful to Bill Fulford and the other editors of this series for the invitation to contribute.

We have been influenced by many individuals over the past few years, in particular those service users who have written about their experiences of distress and of using services. We also want to pay tribute to our professional colleagues in Bradford who have made our work in that city so enjoyable over the past few years. Forward-thinking individuals in Bradford District Care Trust and the University of Bradford gave us the space and encouragement to develop the ideas contained in the book.

Some individuals have made important contributions to particular chapters. Robin Holt offered detailed comments about Chapter 5 for which we are extremely grateful. Much of Chapter 5 would not have been possible without the insights of Ivan Leudar. Chapter 7 benefited enormously from lengthy discussions about the complexity of representation in art and anthropology with Rebecca Thomas, now a doctoral student in visual anthropology at Goldsmiths College, University of London. Sara Maitland's encouragement, enthusiasm and understanding made it much easier for us to write the short stories that are scattered through the text.

But most of all we acknowledge the love and support of our families, especially Joan and Stella, who patiently listened, read and argued with us, and so often put us right. We are grateful to the Ovion Publishing group Ltd., for their permission to quote two lines from 'The Old Language'—a poem by R. S. Thomas, published in *Collected Poems*—at the end of *Doing their best*, (p 26).

Lastly, we would mention the New Beehive public house in the centre of Bradford. It served as our local pub for many years and was where we originally knocked around the idea of postpsychiatry.

Contents

Introduction

'The times they are a changin'

We live through exciting times. Across the world, new ways of thinking about mental health are opening up, ways which few would have thought possible even 10 years ago. Everywhere, groups of service users[1] are coming together to challenge prejudices in the system and to raise demands for more thoughtful forms of support. This user movement is here to stay. Its voice is loud and will not be silenced.

In the preface to his book *Madness and Civilization*, the French philosopher Michel Foucault famously wrote that, since the time of the European Enlightenment, 'the language of psychiatry (has been) a monologue of reason *about* madness' (Foucault 1971, xii–xiii). However, at the dawn of the 21st century, there are signs that real *dialogues* are beginning to take place between those who experience episodes of madness and dislocation and the society in which they live. 'Voluntary sector' or 'non-governmental organizations (NGOs)' which represent the views of service users and/or carers are playing an increasingly important role in both the economically advantaged (EA) and economically disadvantaged (ED) countries. Although these organizations all work to different agendas, they are beginning to provide interventions that are very different in form and orientation from those in the hospitals and clinics of more traditional statutory services.

The winds of change are also beginning to blow through the professional sector. Many mental health nurses, psychologists, occupational therapists, managers and social workers, who have long argued for user involvement in the planning and development of services, are now being joined by a growing number of psychiatrists who are waking up to the positive benefits of working in collaboration with users and carers, and are joining the call for change. Many professionals have been genuinely appalled by the stories of service users and their suffering within 'the system', and want to make services more accountable.

Before we are accused of hopeless optimism, let us quickly say that we are acutely aware that there are other forces working to steer the mental health agenda in a very different direction. The power and wealth of the pharmaceutical

---

[1] We use the terms 'service user' 'user' 'client' 'patient' and 'survivor' interchangeably throughout the text. We are aware that there is an on-going debate about the significance of different forms of terminology.

industry has pushed a great deal of academic psychiatry down a very narrow path. Independent scientific research on the biology of distress is increasingly hard to come by, as medical schools and universities across the world dance to the tune of corporate sponsors. In some countries, sections of the media seem very keen to portray users of mental health services as a 'threat to society', and unfortunately some politicians have been happy to jump on board this particular bandwagon. Some governments are intent on legislating for more coercion. Professionals often feel overburdened with bureaucratic paperwork and are intimidated by a 'blame culture' which is very prevalent in many sections of the public service. Adequate funding for the sorts of interventions that allow people with mental health problems to participate fully in society is hard to come by.

Nevertheless, we are convinced that change is happening and new possibilities are beginning to arise. We hope that our book will contribute to this process. Although we are psychiatrists and our focus is on the fundamental assumptions of our own discipline, our intention is to make what we write of interest to users, carers, managers, other professionals, indeed to anyone who feels that the ways in which we look after one another in times of distress is something that concerns us all.

We do not propose a new 'model' for mental health work; there are plenty of these around already. In fact, we find that our professional models, agendas and frameworks are sometimes part of the problem. We want to expose the ways in which the formulations and interventions of psychiatry can serve to silence any other debate. In the past 10 years, we have had the privilege of working closely with service user organizations mainly in England, Wales and Ireland, but also internationally. We have developed a profound respect for the sort of agendas emerging within this movement. We believe that this is where the future lies. If postpsychiatry means anything, it means an end to the 'monologue of reason about madness'.

In the rest of this introductory chapter, we will first introduce the basic thrust of our analysis and then give a brief chapter by chapter account of the book's contents. We expect that few people will read the book from cover to cover. Indeed, we intend it more as a book that people might come back to from time to time. Likewise, we expect that different readers will find some chapters of more interest and use than others. We expect that few will agree with everything we write! At the same time, we are hopeful that our arguments will stimulate discussion, debate and change.

An emerging contradiction between clinical and academic psychiatry

We first used the term 'postpsychiatry' as the header for a series of articles written for the UK mental health magazine *Open Mind* at the end of the 1990s. We do not claim to have originated the word. Peter Campbell first used it in a chapter in the anthology *Speaking Our Minds*, published in 1996[2]. While we had learned a great deal from the various forms of antipsychiatry and critical psychiatry that emerged between the 1960s and 1980s, we wanted to show how our approach differed from these. We described it as something positive: an attempt to imagine a form of medical encounter with states of distress, alienation and madness, which did not operate with the central assumptions that had guided psychiatry through the 20th century[3].

In these articles, we questioned traditional psychiatric ideas about the nature of knowledge and expertise, and such things as diagnosis, treatment and the social position of psychiatrists. Our critique had the explicit aim of opening up spaces in which other voices could be heard. We repeatedly made the point that service users (individually and in partnerships) had the answers themselves. They were developing new ways of understanding states of madness and distress and had clear ideas about how professionals could help or hinder. Our primary task was to listen to and support this emerging discourse. Feedback on the articles we wrote was generally positive and a number of people asked us to elaborate on the idea of 'postpsychiatry'. We did so in a paper published by the *British Medical Journal* in 2001. This paper generated a good deal of controversy, and from it the idea for this book came into being.

Since 2001, we have been asked to address psychiatrists throughout the UK and have had positive contacts from many others in North America, Europe, Australia and New Zealand and a number of ED countries. While our ideas are still controversial and by no means mainstream, a growing number of our colleagues are telling us that the things we are saying resonate with their own experiences. As we write, a session on the theme of postpsychiatry is scheduled for the next AGM of the Royal College of Psychiatrists, to be held in Edinburgh in June, 2005, in a day devoted to critical psychiatry.

Interestingly, we have found that psychiatrists who work mainly in clinical settings are more interested in (and open to) the challenges we present. In general, academic colleagues[4] appear less prepared to doubt and to question their assumptions. In the UK and other countries, an increasing number of clinical psychiatrists work in multi-disciplinary teams and are actively involved in planning and developing services. Increasingly, they are working outside hospitals, and in their day-to-day work they meet with user groups and other non-medical organizations. Through such encounters, they have become sensitized to the

---

[2]Campbell (1996).

[3]In this sense, postpsychiatry means 'after psychiatry'. However, we also wanted to connect our work with the insights of a number of postmodern thinkers such as Michel Foucault and others. These connections will emerge in the text.

[4]There are notable exceptions here. We are aware of the important stand taken up by Alec Jenner who, for many years as professor of psychiatry in Sheffield, maintained and fostered an interest in philosophy. His pioneering work resulted in the birth of the radical mental health magazine *Asylum* (http://www.asylumonline.net/index.htm) which involved many local service users in writing for and producing the magazine. Today, our colleagues Joanna Moncrieff, Mike Crawford and Jonathan Bindman are now senior academics working in London.

ways in which many users of mental health services have experienced psychiatry as oppressive. Until recently, contact between doctors and patients only happened in clinical settings, and the power differential in these meant that the patient's views were often silenced.

The changes in the way that psychiatrists encounter service users in their daily work has led to more and more psychiatrists wanting to examine the assumptions behind their work. This is reflected in the fact that the Special Interest Group in Philosophy and Psychiatry is one of the largest of such groups in the UK Royal College. Other large Special Interest Groups are dedicated to spirituality, religion, history and transcultural issues. These groups are made up of ordinary working psychiatrists who are questioning the outlook of psychiatry in an open and exciting manner.

At the same time, increasing numbers of psychiatrists are participating in the Critical Psychiatry Network (CPN)[5]. This is a loose grouping of psychiatrists in the UK who are attempting to prevent any extension of the coercive side of psychiatric practice while also struggling to expose and limit corporate (largely pharmaceutical) influence on the discipline. At the time of writing, there is much interest in developing similar networks in other countries, such as the USA. Although we are aware that there are still many psychiatrists who prefer to hold on to traditional ways of practising and are not prepared to question these, we are also increasingly aware of those who want to work closely with service users to develop different sorts of services, with different goals and priorities, and as a result are interested in examining the role and values of psychiatry in a non-defensive manner.

However, whilst these developments have been taking place, as reflected in developments in the UK Royal College and elsewhere, much of *academic* psychiatry has been moving in a very different direction. In parallel with other branches of medicine, psychiatry has been a major growth area for the pharmaceutical industry[6]. Many medical academics have close links with the industry and there is evidence that many prominent research agendas have been developed on the back of these links. With a few notable exceptions, most university-based psychiatrists are involved in some form of biological research (particularly genetic or biochemical), as reflected in the types of articles that are published in the British and American Journals of Psychiatry. Some academics are even showing frustration with the increasingly divergent

---

[5]http://www.critpsynet.freeuk.com/. The Critical Psychiatry Network first met in Bradford in January 1999, when a group of consultant psychiatrists met to express their opposition to government plans to extend compulsory treatment into the community. The group is also opposed to attempts to widen the definition of mental disorder. It is also campaigning against the growing influence of the pharmaceutical industry on the psychiatric profession. As well as its campaigning functions, the group is also an important source of mutual support for colleagues who dare to think differently in these days of uniformity. Increasingly, the group offers informal advice to young doctors contemplating a career in psychiatry, but who are concerned about the contradictions involved.
[6]Moncrieff (2003); see also more extensive discussion in Chapter 6.

concerns of many of their clinical colleagues. In the UK, this frustration is often directed at colleagues in the Royal College of Psychiatrists. In a recent interview, one prominent academic, a professor of clinical neuropharmacology, was asked: 'what is the greatest threat (facing psychiatry)'. He replied: 'The Royal College of Psychiatrists and all the spawning self-serving bureaucracies in medicine that give medical men respectability when their enthusiasm for research or patient contact dries up' (Kerwin 2004: 313).

Such a strident dismissal of the College, its debates, concerns and priorities, by such a prominent academic is striking. We believe that it reflects an emerging gap between the interests and priorities of clinical and academic psychiatrists. While we do not wish to exaggerate this division, we believe that unless there is a major shift in the thinking of academics, the division will grow over the course of the next decade. At the heart of it are, we believe, two fundamentally different views about the identity of doctors who work in the realm of madness and distress, and about how medicine should be related to this realm.

This book is centrally concerned with these differences. Put simply, we believe that until now, most psychiatrists wanted to hold on to an identity centred on the idea that they were delivering science-based technologies to patients suffering from certain identified illnesses. This continues to be the governing ideology of many academics: that the authority of psychiatry is based on its identification with science and technology. As such, psychiatry is very much a modernist venture. Its *primary* discourse is scientific, mainly around biology and positivistic[7] versions of psychology. Issues such as meanings, values and assumptions are not dismissed but they are relatively unimportant, *secondary* concerns.

However, the search by a growing number of clinical psychiatrists for a new identity reflects a new framing of the relationship between knowledge, power and expertise. We identify this as a move beyond modernist psychiatry, hence the idea of *postpsychiatry*. It is an explicit attempt to redefine a discourse about meanings, relationships and values as *primary*. It is not anti-science. Enterprises such as psychopharmacology and cognitive psychology are still important but will get their direction from this discourse. Whatever this is called, at its heart is an attempt to reach beyond the traditional modernist understanding of our role as doctors.

However, modernism, and with it a belief that science and technology are the main way forward, is not the sole preserve of psychiatrists. Many other professionals and service managers are also keen to assert that the way forward will involve technologies such as pharmacology, genetics, cognitive interventions, service frameworks, and so on. Some service user organizations are

---

[7]Positivism is associated with the work of Auguste Comte, who in the mid-19th century proposed that human thought evolved through a series of stages, the religious, metaphysical and scientific. Positivism stressed the unity of natural and human sciences, with the implication that human experience and human problems are best approached through the formal methods of scientific inquiry.

happy to define their problems in medical terms and look to medical science for solutions.

Postpsychiatry has implications way beyond the profession of psychiatry. In the next section, we attempt to spell out these issues a little further. We will then provide an overview of the content of the various chapters.

Psychiatry as a modernist enterprise

Our argument rests on the idea that 'psychiatry' was a creation of the European Enlightenment and the sort of modernist culture and ideas which ensued from this. Two central themes preoccupied the thinkers of the Enlightenment.

First was the idea that the path to discovering *truth* was by way of human *reason* rather than by religious revelation or the veneration of ancient civilizations. This was a U-turn from the ways of thinking of the medieval and renaissance periods. Enlightenment thinkers believed that by the use of reason we would overcome our superstitions and begin to 'assert our natural superiority' over the rest of nature. Rationality was valued in itself. Proponents of this idea maintained that all the problems of our lives on this planet would ultimately yield to scientific investigation and to the application of one sort of technology or another.

Secondly, there was a concern to explore different aspects of what it was to be a person. The idea of human rights and the primacy of the *individual* came into being. As a result of this, the exploration of motives and individual personalities became a central concern in art and literature.

In a similar way, the impetus for a 'mental science', and hence psychiatry, grew out of this. Most historians of psychiatry (even those who defend the discipline against the critique of Foucault, Scull and others) would agree that, unlike the history of Western medicine which dates back to Hippocrates and the ancient Greeks, the history of psychiatry would not, and could not have come into being had it not been for the Enlightenment.

Our challenge to modernist psychiatry is reflected in a wider intellectual questioning of the ideas engendered by the Enlightenment, which has gathered strength over the past 30 years. The notion that human reason could lead us to the truth led to discourses as diverse as Marxism, liberalism and psychoanalysis. Each of these grand narratives claimed to be a path to truth, each claimed to have some foundational and universal insights into the 'human condition'. However, many philosophers are now questioning the possibility of such foundational truths. This is broadly what postmodernist thought has been about[8]. The term postmodernism has been used in different ways, but we use it in this book to refer to a coming to terms with the downside of the modernist

---

[8]See Bracken (2003), Lewis (2000), and Laugharne (2004) for overviews of postmodernism and psychiatry.

Enlightenment dream: a world ordered according to the dictates of reason; a world shaped by science, technology and the primacy of efficiency. As Barry Smart writes, postmodernity involves:

> ... a form of reflection upon and a response to the accumulating signs of the limits and limitations of modernity. Postmodernity as a way of living with the doubts, uncertainties and anxieties which seem increasingly to be a corollary of modernity, the inescapable price to be paid for the gains, the benefits and the pleasures, associated with modernity. (Smart 1993: 12)

To us, postmodern thinking does not involve a *rejection* of Enlightenment values and ideals, but instead reflects a concern to understand their limitations. When it comes to developing a critique of our social realities, postmodernism does not reject the insights of discourses such as Marxism, liberalism or psychoanalysis. It simply rejects their claims to be foundational and *universally valid*. It does not dismiss their insights into the contradictions of our personal and cultural worlds, but posits their truths as partial, contingent and local.

In Fig. 1, we have linked the Enlightenment to psychiatry by three sets of arrows. These represent three basic orientations that lie at the heart of psychiatry. They provide the framework for our analysis of psychiatry's identity and provide the basis of the postpsychiatry way forward.

Psychiatry developed as a separate area of medical practice in the 19th century. It emerged with these assumptions in place. We believe that while challenges were presented to these assumptions during the course of the last century, they

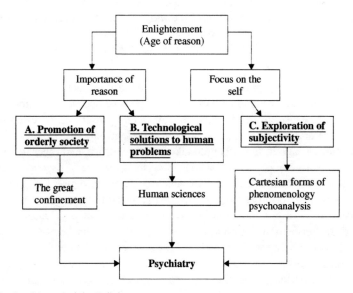

Fig. 1 Psychiatry and the Enlightenment.

continued to guide the basic orientation of the discipline throughout this period.

Madness and distress need to be excluded and controlled: the growth of professional expertise and authority

With its focus on reason and order, the Enlightenment spawned an era in which society sought to rid itself of 'unreasonable' elements. As the historian Roy Porter writes:

> ... the enterprise of the age of reason, gaining authority from the mid-seventeenth century onwards, was to criticise, condemn and crush whatever its protagonists considered to be foolish or unreasonable .... And all that was so labelled could be deemed inimical to society or the state—indeed could be regarded as a menace to the proper workings of an orderly, efficient, progressive, rational society. (Porter 1987: 14–15)

Hence 'unreasonable people', such as the insane, were incarcerated in institutions. Historians have pointed out that the emergence of such institutions was not in itself a 'progressive' or medical, venture; it was simply an act of social exclusion. According to Foucault, doctors became involved with them initially in order to treat physical illness and offer moral guidance, not as experts in disorders of the mind. Scull has shown how the involvement of the medical profession changed, after doctors fought a successful battle for control of the insane against lawyers and the lay sector, and began systematically to order and classify the inmates (Scull 1979). Roy Porter writes:

> ... the rise of psychological medicine was more the consequence than the cause of the rise of the insane asylum. Psychiatry could flourish once, but not before, large numbers of inmates were crowded into asylums. (Porter 1987: 17)

In the 20th century, psychiatry's promise to control madness through medical science went hand in glove with the increasing social acceptance of the role of technical expertise. In most countries, substantial power was invested in the profession, and psychiatrists were given the right and the responsibility to detain patients and to force them to take powerful drugs, and other treatments such as electro-convulsive therapy (ECT). The discourse of psychopathology became the accepted framework in which coercive medicine was practised. In spite of the enormity of this power and responsibility, until recently there has been little discussion about the coercive aspects of psychiatric practice within the profession. Psychiatrists have generally been keen to downplay the differences between their work and that of their medical colleagues. There are echoes of this in contemporary writings about stigma, in which professionals seek to educate the public about the equivalence of psychiatric and medical illness. However, patients (and the public) are well aware that a diagnosis such as diabetes does not lead to compulsory detention in hospital, whereas the label schizophrenia is a major risk factor for this.

Mental and emotional problems are best framed through a technical idiom

The Enlightenment focus on reason also gave birth to various human sciences such as psychology, sociology and anthropology. These set out to discover the universal laws underlying human behaviour and to develop causal accounts of how these laws operated. Psychiatry attempted to do something similar with regard to madness and distress. One important promise of the Enlightenment was that human pain and suffering would be overcome by the advance of rationality and science. To this end, psychiatry has attempted to replace spiritual, moral, political and folk understandings of madness with the framework of psychopathology and neuroscience. The culmination of this was the recent 'decade of the brain' when it was firmly asserted that the causes of madness are to be found in neurotransmitter abnormalities. These abnormalities are then targeted with drugs of different sorts. Other interventions, such as cognitive therapy, are only accepted as long as they work within the same technical idiom.

Perhaps the best example of this technical framing of our mental and emotional problems is the ever-expanding Diagnostic and Statistical Manual (DSM) of the American Psychiatric Association. Over 300 different mental illnesses are now described by the DSM, the majority 'identified' in the past 20 years. In a recent critical account of this expansion, Kutchins and Kirk wrote that:

> DSM is a guidebook that tells us how we should think about manifestations of sadness and anxiety, sexual activities, alcohol and substance abuse, and many other behaviours. Consequently, the categories created for DSM reorient our thinking about important social matters and affect our social institutions. (Kutchins & Kirk 1999: 11)

Madness and distress are located 'inside': methodological individualism

The Enlightenment concern with the individual and the quest to explore the nature of subjectivity (the 'internal world' of human beings) ultimately led to movements such as phenomenology and psychoanalysis.

Phenomenology is a subject that we shall meet at various points in this book. We shall not explore its various philosophical and psychological meanings here but will do so at some length in Chapter 4. At this stage, we simply want to make the point that in the hands of the German philosopher and psychiatrist, Karl Jaspers, phenomenology became primarily concerned with the identification of psychiatric symptoms in the individual patient. Jaspers provided detailed definitions of individual symptoms and a way of classifying them, which has lasted to this day. Importantly, he sought to distinguish the *form* of a mental symptom from its *content*. For Jaspers, the *forms* of psychopathology were universal and arose because of phenomena happening inside the individual. The *content* of psychiatric symptoms was influenced by the social and cultural context, but this was very much of secondary importance. For example, if a person hears voices speaking about them in the third person such as 'look at what she's doing now', this is described by the Jaspersian psychopathologist as a *third person auditory hallucination*. This is the *form* of the symptom. According to this view, the fact that a person in one part of the world hears an ancestral spirit talking about them, while in another part it is an alien voice from another planet, depends on the person's culture. This is the *content* of the symptom; it relates to the context of the person's life and is of secondary importance.

Jaspers' influence on European psychiatry was profound. The prominent British psychiatrist, Aubrey Lewis described his *General Psychopathology* as 'one of the most important and influential books there are in psychiatry' (quoted by Beaumont 1992: 544). Psychiatry continues to separate mental phenomena from background contextual factors. Distress, dislocation, feelings of persecution and other experiences are understood at the level of the individual, and social and cultural issues are external 'factors' which may or may not be taken into account[9]. Although some changes are happening, most psychiatric encounters with patients still occur in hospitals and clinics, and the therapeutic focus is on the individual, with drug treatments or psychotherapy. Biological, behavioural, cognitive and psychodynamic approaches all share this conceptual and therapeutic focus on the individual self. Even social psychiatry has been dominated by an epidemiological approach, which sees its job as the identification of disordered individuals in populations.

Psychoanalysis is probably the best example of a discourse concerned with the 'exploration of subjectivity'. In our diagram representing the Enlightenment (Fig. 1) above, we show the focus on the individual as a 'search for individual truth'. Freud himself hoped that psychoanalysis might one day merge with biology and was committed to positivism. During the course of the 20th century, various schools of humanistic and interpretive psychotherapy emerged which rejected the idea that human reality could be grasped in a technical idiom. In books such as *The Divided Self*, R.D. Laing (1965) provided a brilliant critique of positivism in psychiatry. As an alternative, he essentially developed an approach centred on a modified form of psychoanalysis. While recognizing the importance of family dynamics, the focus was still very much on 'the self' and interventions that involved psychotherapy. Similarly, David Ingleby provided a powerful analysis of positivism and reductionism (see below) in the introduction to his book *Critical Psychiatry*[10] published in 1981. However, he also turned to Freud and psychoanalysis in an effort to develop an alternative. The American

---

[9]See Samson (1995) for a discussion of this.
[10]See Ingleby (1981).

Joel Kovel advocated a similar approach (Kovel 1988). While we are sympathetic to the analyses of Laing, Ingleby and Kovel, we regard psychoanalysis as a flower of the Enlightenment, saturated with assumptions about the inner depths of subjective experience, and falling prey to the problems of methodological individualism that downplay the importance of contexts in shaping and giving meaning to experience. We see it as a part of the problem, not the solution[11].

Postmodernity, postpsychiatry, and a new direction for mental health

At the dawn of the 21st century we believe that there is a need to interrogate these three assumptions. As we have already stated, postmodern thought does not involve a *rejection* of reason, science or technology but instead challenges the idea that these should be social goals *in themselves*. Moreover, postmodern thinkers argue that science and technology are not neutral and disinterested activities but instead are deeply imbued with values and assumptions[12]. The postmodern approach is to *begin with* a democratic debate about the goals, the methods and the applications of science. For example, in the field of agriculture and food production, the organic movement rejects the idea that 'efficiency' should be a goal in itself. It seeks a different form of food science, one that is built on a different way of understanding the relationship between human beings and the natural world. Postmodern thinkers also question the idea that the individual self is some sort of universal 'given'. Instead, they note the many different ways in which selfhood is constructed and experienced transculturally and across different historical periods.

For us, postpsychiatry is about a realization that the three guiding assumptions of modernist psychiatry are only that: assumptions. They are the products of a particular cultural change, and as we move beyond the embrace of that culture we need to interrogate those assumptions and seek new ways of understanding and relating to experiences of madness and distress. The following are some of the questions that we believe emerge from this analysis:

- If psychiatry is the product of the institution, should we not question its ability to guide the sort of care that we want to deliver in the post-institutional era?
- Can we imagine a relationship between medicine and madness which is different from that forged in the asylums and hospitals of a previous age?

---

[11]David Ingleby's analysis is in part inspired by Foucault's early work, but it is limited by virtue of the fact that *Critical Psychiatry* was published before Foucault's later writings about power and subjectivity really began to have an impact on critical thinking in mental health. This influence is apparent in the first two chapters of Nikolas Rose and Paul Miller's book, *The Power of Psychiatry*, which in many respects provide a starting point for our analysis. For an account of these two books and the development of critical psychiatry, see Thomas and Bracken (2004).

[12]Jerry Ravetz has used the term 'postnormal science' to indicate emerging scientific discourses that are grappling with these issues. The idea of 'normal' science comes from the work of Thomas Kuhn (1962).

- Can we begin to imagine different forms of mental health care which do not rely on psychiatry at all?
- If psychiatry is the product of a culture which was preoccupied with rationality and the individual self, what sort of mental health care is appropriate in the postmodern, multi-cultural world in which many of these preoccupations are losing their dominance?
- The Enlightenment understanding of rationality was dominated by a very (White) male perspective. Should we not attempt to develop a discourse about distress that incorporates insights from more than 30 years of feminist and postcolonial thinking and writing in this realm?
- Is Western psychiatry appropriate to cultural groups which do not share Enlightenment preoccupations, but instead value a spiritual ordering of the world and an ethical emphasis on the importance of family and community?
- How can we separate mental health care from the agenda of social exclusion, coercion and control to which it became bound in the last two centuries?

We believe that if we do not face up to these questions, we will replicate the failures of the last century as we move forward. For these reasons, we propose that mental health care should seek to unshackle itself from the three basic assumptions of modernist psychiatry in something like the following ways.

Rethinking the politics of mental health

Contrary to the path followed in the 20th century where the medical profession took a lead role when it came to controlling madness, we believe that the time has come for doctors to move in the opposite direction. This is not to say that *society* should never remove a person's liberty on account of mental disorder, but that the medical profession should not be making the key decisions. In place of medical authority, we envisage increased lay involvement (voluntary sector organizations and self-help groups), and the use of advance statements[13] (i.e. service users giving directions as to how they wish to be treated when they become unwell) and advocacy. The medical profession would have powers and responsibilities commensurate with its knowledge and would be able to provide advice if necessary. However, we believe that if genuine trust is ever to be established between the medical profession and those who suffer episodes of madness, there needs to be a substantial weakening of the link between treatment and coercion[14].

---

[13]Thomas Szasz (1982) was one of the earliest advocates of the advance directive (advance statement or 'living will') in psychiatric care.

[14]There are signs that a growing number of psychiatrists are unhappy with the prominent role given to them in involuntary interventions. As we write, under the leadership of Dr Mike Shooter, the Royal College of Psychiatrists has joined with other mental health organizations to oppose any extension of coercive treatments in the new Mental Health Bill in Britain.

However, psychiatric power is about something much wider than simply coercion; in fact, the psychiatric interventions that most patients experience are on a voluntary basis. To understand the power of psychiatry is to understand how something like the provision of a psychiatric diagnosis can in itself be experienced as destructive and controlling by service users. In addition, postpsychiatry is keen to point out that psychiatric knowledge shapes the way we understand ourselves, and the relationship between this understanding and the interests of the global pharmaceutical industry.

Ethics before technology

The major current concern of medicine is with 'clinical effectiveness' and 'evidence-based practice': the idea that science should guide clinical practice. It proposes that substantial progress would be made if clinical practice was guided by the research literature about the effectiveness of treatments and procedures. Psychiatry has embraced this agenda, and many in the profession believe that the 'evidence-based practice' framework holds the answer to many of the discipline's current problems. The difficulty with this is that the clinical effectiveness framework tends to ignore the role of values in research and practice. However, our argument is that because psychiatry is premised on certain assumptions about the nature of the self and the world (as is Western biomedicine generally), values are *built into* its diagnostic categories. This emerges in the historical work of Foucault (discussed above) as well as that of medical anthropologists (e.g. Gaines 1992), philosophers (e.g. Fulford 1994) and, more recently, psychiatrists themselves (e.g. Sadler 2005).

We believe that it is possible to practise good medicine in the area of mental health without a primary focus on questions such as, 'What is the diagnosis?' We have both worked with teams[15] for whom the primary questions were, 'What does this person, and this family, need at this stage?', 'How can we help this person cope with this crisis without a loss of dignity?' and 'How can we help this person avoid coercive interventions?' In addition, while these teams were acutely aware of the pain and suffering involved in states of madness, they also attempted to avoid the assumption that everything to do with madness was negative or meaningless.

Recognizing the importance of social and cultural contexts: methodological holism

In contrast to the dominant tendency in psychiatry to relegate issues of context (in terms of social, political, cultural and temporal locations) to secondary

---

[15]For example: the work of the Bradford home treatment team (Bracken and Cohen 1999) and the work of Ian Murray and colleagues in Dryll y Car, a crisis house set up in North Wales in 1992 (Williams *et al.* 1999).

status, we propose that they should be central to our understanding of distress and madness. A context-centred approach seeks to understand experiences of sadness, paranoia, self-harm, suicidal thoughts and all the other phenomena we lump together as 'psychiatric' not only in terms of what is happening in the individual at one moment in time but in terms of other dimensions of the person's reality. For example, one of us (P.B.) has argued that we can only understand how any particular individual will respond to traumatic events in their life if we understand the way of life of that person. Furthermore, helping someone recover from trauma is often more about helping to re-establish that way of life rather than any particular intervention on an individual level (Bracken 2002).

Two diagrams. Beyond reductionism and towards a medical practice based on hermeneutics

In the past 20 years, as academic psychiatry has become ever more focused on biological research, this has been accompanied by a profound ideological commitment to what is known as reductionism. Reductionism is the belief that all sorts of events that happen at different levels of reality can be explained in terms of (i.e. reduced to) one type of knowledge. In psychiatry, reductionism involves the assertion that aspects of meaningful human behaviour (such as our worries, regrets, fears, beliefs, hopes, loves and doubts) can be fully explained in terms of 'non-meaningful' entities such as genes, neurotransmitters and ultimately atoms and molecules.

Reductionism is now the ruling ideology of mainstream academic psychiatry. It is very much a modernist idea. While the discipline may have flirted with interpretive and humanistic approaches to psychotherapy in the 1970s and 1980s, these have long been rejected. Cognitive psychology is acceptable as long as it is framed as a positivist science that also seeks to explain complex aspects of human life in a reductive manner[16]. In Fig. 2 we present reductionism as a central theme in late 20th century academic psychiatry; this also relates it to the analysis presented in Fig. 1 earlier.

We use hermeneutics as a way to to get beyond reductionism. Like phenomenology, the term 'hermeneutics' has many meanings[17]. Originally, hermeneutics referred to the science and methodology of interpreting texts, especially the books of the Bible, but in the past century it has come to refer to approaches to human behaviour and social organization that prioritize questions of meaning. In our attempt to think of ways in which medicine can engage appropriately with people in states of madness and distress, we put forward hermeneutics as a possible organizing principle.

---

[16]See Chapter 5 for a more extensive discussion of cognitive psychology.

[17]See Philips (1996) for a good discussion of hermeneutics in relation to psychiatry.

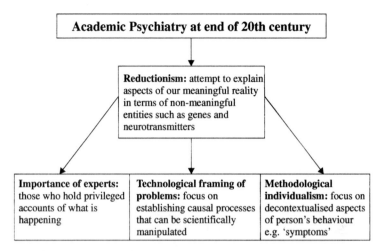

Fig. 2 Reductionism and Academic Psychiatry.

To us, reductionist approaches simply cannot account for the sort of problems we encounter in our day-to-day practice. In our understanding, the problems people bring to us as psychiatrists are essentially 'mental' as opposed to 'physical'. Neurologists deal with nervous system conditions that are primarily organic (physical) in nature. While not wanting to be too prescriptive, we think the word 'mental' usually denotes something to do with that aspect of the world in which meanings play a role. When we talk about 'functional impairment', we are already in a world of judgements, perspectives and values[18]. For the most part, these are problems that make sense only in a world structured by such things as language, cultural assumptions, personal roles, relationships, boundaries, moral dilemmas and priorities.

We maintain that attempting to understand phenomena such as hearing voices, sadness, withdrawal, euphoria, obsessionality, self-harm, suicidal ideation, fearfulness, and so on by reference to neurotransmitters and DNA alone is akin to someone attempting to understand a painting by an artist such as Picasso by analysing the chemical composition of the pigments on the canvas. To do so would give only a very limited and narrow interpretation of the process of Picasso's art. To have a greater understanding of the work, we need to know something about the artist: his life and outlook and his approach to art. We may want to compare it with other works by Picasso. We also need to look beyond the individual artist to what is happening in the world of art and culture more generally. This process of interpretation in order to make sense of things is what we mean by 'hermeneutics'. In Fig. 3, we present this as a central organizing principle of postpsychiatry.

---

[18]A discourse of 'values-based medicine' has recently emerged from this insight, see Fulford (2004).

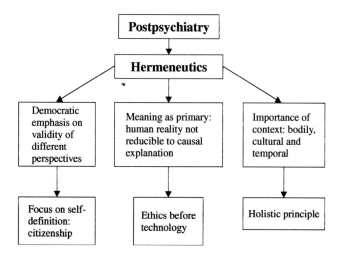

Fig. 3 Postpsychiatry and Hermeneutics.

Rather than investing an individual professional with the 'expertise' to interpret symptoms and to diagnose diseases, hermeneutics insists that a variety of different perspectives be brought to bear and insists that the service user has the right to negotiate how his/her reality is defined. It resists the impulse to reduce our actions to biochemical explanations and refuses the idea that technological interventions are neutral and value-free. Just as we never reach the 'correct' interpretation of a painting or a play, hermeneutics insists that human reality is something open, full of potential and unyielding to formulae or models. Meaning cannot be fixed. Central to hermeneutics is context. The interplay of our culture, our social world within that culture, the historical moment in which we live and the myriad other influences which have shaped and continue to shape our lives are what invest them with meaning. Only by looking at all these elements 'holistically' can we begin to try to understand the meaning of madness and distress.

Outline of the book

We appreciate that most people are unlikely to pick up this book up and read it from cover to cover. However, we hope that while dipping into the book people may find ideas or examples that suit their own purposes, rather along the lines of Gilles Deleuze's proposition that theories can be used like tools from a toolbox[19]. The book is *not* meant as some sort of blueprint or manifesto; it is *not* a guide to what should be done. Rather we hope that by developing

---

[19]'A theory is exactly like a box of tools.... It must be useful. It must function.... it was Proust who said it so clearly: treat my book as a pair of glasses directed to the outside; if they don't suit you, find another pair' (Deleuze; quoted in Foucault 1977*b*: 208). This quotation is from an article called 'Intellectuals and Power'. This is essentially the transcript of a 1972 discussion between

a critique of some of the fundamental assumptions underlying psychiatric theory and practice, we will help to open up spaces in which different sorts of dialogues and discourses might flourish.

This book is structured in three broad sections. The first (Chapters 1 and 2) examines the real contexts in which service users live their lives and use mental health services, and in which mental health professionals work to deliver those services. **Chapter 1** begins with a brief examination of the World Health Organization's global project to try to persuade the governments of all the countries of the world to prioritize the development of services for people who experience madness and other states of distress[20]. We then move on to consider the British Government's attempts since 1997 to change the ethos of the National Health Service. We recognize that this is a singularly local context, but it is the one in which we have worked as clinicians for many years. In any case, our view is that there are certain underlying commonalities in the way that advanced liberal democracies are currently thinking about psychiatry. One of the things we find particularly striking is the chasm that has opened up between the rhetoric of government policy on the one hand, and responses of policy makers and professional groups to that rhetoric on the other.

This book would not exist were it not for the courage of the growing number of mental health service users and survivors who have written about their experiences. In the last 10 years or so, this has evolved into a recognizable body of personal testimony and narrative. This includes what is now known as 'user-led research'. In **Chapter 2**, we examine some of this literature. We discover a remarkable diversity of experiences and views. Yes, there are attitudes that some might regard as 'anti-psychiatry', but there are also people who write in positive terms about their experiences of diagnosis and treatment within psychiatry. The majority of the views expressed fall somewhere in between these two extremes. People recognize that psychiatry has brought some benefits into their lives but there are personal costs to be borne. In addition, many people describe a deep sense of ambivalence about the significations and meanings attached to psychiatry, and particularly psychiatric medication. In this chapter, we are trying to re-establish contact with the voices that are customarily excluded from debates about madness.

Deleuze and Foucault. In the same article, Foucault says: 'the intellectual's role is no longer to place himself "somewhat ahead and to the side" in order to express the stifled truth of the collectivity; rather, it is to struggle against the forms of power that transform him into its object and instrument in the sphere of "knowledge", "truth", "consciousness", and "discourse" (pp. 207–208). This was Foucault putting some distance between himself and Marxist intellectuals of the 1970s who claimed to be in the 'vanguard of the masses', believing that their analysis gave them a guide to how social change should proceed.

[20]We use expressions such as 'madness', 'states of distress' and 'alienation' throughout the text. We also use terms such as 'psychosis' and 'mental illness' at times. While attempting to use a non-medical language as much as possible, we are aware that medical terms are now part of the vernacular vocabulary of distress.

The second section deals at length with the underlying philosophical issues that we have found valuable in helping to orientate ourselves to the problems and conflicts implicit in mental health practice. It deals specifically with the three key elements that we described earlier: the power of psychiatry and its role in social exclusion (Chapter 3), methodological individualism (Chapters 4 and 5) and psychiatry as a technical idiom of distress (Chapter 6).

In **Chapter 3**, we examine the first theme of postpsychiatry: the relationship between psychiatry, exclusion and coercion. At issue here is the nature of power and the role of professionals in the lives of service users. We draw attention to the work of members of groups such as Mad Pride, Mad Women and the Hearing Voices Network, who refuse the psychiatric way of framing their experiences as 'symptoms'. We examine the idea of citizenship in the field of mental health. In recent years, citizenship has become a fashionable idea in advanced liberal democracies, and it is not surprising to discover its influence in liberal discourses about mental health. However, we argue that 'a citizenship agenda' has real value in helping mental health professionals to think outside their biological or psychosocial frameworks, and to consider issues that are of greater concern to mental health service users.

In many respects, **Chapter 4** is at the heart of the book. This is centrally concerned with what we might call the 'gaze' of psychiatry: how it 'sees' or encounters the problems people bring to it. This is a complex issue involving questions of diagnosis and framing, as well as power and priorities. We have already mentioned the work of Karl Jaspers and his understanding of phenomenology. In Chapter 4, we argue that this version of phenomenology is deeply Cartesian[21]; it presents phenomenology as a rigorous science of human experience, which we believe to be problematic. It also tends to separate the person's experiences from the human contexts that render them meaningful, and from the body, through which any experience is brought into being. In the second half of the chapter, we spell out how the philosophy of Martin Heidegger serves to challenge this Cartesian viewpoint and thus opens up the possibility of very different starting points for psychology and medicine.

In **Chapter 5**, we continue to develop some of the themes that emerged in Chapter 4, this time with regard to cognitivism and the relationship between mind, language and meaning. We trace the common roots of cognitivism (and its therapeutic offshoot, cognitive therapy) and psycholinguistics, through the theories of George Miller and Noam Chomsky. Cognitivism and psycholinguistics have played an important role in recent theories of psychosis, especially the experiences that are associated with the diagnosis of schizophrenia. We consider the theories of Chris Frith as an example of this. The second half of this chapter mounts a critique of this work using the later philosophy of Ludwig Wittgenstein.

---

[21]That is shaped by the outlook of the philosopher Rene Descartes.

Chapter 6 marks the end of the central section and also starts the process of opening up some of the implications of our analysis for the world of mental health practice. If postpsychiatry is to be remembered by an aphorism, then that aphorism would be 'ethics before technology'. In Chapter 6, we dwell in detail on this. Our most important proposition here is that, despite claims to objectivity and neutrality, the technology and evidence on which current mental health practice are based are laden with assumptions and particular interests. Our position is that there is no such thing as a truly objective human knowledge or understanding, and that the sooner we recognize this and start attending to issues of transparency and accountability, the better for all concerned. We start by challenging the way that the profession conventionally interprets the evidence (from randomized controlled trials) for the effectiveness of psychotropic medication. Related to this, we consider the cultural significance of the 'Prozac phenomenon' and the highly problematic links between academic psychiatry and the pharmacological industry. We propose that, to a large extent, the effectiveness of drugs used in psychiatry is to be understood in terms of their cultural significance. This is an important issue that we return to in the final section of the book. At the end of Chapter 6, we argue the case for the priority of ethics in mental health practice and examine a key event in the history of psychiatry: the opening of the York Retreat at the end of the 18th century.

The final section tries to develop some of the understandings gained in the middle section in relation to the world of mental health practice. We begin with an attempt to foreground the issue of ethics by turning the moral gaze on ourselves as writers. In **Chapter 7**, we explore the historically important role of case histories in medicine as a prelude to a more detailed consideration of case history as narrative. Using the work of the psychiatrist and anthropologist Robert Barrett, we examine critically the idea of 'case' in psychiatry, and how psychiatric writing in case notes and other clinical material serves to describe much more than illness; it becomes a way of constructing a person. These days, the role of case history as one of the principal begetters of evidence has been replaced by evidence-based medicine, but this move has been partly offset by recent interest in what is called 'narrative'. We are sympathetic to the idea of narrative-based medicine, but we also consider it important to expose narrative to the same type of critical scrutiny as that to which we subjected phenomenology and cognitivism.

Chapter 7's critical approach to narrative is directly relevant to the notion of 'recovery' that we expound in **Chapter 8**. Recovery is a buzz word at the moment. We believe that, in general, the recovery movement is a very positive development. Essentially it involves professionals and service users working together in a spirit of hope. It involves people seeking different ways of moving forward, different ways of establishing a life independent of services and labels. However, across America and, to a lesser extent, in Britain, so-called experts in recovery are developing 'recovery training packages'. We are deeply sceptical at this turning of recovery into a commodity, to be marketed, sold and turned into profit. Instead, we look to some recent qualitative studies of recovery, most of which have relied on the methodology of service user-led research, or have been undertaken from a service user perspective. We summarize some of the principal relevant findings.

This leads conveniently to the final perspective on recovery. In Chapter 7, we argued that we should not consider *narrative* apart from its ethical and moral dimensions. We apply this principle to recovery, with reference to Susan Brison's book *Aftermath*. This is a powerful and moving account of her personal experiences of recovery from a life-threatening sexual assault. One of many important themes to emerge from her writing is the idea of recovery as a moral process. We consider the implications of her ideas for our own engagement with suffering, as doctors.

In **Chapter 9**, we try to describe how our ideas have influenced our work as psychiatrists. Postpsychiatry, as we have said already, is not a new form of 'therapy'. We are not attempting here to describe 'cases'. Instead we focus here on the broader, community-based aspects of our work in Bradford. We begin by describing the city, its history and origins, and the important historical role played by migrant workers in the last 200 years of the city's history. We outline the work of *Sharing Voices Bradford*, which demonstrates the value of community development in creating safe spaces (or 'ethical' spaces) in which different understandings of, and responses to, madness and distress can be articulated. We believe that such an approach has the potential to bring particular benefits to Black and minority ethnic communities. But it does not stop there. The idea of safe spaces in which people can explore their own understandings of madness applies to all communities. This is amply demonstrated by Rufus May's work with *Evolving Minds*, in the Pennine town of Hebden Bridge. We revisit the concept of citizenship and describe how Bradford District Care Trust has set about working towards a *citizenship agenda*. This is a courageous endeavour, but one fraught with difficulties and problems.

In **Chapter 10**, we return full circle to some of the issues that we began with—the contexts, national and international, in which we live and work. This gives us the opportunity to look at some work that we regard as important, for example that of the late Loren Mosher. The latest twist in the context of British policy is the realization that the country cannot go on spending on health at the rate it has been doing for the last 10 years. Politicians and policy makers are realizing that the benefits to be gained by endless spending on technology in health must be questioned. In our view, this debate has to be set against a global context in which gross disparities exist between the resources available to EA and ED countries. This shows that the ideas we developed in the central sections of this book, dealing with the ways in which we would want to be cared for were we to experience madness (promoting the importance of contexts and ethics and the meaningfulness of human relationships and community), help us to begin the task of thinking through these complex issues in ways that are ethical and sustainable.

There is one last point we want to make. Whenever clinicians write books about their work, they feel obliged in some way to describe 'cases'. What point is there writing about clinical practice without presenting examples? Everyone is curious to find out how you do it. We debated the pros and cons of presented case examples, and Chapter 7 reflects the debates we had with ourselves (and friends and colleagues too). We decided that writing case histories based on our clinical work with Bradford's Home Treatment Service or Assertive Outreach Team would be unsatisfactory. How would we decide which cases to represent, on what basis and for what purpose? How would we handle the issues of confidentiality, of consent and editorial control? In any case, how would others interpret such representations? Would people regard them as a form of therapy? We would certainly hope not! Had we written just one case history, it would merely have represented selected scenes from an individual's life. The issues of power and representation in such narratives are so all-encompassing that in our view, we cannot justify the use of case histories in a work like this. As discussed in Chapter 2, service users are writing their own stories and doing their own research.

Nevertheless, we still wanted to convey something of the world in which we work. In the end, we decided that the best way to do this was through the medium of short stories. Scattered throughout this text are six fictional narratives, set in italics to separate them from the main text. They are placed at certain points in the text in order to emphasize certain points in the adjacent chapters. They are deliberately set to disrupt the calm rational flow that normally takes us through an academic text. The characters and situations are imaginary, although it would be disingenuous to propose that that they are unrelated to our experiences as clinicians. The great advantage of writing fiction in this way is that it enables us to negotiate a complex manoeuvre—that of relinquishing the privileged, all-encompassing, omniscient narrative voice from nowhere and everywhere, and of putting the story-telling into the voice of the main protagonist. Besides, the act of engaging with a piece of fiction means we enter different worlds, and that is exactly what we are striving to achieve in writing this book.

Doing their best

In the summer, we would spend hours together on the crags overlooking the valley. You loved to watch the birds spin beneath your feet. Sometimes you would lie on your back in the warm sun, losing yourself in the vast sky. What were you thinking of? I remember you looking down into the deep pools below, watching a dipper skim the surface. You were deeper than those pools, far deeper than any of us knew. Sometimes you would write, nothing much, a few notes, scraps perhaps. But later, when the autumn gales howled and night drew on, you would weave those notes and scraps into a web of words so fine that it lay gently on my soul, caressing me with that summer sun.

I have lost count of how many times I have made this journey, through the heart of Snowdonia to this house by the sea. Today it is a grey listless sea, frozen under the bleak sky, and they gave me his suitcase. At home I opened it and found beneath an old check flannel shirt with frayed dirt grey cuffs the pen I bought him for his 50th birthday. He said he wanted to write. It was the first time that he had shown any interest in writing for over 30 years. They had just moved him to the sea side. A halfway house they called it. He had his own room there. It was much better than the old ward with 32 beds standing to attention along the walls. It seemed to bring back a spark in him, at least for a few weeks. Before when he used to write he would craft his poems with such precision and love. The physical act of holding a pen and of writing turned his body into a servant to his art. Only the best tools suited his ceremony. He wrote poems in the Old Language that were so full of love and of life. I hoped that the pen might help rekindle the fuse that drove him to write. But the devils returned and he fell silent again.

Long ago now, I remember nurses in uniforms and caps, doctors in white coats. In his first summer, I took him to the carnival in the grounds. How strange, he said, that they should have this here. But then it is a mad house, he added.

Doctor Griffiths didn't want him to go to that place. Neither did we. He said that it was unusual for anyone to leave once they were in, so it had to be a last resort. He tried, as did we all. We tried as long as we could to look after him at home. His roots were on that hill, in the woods overlooking the Wnion. The last thing we wanted was for him to be uprooted. Doctor Griffiths was right. Perhaps if we had tried a bit longer he would have pulled through. Who knows? Perhaps with mam's strength, if she had lived, we might have seen it through.

On his first day in the old hospital I remember the nurse taking his clothes. She said he could have new ones after he had had a bath. He had to be clean to be examined. Then the doctor saw him. He spent an hour questioning him, checking him, examining him, writing about him. Then he spoke to me. He was kind. If I remember correctly he was English, from London. He told me it was an illness, schizophrenia I think. He was excited because they had just managed to get a supply of a new pill. It had been discovered in France a few years earlier. It was the first time that they had had something that could cure the illness. He would be cured completely. He filled our hearts with hope. He said

> it has been possible to relax security arrangements; and physical restraints have been almost abolished. Patients who previously would have needed admission to a mental hospital can now be taken into the open wards of general hospitals, with the sense of freedom given by ready access to the coming and going in the corridors and in the street outside. It is particularly gratifying to be able to treat the young patients, with a sharp attack of illness and good chances of full recovery, in such a benign environment.

It would bring him back too, he said. He started the pill; time passed by. There was no change. He just got heavier by the day, drooling like an imbecile and shuffling like an old man. I wondered.

A couple of years later they said that he was a chronic case, incurable. They moved him to another ward, a large dusty hall full of men's sweat and silence. It faced north towards the hills; no light found its way there. A new doctor took over his care. He told us that a different treatment would help. It was a well-established treatment that had been used many times before in similar cases with success. There was pity in his eyes when he warned us not to build up our hopes.

> The idea seemed bizarre, but it was found to work

he said, and he promised they would start carefully. They would begin with a very light form of the treatment, every day for weeks and weeks it continued, even on a Saturday when I visited. I can remember seeing him lying on his bed. The therapy was taking something out of him; he would lie there still and quiet. He always looked so pale after it, a fine dew of sweat clinging to his brow. So I gently patted his brow; I wanted him to know I was there. Did he? Did he sense my presence? I hope he did.

> Only if this proves insufficient is sopor or full coma treatment possibly required; and often additional light sopors will be sufficient

is what the new doctor told me, so they had to deepen his therapy. Everybody was concerned because he seemed not to be making any progress. Back home we were frightened, Tad, Dafydd, Anwen and me. Then the hospital in Rhyl phoned. Come immediately, they said. Mr Roberts the minister took us in his new motor, across the moors at dawn. When we arrived, breathless, he was grey and close to death. In the stifling room, he was alone. We feared that he was lost. The coma had gone too deep, the nurse whispered, and the treatment had damaged his brain. But even then his body pulled him through, and he recovered. He was made of granite; he was quarried, not born. His strength *carried him through it, but still he could not speak; the devils still assailed him. And when they sent him back to the old hospital they continued the therapy, gently this time, a modified coma they called it. How was it the doctor described him? Refractory? That's it; a refractory case is the expression he used. I'd never heard of it before. Can you say it in Welsh I asked? But he didn't speak Welsh. Later I found out that it meant stubborn, resisting their attempts to treat him. So they added a new treatment.*

> *If insulin and ECT are combined in the early weeks of treatment, both types of symptoms, paranoid and depressive, will improve together, and better results will be obtained*

and so they added the shock treatment to the insulin therapy. It was no use. They tried their best, but it served him no benefit. Still and silent he remained, deeply submerged in his pool. Stubborn? A strange kind of stubbornness that kept one so young away from life. With the new treatment, his slowness increased. He became more distant. He used to hold his hand up for me to take, just as he did when he was a small boy and he wanted to go to the forest to hear the birds. But he lost the urge to cling to my hand when I visited. Each week as that new treatment progressed, he slipped further away. Then one day I came and his hand was motionless, a thing of soft warm marble. Still, I sat there and held his mute limp hand.

I want to hold your hand was on the radio when the doctor called me in. It was number one. He had something important he wanted to discuss. Have you spoken to him about it, I asked? There was little point, he said, because he never spoke to them. Besides, they thought that he was incapable of understanding it. They thought I might be able to get through to him. The doctor told me that

> *the point has now been reached where the swing towards conservatism has gone too far. The tranquillising drugs have not enabled many chronic patients to be brought out from the back wards of mental hospitals; too often they have succeeded only in muffling the cries for help coming from these wards, where the patients may now accept their chronic state more placidly.*

He tried to explain what they wanted to do, but I found it difficult to follow. They wanted to remove some of the nerves from his brain. The operation was quite safe, and some people did remarkably well afterwards

> *. . . over 30 per cent of all schizophrenics operated upon were able to leave their hospitals*

I was told. Tad was against it. He didn't think it was right, that it wasn't natural interfering in things like that. Dafydd and Anwen thought the same as I; we were desperate to see him better. That night we prayed at home together, and at Chapel the next day. Mr Roberts came. He reminded us about the raising up of Lazarus. He said that we must put our faith in our Saviour and in the doctors' skills. Then he would be delivered back to us. It's miraculous the things they can do these days, he told us; the doctors will have spent years perfecting this treatment. We must pray for guidance and have faith. Dr Griffiths wasn't sure. It was the most difficult decision we have ever had to make. In the end, we thought that if there was the slightest chance of some improvement for him then the doctors should go ahead. I could not have lived with myself knowing that there might have been a chance that it would have made him better. As things stand I have not been able to live with myself anyway.

In the early weeks after the operation we held our breaths. We dared not to hope; we could not even speak about it for it seemed that he had turned a corner. He started to speak, and he greeted us for the first time in years when we visited. It seemed to me, though, that the devils—for that remains the only way I can talk of them—still visited him. But he was less perturbed; his worries had eased. How is Mam, he asked one day? He had forgotten that she had died the year before he came into hospital. Never mind, he said without a glimmer of sadness, did you bring chocolate? And he left the room; he ran out and did something that he had never done before. Oh dear God, I shall never forgive myself for allowing them do this, this awful thing to him. He went into the town, to the Hope and Anchor halfway down the hill, and he drank. The phone was ringing when we got home. We can't control him; he's raging about the ward, they said; we'll have to put the jacket on him, put him in the cell. I was ashamed of myself for allowing them do this awful thing to him. They were doing their best; they did this thing to him because they really believed that it would help him. But how can he ever forgive me for allowing it to happen?

> After operation these paranoid patients are much more amenable to taking maintenance drug therapy, and are much more willing to continue under follow-up care, so that for the first time they can be kept under control outside hospital. Those who at this date are content to leave permanently 'tranquillised' in the back wards of their hospitals, patients who are capable of recovery with a modified leucotomy, should remember the principle that we should always treat our patients as we would wish to be treated ourselves, if we were so placed.

And now your case is empty. Your pen I shall keep, and the anthology I bought you for your 21st birthday. It was at the bottom, and must have lain there unopened for years. But on the title page you had written

> When spring wakens the hearts
> Of the young children to sing, what song shall be theirs?

1 Values, evidence, conflict

In March 2002, psychiatrists working in England received promotional material from the drug company Eli Lilly. There is nothing unusual in this; doctors receive glossy brochures from drug companies every day. But this was different. The small, insignificant card that fell through our letter boxes asked the question; 'What will be the impact of the NICE guidance for your patients with schizophrenia?' On offer was a summary of the National Schizophrenia Fellowship's[1] survey on patients' views about the management of schizophrenia. Also on offer was a 'NICE into Action' pack, containing information on how psychiatrists could implement the National Institute for Clinical Excellence (NICE) guidance on the use of atypical neuroleptics, all this coming 2 months before the publication of the NICE guidance on the use of the atypical neuroleptics for the treatment of schizophrenia. Lilly of course manufacture the atypical neuroleptic olanzapine (zyprexa), and have a clear interest in the promotion of guidelines that advocate for the use of these drugs. A few days later, there was a second mail shot from Lilly proclaiming the benefits of olanzapine over its rival, risperidone (risperdal). A month earlier, Janssen-Cilag, the manufacturers of risperidone, had sent out promotional material offering a free booklet reviewing proposed changes to the mental health act. The booklet dealt specifically with the framework for determining when patients could be treated without consent, '. . . even outside the hospital setting.' Recent pharmaceutical company promotional material has also included guides to the National Service Framework for Mental Health (Lilly, Janssen-Cilag and Organon), and the housing needs of people with mental health problems (Janssen-Cilag). There have even been publications jointly between the National Institute of Mental Health in England[2] and the pharmaceutical industry (through the Mental Health Partnership of the Association of the British Pharmaceutical Industry, which includes 10 leading pharmaceutical companies), examining the possibilities of partnership working to support the implementation of mental health policy.

Evidence, and the research upon which it is based, is not neutral. Investigators perform research from a particular viewpoint or perspective. In doing so, they are driven by a variety of interests and concerns. Some of these may be understood in terms of scientific curiosity, or terms of a commitment to extending knowledge in order to help others. In Chapter 6, we will describe

---

[1]Now known as *Rethink*.
[2]National Institute of Mental Health in England (2000).

how other interests shape and influence scientific knowledge. We will see that the pharmaceutical industry has created a grey area in which its interests are paraded around disguised as science. In this chapter, we shall consider the agendas that have informed the development of mental health services in the last 10 years. One of the points we want to make in doing so is to draw attention to a conflict between two sets of fundamentally different values.

Psychiatry: the global policy context

In August 2002, the Twelfth World Congress of Psychiatry organized by the World Psychiatric Association (WPA) took place in Yokohama. There were many satellite symposia organized by pharmaceutical companies at this prestigious gathering. Some dealt with the transcultural aspects of diagnosis: 'Psychiatric treatment of mental health disorders across populations—do east and west meet?' (Pfizer), 'Transcultural aspects of depression and anxiety disorders' (GlaxoSmithKline), 'Recognition and treatment of depression: differences between American, European and Japanese practices' (Janssen), 'Eye on Asia: deducing the socio-economic burden of depression' (Wyeth). Others dealt with the management of psychosis 'Raising the level of schizophrenia care' (Janssen-Cilag) and 'Optimising patient outcomes in schizophrenia' (Pfizer). At national and international levels, it appears that the concerns of psychiatry and the pharmaceutical industry are becoming woven ever more closely together.

Psychiatry has become a powerful global force that shapes how we are able to talk about ourselves, our emotions and the way we think. This can seen in the work of the World Health Organization. The WHO's mental health Global Action Plan[3] (mhGAP) argues the need for a 'new approach' to mental health. The purpose of this 5-year plan is to make governments more aware of mental health problems, and to get them to devote more resources to psychiatric services and mental health promotion strategies aimed at educating and persuading hundreds of millions of people across the planet about their mental health. The case for the programme is made in the following terms. It asserts right at the outset that psychiatric disorders are universals[4]:

> 450 million people suffer from mental disorders in both developed and developing countries
>
> One in every four people . . . develop one or more mental disorders at some stage in life

It identifies depression, schizophrenia, substance abuse and dementia as the most common disorders, especially in the poor, and draws particular attention to the economic impact of these disorders. Those who suffer from mental

---

[3]World Health Organization (2002).
[4]World Health Organization (2002: 2).

health problems, and their families, experience 'reduced productivity', loss of income, and face 'catastrophic' health care costs (World health organization 2002: 2). In the USA alone, estimates of the total economic burden have been calculated at US$148 billion per annum.

In turn, the WHO ties economic loss and disability associated with mental disorder to stigma. The victimization of those suffering from mental disorders is a global problem, and as a result they experience discrimination, especially in the fields of housing and employment. Their ability to fulfil other normal social roles is also compromised. Stigma, it is claimed, is maintained by inaccurate societal and cultural attitudes towards mental disorders, such as the belief that people who experience them are bewitched, or prone to violence, or that their conditions are untreatable. The WHO asserts that the progress of science, and growth of knowledge and understanding about the true nature of mental disorder, will rectify this, bringing new hope through treatment advances, dispelling ignorance and thus stigma[5]:

> We know that mental disorders are the outcome of a combination of factors, and that they have a physical basis in the brain.

The WHO claims that effective treatment can result in successful symptom control in 70% of cases of depression and schizophrenia, and the continuation of treatment substantially reduces the risk of recurrence. It points out that drug treatment is cheap in many countries; it costs US$5 a month to treat schizophrenia and US$2–3 for depression. It proposes an anti-stigma campaign to change public attitudes, aimed at[6]:

> ... consumers, families and their organisations, *who need to be sensitized about mental disorders, available treatment*, and their rights in the service system.

Across the face of the planet, the initiative argues, only a small proportion of those in need receive even basic treatment for their problems. The WHO Project ATLAS 2000–2001 surveyed information from 185 countries covering 99.3% of the world's population. The governments of two-fifths of the countries surveyed had no mental health policies. In more than a quarter, patients had no access to basic psychiatric drugs at a primary care level. More than 70% of the world's population had access to less than one psychiatrist per 100 000 people. Thus, the mhGAP initiative aims to set up partnerships with other groups, including United Nations (UN) organizations, the World Bank, private industry, academic institutions and non-governmental organizations (NGOs). The purpose is to ensure that all governments have strategies to increase the availability of psychiatric treatment in primary care, improve public education about psychiatric disorders and establish national policies and programmes in mental health.

---

[5]World Health Organization (2002: 4).
[6]World Health Organization (2002: 18; emphasis added).

A similar programme has emerged in the USA. In 2002, President Bush set up the New Freedom Commission to undertake a fundamental review of US mental health services. The report, published in 2004[7], advocates for the full integration of psychiatric patients in the community rather than institutional care. It argues for whole population screening for mental disorders on the grounds that they are very common and frequently go undetected. Lenzer (2004) points out that this screening, which would start with pre-school children, would also include 'state-of-the-art' treatment interventions based in the Texas Medication Algorithm Project (TMAP). TMAP is an evidence-based model for drug treatment that has been claimed to generate better outcomes. However, Lenzer points out that concerns have been raised about links between the pharmaceutical industry and the Texas project. Her article outlines the links that exist not only between the project and the industry, but also between the Bush family and the industry. In other words, the suspicion is that what is presented as a scientific attempt to improve the quality of mental health services is in reality an alliance between politicians and the pharmaceutical industry.

Psychiatry: the policy context in England

The development of community care in England has occurred against a cultural background in which the values of health care, and the relationships between participants involved in it have changed profoundly. For the first 25 years of its life, the NHS was organized around the principle of beneficent paternalism. Patients were expected to defer to the authority and wisdom of medical practitioners. The ideas of Illich (1976) and Kennedy (1981), coupled with the rise of consumerism in health, signalled profound changes in the relationship between the medical profession and patients. 'Consumerism' implies that we may think of ourselves as consumers of health care. It implies that we have choices to make as far as our health is concerned. It assumes that we are free to make these choices and that as citizens we have the right to make them. Consumerism originates in Western capitalism, which in turn has its own assumptions about the organization of society and the relationships we find in it. Health care can be thought of as a commodity to be advertised, sold, traded and bought, as is the case with any other commodity. In this view, markets (we have gained and lost a 'free market' in the NHS) involve purchasers, providers and patients as consumers, all metaphors drawn from capitalism. This shift in health care values has led to successive governments following policies that have emphasized the importance of consultation with and the involvement of patients in service development and planning, the

---

[7]Available on http://www.whitehouse.gov/infocus/newfreedom/newfreedom-report-2004.pdf accessed February 24, 2005.

processes of delivery of individual care programmes, and research. This is reflected in a number of government policy documents, such as the White Paper *Caring for People* (HMSO 1989), the NHS and Community Care Act of 1990, *The Health of the Nation* (HMSO 1992) and the Department of Health's *Patients' Charter*. All these place the concerns and interests of patients in a position of central importance in health care.

On its election to power in May 1997, the Labour government set about a series of major reforms of health care in England, many of which were intended to improve the quality of services through the investment of additional resources. But, in doing so, the government was determined to forge a new relationship between patients, the professions and the public. These reforms were driven by three principles. The first was reciprocity; that if the quality of services was to improve, then staff had to be adequately resourced. The second was accountability; providing adequate resources meant massive investment, realized through public taxation. Thus the public, as tax payers, became key stakeholders in the NHS and, as patients, had the right to a prominent voice in decisions about health care, both locally and nationally. The third principle was responsibility; the public were encouraged to see themselves as lessening their dependence on professional staff, and accepting more responsibility for their own health. Related to these principles was a commitment to tackling health inequalities. This was to be brought about by improving the quality of health care, steps to tackle poverty, especially child poverty, and encouraging greater personal responsibility for health. All these changes were set out in detail in the NHS Plan (HMSO 2000). An important feature of the Plan was a commitment to improving standards in the NHS. This commitment was to be delivered by National Service Frameworks (NSFs) and NICE. The NSF for Mental Health was one of the first frameworks published. In addition, the government set up the National Institute for Mental Health in England (NIMHE) at the end of 2001 to take forward the changes proposed by the NHS Plan and NSF for Mental Health.

There are two aspects of the NHS Plan to which we want to draw attention. These are its democratic ideals, which stress the importance of accountability and the involvement of the public as citizens, and, secondly, the importance it attaches to the social contexts of health care. Although, as we shall see, health care technologies dominate the NHS Plan's attempts to improve the nation's health, it also places patients' interests at the heart of health care. It came into being after extensive consultation to elucidate public concerns about the NHS, and to find out what changes people thought were necessary. Public opinion was that the needs of the system rather than those of the patient dictated much of the work of the NHS:

> While people continue to show real faith in the integrity and professionalism
> of NHS staff, they see problems in some staff attitudes. Patients feel talked
> at too much and listened to not enough. (HMSO 2000: 135)

There was a need to see different ways of working in the NHS with a much greater focus on patients' interests:

> For the first time patients will have a real say in the NHS. They will have new powers and more influence over the way the NHS works . . . (HMSO 2000: 12)

To achieve this, the Plan set out the government's intention to ensure that patients would have more information to enable them to look after their own health, through extending the 'Expert Patient' programme. Patients would also have the option of greater information about the treatment planned for them, for example by having the right to have copies of letters between clinicians about their care. A Patients' Forum and a new Patients' Advocacy and Liaison Service would be established in each hospital to represent the interests of patients. At a wider level, the Plan recognized that there was a need for much greater professional accountability to the public, who would be given greater influence over the regulation of the professions, especially the General Medical Council. In other words, the government was seeking a different type of relationship between the public and the medical profession. In particular, there were concerns about existing mechanisms whereby consent was sought from patients and relatives:

> We need to change the culture to recognize the central importance of the rights of each patient. (HMSO 2000: 93)

Overall, the Plan stresses the *rights of patients as citizens*:

> Patients and citizens have had too little influence at every level of the NHS. (HMSO 2000: 94)

and:

> There will be major increases in the citizen and lay membership of all the professional regulatory bodies, including the General Medical Council. (HMSO 2000: 95)

'Citizen and patient representatives' would constitute one-third of the membership of the new NHS Modernization Board. The Commission for Health Improvement would include 'citizen and lay inspectors' on its inspection teams. The NICE would be advised by a new 'Citizens Council'. The word 'citizen' or its derivatives appears 19 times in the Plan. Citizens, it seems, are to play a central role in the reforms of the NHS.

The second feature of the NHS Plan that we want to highlight is the importance it attaches to social contexts and health. We can see this in the way it draws attention to health inequalities and the impact of poverty on health. There is nothing new here. The Black report (Black *et al.* 1982) drew attention the failure of the NHS in its first 25 years to close the health gap between the wealthiest and the poorest in society, an exercise that was repeated in

Variations in Health (Department of Health 1995). But, in the *NHS Plan*, the government's references to health inequalities play a key part in plans to reform the NHS. The *NHS Plan* talks about health inequalities in terms of 'injustice' that must be tackled by dealing with their fundamental causes. This means:

> ... tackling disadvantage in all its forms—poverty, lack of educational attainment, unemployment, discrimination and social exclusion. *It means recognising the specific health needs of different groups, including people with disabilities and minority ethnic groups.* (HMSO 2000: 106; emphasis added)

A number of proposals for tackling these injustices are set out. They include targets to tackle infant mortality, tied in to government targets to abolish child poverty, and new ways of deciding on the allocation of NHS funding to ensure that resources go to the communities with the greatest need. In this view, social exclusion is not simply associated with poorer health and health inequalities, *but poor health is directly tied to the experience of social exclusion and is brought about by it.* The Plan implies that investment in more scientific research and better health care technology, and that treatment is insufficient to improve the health of all members of society.

In our view, this is an important moment in the history of health care. The Plan sets out an enlightened and compassionate programme to reform the NHS. It places the interest of citizens (in the role of patients) ahead of professional interests. It has democratic ideals and values at its heart as it sets out the health services' role in understanding and tackling the effects of social exclusion on health. Most important of all, it acknowledges that science unaided will not improve the nation's health. Science must be matched by a commitment to understand and change the wider social contexts in which health care takes place. Nowhere is this more important than in psychiatry. As far as the technologies of health care are concerned, the Plan contained two components that were to play an important part in improving the nation's health, the NSF for Mental Health and the NICE. How do they measure up to the ideals set out in the Plan?

Democratic ideals or control and coercion?

National Service Framework for Mental Health

The government published its NSF for Mental Health in 1999, having first set out its plans to invest an extra £700 million to reform and improve services in *Modernising Mental Health Services* (Department of Health 1998*a*). The language used in this ministerial statement of intent and the accompanying press release is revealing. We breathe the air of another planet as we leave behind the rhetoric of citizens and partnership. The need to increase resources to improve services is couched in terms of the failure of community care, the risk posed by the mentally ill, and the need to improve public confidence in the mental health care system;

> Care in the community has failed because, while it improved the treatment of many people who were mentally ill, it left far too many walking the streets, often at risk to themselves and a nuisance to others. A small but significant minority have been a threat to others or themselves. (Dobson 1998)

and

> This is where the policy of care in the community has failed. Its failure to deal effectively with the most severe cases has dealt a blow to all mental health efforts and lost the confidence of the public. (Department of Health 1998*b*)

We see a schism opening up between the vision of the NHS Plan, and the new world of community care. These two documents go on to outline the key elements in the government's strategy for mental health, which included reforms to the mental health act to:

> . . . ensure that patients who might otherwise be a danger to themselves and others *are no longer allowed to refuse to comply with the treatment they need.* (Dobson 1998; emphasis added)

and

> . . . changing the law to permit the detention of a small group of people who have not committed a crime but whose untreatable psychiatric disorder makes them dangerous. (Dobson 1998)

The stated aim of the NSF (Department of Health 1999) was to improve quality by removing unacceptable variations in the standards of care across the country. It sought to achieve this by setting national standards and defining service models for people with mental health problems, and setting up mechanisms for local implementation with performance indicators for review. It set out standards in five areas; mental health promotion (1), primary care and service access (2 and 3), effective services for people with severe mental illness (4 and 5), carers needs (6) and suicide prevention (7). The Framework was developed with advice from an External Reference Group (ERG), whose members were drawn from health and social care professionals, service users, carers, managers and the non-statutory sector. A statement of values figures prominently in the introduction to the NSF. Amongst other things, those who experience mental health problems can expect that services will involve users and carers in the planning and delivery of care. Services will be non-discriminatory, and will offer choices and promote independence. They will be properly accountable to the public, service users and carers. The introduction also values partnerships between NHS, social care organizations and their partners, with a focus on local health and social care communities. We will consider Standards 4 and 5 (services for people with serious mental illnesses) in greater detail, so that we can be clear about the assumptions that underlie the NSF as far as this group of people is concerned.

The purpose of Standards 4 and 5 is to ensure that people with severe mental illness receive the range of services they need. Standard 4 indicates that all service users on the care programme approach (CPA) receive care that optimizes engagement, reduces risk and prevents crises. They should have a care plan specifying how this is to be achieved. Standard 5 deals with what should happen if the person needs care away from home, which should be in the least restrictive environment necessary to protect the public and themselves, and as close to home as possible. The management and disposal of risk are central to the aims of both standards, and is expressed in terms that echo Frank Dobson's statements:

> Some people with severe and enduring mental illness find it difficult to engage with and maintain contact with services, posing a risk to themselves or to others. (Department of Health 1999: 43)

and

> Assessment should cover psychiatric, psychological and social functioning, risk to the individual and others, including previous violence and criminal record . . . (Department of Health 1999: 43)

and

> All staff involved in performing assessments should receive training in risk assessment and risk management, updated regularly. (Department of Health 1999: 43)

Standards 4 and 5 deal primarily with professional interventions and services. They attach importance to the role of neuroleptic medication that has '. . . a proven reduction in rate of relapse', and:

> The development of new and atypical drugs, with a different range of side-effects, (that) may offer scope for improving the effectiveness of treatment and reducing the impact of side effects. Clozapine may be effective in those who have not responded to the older drugs. (Department of Health 1999: 45)

They stress the importance of ensuring that people stay on medication, through written information and 'compliance therapy'. The effectiveness of psychological interventions such as cognitive therapy for psychosis and anxiety management techniques is also stressed. Particular attention is drawn to those service users who are 'difficult to engage', and who are:

> . . . more likely to live in inner city areas, to be homeless, and to be over-represented in suicide, violence and homicide. (Department of Health 1999: 46)

The issue of risk also figures prominently in the NSF's discussion of this group's problems:

> If personal and public safety and well-being are to be assured, it is essential that mental health services stay in contact with people with severe and enduring mental illness, especially individuals who are assessed as at risk of harm themselves or of posing a risk to others. (Department of Health 1999: 50)

The Framework proposes that assertive outreach services provide a means of responding to these issues.

The National Institute for Clinical Excellence

NICE was set up as a special health authority in 1999 to provide expert technical guidance in the form of clinical practice guidelines on the effectiveness of different therapies. In 2002, it published its technical assessment on the use of atypical neuroleptic drugs (NICE 2002*a*). NICE considered diverse sources of evidence, which included a systematic review of atypical neuroleptics from the NHS Centre for Reviews and Dissemination in the University of York, submissions from patient and other groups (which included the Zito Trust and SANE), professional organizations (the Royal College of Psychiatrists) and the pharmaceutical industry. The guidelines begin by pointing out that although the aetiology of schizophrenia remains poorly understood, we are nevertheless to understand the effectiveness of atypical neuroleptics in terms of a modified dopamine theory. Although the NICE guidelines on the management of schizophrenia (NICE 2002*b*) point out that the management of the condition should address the person's emotional and social needs, the implication is that the pharmacological management of schizophrenia is *a priori*, and without it psychological and other interventions may be ineffective:

> Antipsychotic drugs are an indispensable treatment for most people in the recovery phase of schizophrenia . . . Drugs are also necessary for psychological treatments to be effective. (NICE 2002*b*: 17)

The technical paper on atypical neuroleptics also points out that although psychological and social interventions are important, the pharmacological treatment of schizophrenia accounts for <5% of the total health care costs for the condition (NICE 2002*a*: 3).

NICE surveyed 172 randomized controlled trials (RCTs), with evidence from a further 53 studies in which atypical neuroleptics were compared with typical drugs. The guidelines conclude that the former are at least as efficacious as the latter, and that there is evidence that they may vary in their relative effects on positive and negative symptoms of schizophrenia. All atypicals appeared to have a lower frequency of extrapyramidal side effects than conventional drugs, although there was no evidence favouring any one atypical over the others in terms of overall efficacy. The Appraisal Committee concluded that more widespread use of atypical neuroleptics would benefit individuals with schizophrenia, because of the likelihood of fewer extrapyramidal side effects. To achieve this, the guidelines recommend that all clinicians treating people suffering from schizophrenia should audit their neuroleptic prescribing practice. The audit standard is that 100% of people newly diagnosed with schizophrenia must be prescribed atypical neuroleptics (NICE 2002a: 19).

National Institute for Mental Health in England (NIMHE)

NIMHE was set up towards the end of 2001 with the purpose of improving mental health services by ensuring that the changes advocated for by the NSF and NICE were implemented. It is located within the NHS Modernization Agency, and led by the National Director for Mental Health. It is a 'virtual institute' with regional centres, and it has no core funding. Its work is truly diverse, and it has more than 20 work streams from acute in-patient care to workforce issues, from partnerships with the pharmaceutical industry to values in mental health practice. NIMHE's work stream on the mental health of Black and minority ethnic (BME) communities is of particular importance and relevance to our clinical work in Bradford's culturally diverse population (see also Chapter 9), and to our critique of mental health theory and practice. For these reasons, we shall focus specifically on this aspect of its work.

> There does not appear to be a single area of mental health care in this country in which Black and minority ethnic groups fare as well as, or better than, the majority White community. Both in terms of service experience and the outcome of service interventions, they fare much worse than people from the ethnic majority do. In addition, disease burden associated with mental disorder appears to fall disproportionately on minority ethnic populations.
> (NIMHE 2003: 10)

Over the last 2 years, the NSF has been augmented by a number of consultation and policy documents dealing with the lamentable failure of mental health services to meet the needs of the country's BME communities. Much of this work has stemmed directly from NIMHE's work. Over the last 50 years there have been thousands of research papers written by academics, hundreds of reports, and dozens of inquiries trying to account for the health inequalities experienced by members of our BME communities who use mental health services. Many explanations have been proposed, White stereotypes about Black and Asian people, culturally inappropriate services, stigma; we would not reject any of these. In recent years, there has been a move away from a preoccupation with supposed racial or cultural differences and their role in shaping individual predisposition to mental disorder, to a greater concern with the relationship between racism, injustice and inequality and the social exclusion and stigmatization that disproportionately affect people from BME communities. Increasingly, these factors, not 'racially' based biological differences, are considered to lie at the root of the experiences of distress and psychosis. One of the most important events in bringing about this change in attitude in health was the racist murder of Stephen Lawrence, an 18-year-old Black student who was murdered on April 22, 1993 while waiting for a bus in Eltham, South London. He was attacked without provocation by a racist gang of five or six youths and murdered, dying from two 5 inch stab wounds, one to the chest and the other to an arm. Four years later, the Home Secretary, Jack Straw, announced an inquiry into the murder and the failed police investigation, chaired by Sir William Macpherson of Cluny. The report, published in February 1999, accused the Metropolitan Police of institutional racism in its failure to investigate the murder properly, and to bring the murderers to justice. It made 70 recommendations to end institutional racism in the police. Kwame McKenzie, a Black academic psychiatrist working at the Institute of Psychiatry, wrote as follows in an editorial in the *British Medical Journal* shortly after the publication of the *Macpherson Report*:

> Health disparities are brought about and perpetuated not only by culture, class and socio-political forces external to medicine, but also by the ideology of the medical profession. This ideology leads to ineffective or no action in the face of disparities and to a lack of concerted effort to teach or discuss racism in medicine in undergraduate and postgraduate curriculums. Moreover, the emphasis on the biomedical model undermines the anthropological research which is needed to properly document the perceptions, needs, and aspirations of minority ethnic groups. (McKenzie 1999: 616–617)

The murder of Stephen Lawrence and the death of David 'Rocky' Bennett have had profound implications for government policy and thinking about the interface between BME communities and mental health services. David Bennett was a 38-year-old Rastafarian who died in a medium secure unit on the evening of Friday 30 October 1998, while being restrained by four members of staff[8]. He came from Jamaica to join his family in England in 1968, at the age of 8 years. For 18 of the 30 years he lived in this country, he was under the care of psychiatric services. His sister, Dr Joanna Bennett, describes how his family first became worried about him in 1980, when he appeared to have '. . . problems with his behaviour and his emotions.' He saw a consultant psychiatrist who was 'dismissive', putting his problems down to cannabis intoxication. He was admitted to hospital in December 1984 when subject to a probation order, but discharged himself and, as a result, he was sentenced in January 1985 to 6 months' imprisonment. His sister visited him, and was '. . . horrified at his appearance and behaviour.' He appeared to be very unwell, and was being bullied by those around him. A month after

---

[8]The following account is taken from the independent inquiry into his death published by NSCNHS Strategic Health Authority (2003).

his release from jail, he was readmitted to hospital, where the diagnosis of schizophrenia was made for the first time. This was a difficult admission. The report refers to '. . . unprovoked attacks . . .' by David on other patients and staff. As a result, he was transferred to a private psychiatric facility in July 1985.

Over the next 10 years, he had a series of admissions to hospital. In 1996 he was assaulted and racially abused by another patient in a secure unit. No action appears to have been taken. His sister contacted the ward to say that her brother had complained of being overmedicated, and shortly after this there were concerns about his physical state. He was seen by a cardiologist after an episode of bradycardia and hypotension. At the end of October 1998, a month before his death, he was on 700 mg clozapine daily, 30 mg of haloperidol and 200 mg sulpiride.

On the day of his death, David had appeared settled. Nothing untoward was noticed about his behaviour. Around 10 p.m. he wanted to use the phone, but it was in use by another patient. He returned to ask how long he was going to be. He looked angry and demanded to use the phone. There was a scuffle. He tried to grab the phone, and threw a punch at the other patient. Shortly after this, the other man kicked David's door shouting highly offensive racist remarks at him. He hit David on the chin. Staff intervened, and in the following discussion decided to remove David to a more secure ward because his mental state was 'fragile'. He appeared agitated. He was loud, shouting out that he wanted to kill the other man. When he was told of his move, and that the other patient was staying on the ward, he punched the nurse at least three times in the face. He was restrained by up to four members of staff for a period of 25 min. At first he struggled, but then fell quiet. At some point during this period, someone noticed that he had been incontinent of urine. By this time, he had stopped breathing and no pulse could be detected. Cardio-pulmonary resuscitation was commenced and an ambulance called. He was pronounced dead on arrival at the local casualty department at 12.20 a.m. on Saturday October 31, 1998.

These events add a tragic human dimension to the consultation papers and policy documents that have dominated mental health practice over the last 10 years. Sadly, the death of David Bennett is not an isolated tragedy. In 1984, Michael Martin died in Broadmoor. Four years later, Joseph Watts also died in Broadmoor. The verdict was accidental death. In 1991, Orville Blackwood died of heart failure after being forcibly injected with a combination of promazine and fluphenazine decanoate in Broadmoor. All three men were African-Caribbean. According to MIND (2003), there have been 27 deaths of patients from BME communities in psychiatric care from 1980 until 2003. This list is almost certainly incomplete because no formal figures are kept. Since the end of the 18th century, the history of psychiatry is littered with patient deaths, scandals and abuse. There is no doubt that members of Britain's BME communities, particularly young African-Caribbean men, have experienced the most extreme abuses in what is supposed to be a caring system.

The case of David Bennett is emblematic of a range of painful and problematic encounters between psychiatric patients and mental health services that affect people from many cultural backgrounds. Of course, the tragedy and the irony is that in the great majority of cases, the pain and harm that we inflict upon patients is not intended. We work as doctors, nurses, social workers and psychologists because we want to help people. We care for them.

Following the publication of the Macpherson report, the Race Relations Amendment Act was published in 2000. This placed a specific responsibility on all public authorities to engage positively and proactively with BME communities, and to tackle social exclusion and discrimination. Here lies the first difficulty, because, unlike many local authorities, the NHS has very little experience in dealing with institutional racism. Indeed, there is reluctance on the part of some, especially politicians, to accept that the expression institutional racism applies to the NHS. On at least two occasions, the Health Minister, Jacqui Smith, refused publicly to accept that the term is appropriate to describe the situation in the NHS[9]. Despite this, the government has appeared to take the issue seriously, and has published a flurry of consultation and policy documents. NIMHE's (2003) public consultation exercise, *Inside Outside*, was written following 12 consultation events with Black and African-Caribbean, South Asian, Chinese and Irish communities in early 2003. In addition, the Department of Health (2003) published a consultation paper, *Delivering Race Equality*, which subsequently evolved into an action plan (Department of Health 2005). *Inside Outside* spells out the policy context, the Race Relations (Amendment) Act (RRA), which places a duty on all public authorities to eliminate unlawful discrimination, and to promote equal opportunity and good relations between people from different racial groups. It describes the problems of mental health care experienced by black and minority ethnic groups as follows:

> . . . that there is an over-emphasis on institutional and coercive models of care;
>
> . . . that professional and organisational requirements are given priority over individual needs and rights;
>
> . . . that institutional racism exists with mental health care. (NIMHE 2003: 7)

It argues that:

> Those who use mental health services are identified, first and foremost, as citizens with mental health needs, which are understood as located in a social and cultural context. (NIMHE 2003: 7)

The report sets out three strategic objectives: to end ethnic inequalities in mental health care, in terms of both the experience of services and outcome;

---

[9]The first occasion was in April 2004 when interviewed by Jon Snow on *Channel 4 News*, the second was at a public meeting held in Bradford in December 2004 to launch the Department of Health's *Delivering Race Equality* programme.

to develop a mental health workforce capable of delivering effective mental health services to a multicultural society; and to build capacity within the BME communities and voluntary sector to respond to the communities' mental health needs. It proposes the use of community development workers as a means of building capacity. The emphasis in *Delivering Race Equality* is slightly different. It sought opinions about a draft framework informed largely by the RRA. The areas of concern flagged up by the document were broadly similar to those raised by *Inside Outside*, but focused more specifically on suicide, pathways to care and in-patient facilities. It proposed that three fundamental building blocks were essential to improve service delivery and outcome for people from BME communities: better quality information; more appropriate and responsive services; and increased community engagement. The final action plan of *Delivering Race Equality* published in 2005 after the publication of the independent inquiry into the death of David Bennett also acknowledged the importance of this report. It promised a 5-year action plan with the employment of 500 community development workers to engage local communities and build capacity in them.

Inside Outside and *Delivering Race Equality* stress the importance of engaging communities, and promote community development as a way of achieving this. In Chapter 10, we will describe in detail the work of *Sharing Voices Bradford*, a community development project that has been working with Bradford's BME communities in the broad field of mental health over the last 4 years. Both documents also stress the importance of workforce issues, especially the need to enhance cultural competencies. *Inside Outside* (NIMHE 2003: 30) also points out that critical theory is an important element in helping the workforce to think through issues relating to cultural diversity, as part of the development of cultural competency.

Kam Bhui (2004) and his colleagues have pointed out that these two documents appear to have different emphases. *Inside Outside* stresses equity, whereas *Delivering Race Equality* shifts attention in the direction of organizational change. This is both confusing, and may also give rise to the impression that the views of ethnic minorities have not been fully taken into account right from the outset. In any case, it is difficult to see how organizational change or better quality data are going to make a great deal of difference. Kam Bhui and his colleagues also point out that the emphasis on race as a focus of reform may unnecessarily restrict the potential for improvement. This is because targeting 'race' tends to treat large groups that are heterogeneous in nature as if they are all the same. The appellation 'South Asian', for example, is enormously diverse, and includes many different language and faith groupings. It also ignores the complex range of cultural identities and practices contained within particular communities, encompassed in terms of generation and age. This suggests that a more sophisticated approach is necessary, one that recognizes the complexity of individual cultural identity.

Power, values and interest

At this point, there are several issues we want to raise; all will map onto areas that we will consider in greater detail later on. These concern the contested nature of mental disorder, the undermining of local systems for understanding madness and the implicit values of psychiatry as a form of Western expertise.

The contested nature of mental disorder

Those who advocate for the global relevance of psychiatry or the uncritical application of its knowledge through NSFs and NICE guidelines within our multicultural society overlook the contested nature of mental health theory and practice. The WHO mhGAP initiative takes for granted the concept of mental disorder, and assumes that psychiatric treatments and associated systems of health care are unproblematic. Likewise, the NICE technical document on atypical neuroleptics confidently asserts that schizophrenia is a syndrome characterized by '. . . a broad range of cognitive, emotional and behavioural problems' (NICE 2002a: 3). There is a serious difficulty with such statements; the nature of schizophrenia is contested. Over the last 15 years, the survivor movement has questioned and challenged the assumptions of psychiatry, and its right to interpret their experiences. This is not a local phenomenon. The survivor movement across the world questions the concepts of psychiatry, its theories and treatments. In the next chapter, we shall examine the diverse interpretations and meanings attached by service users to their experiences. Elsewhere, the problematic status of the scientific basis of schizophrenia has been described by several commentators (Bentall 1990, 2003; Boyle 1993; Thomas 1997; Johnstone 2000). Recent critiques have extended these arguments to attention deficit hyperactivity disorder in children (Timimi 2002).

Historically speaking, the categorical view of illness has been a key element of the biomedical model, and has played an important part in shaping the way psychiatrists understand psychosis. However, there is increasing evidence to support a dimensional view of psychosis. This proposes that there is a general predisposition to psychosis to be found in the population at large (Meehl 1962). Those diagnosed as schizophrenic are simply those who present with the most severe expression of traits that are to be found subclinically in the community. There is now considerable evidence to support this view, both for auditory hallucinations and for paranoid delusions. Sidgwick undertook a large-scale general population survey of 17 000 subjects, almost 4% of whom had heard voices (Sidgwick *et al.* 1894). This figure is remarkably similar to that obtained in a recent epidemiological study by Tien (1991). Subjects were interviewed with a diagnostic schedule devised by the National Institute of Mental Health, and widely used in psychiatric research. Between 10 and 15% of the sample of 18 500 admitted to hallucinations of one or more sensory modalities, and 2% of the sample admitted to hearing voices. In this country,

Johns *et al.* (2002), using data from the Fourth National Survey of Ethnic Minorities, found that 4% of the White population said they had experienced verbal auditory hallucinations. African-Caribbean people were two and a half times more likely to have had the experience than White people. A quarter of all those who heard voices met the criteria for psychosis on the Psychosis Screening Questionnaire. Other, non-epidemiological, studies have found that the experience is not restricted to adults. In The Netherlands, Escher *et al.* (2002) identified a group of 80 children through the media who heard voices. About half the sample were not in contact with children's mental health services. When followed up over 3 years, 60% of the children's voices had ceased. Other studies that have identified verbal auditory hallucinations in non-clinical populations include those by Posey & Losch (1983), Romme & Escher (1989) Barrett & Etheridge (1992) and Leudar *et al.* (1996). Recent studies have also shown that paranoid delusions are to be found in non-clinical populations (Fenigstein & Vanable 1992; van Os *et al.* 1999; Martin & Penn 2001; Ellett *et al.* 2003).

The question that arises here is how should we think of those people in the community who have psychotic experiences and who meet the criteria for psychosis. Are we to think of them as undiagnosed patients in need of the panoply of NSF and NICE guidelines, including assessment, treatment and care plans? Or are we to think of them in some other way, perhaps as people who have unusual experiences, but who have accepted those experiences, are comfortable with them and live their lives alongside them without difficulty? These questions are important given the current vogue for early intervention in psychosis. It is claimed that services designed to intervene promptly and treat schizophrenia in its earliest stages can help to prevent deterioration in cognitive function (Amminger *et al.* 2002), the so-called defect state, and prevent treatment resistance (Edwards *et al.* 1998). The continuum view of psychosis poses difficult questions for those who advocate for early intervention for psychosis. How are we to regard people in the community with non-clinical voices or delusions? Should we consider them to be 'pre-schizophrenic'? Are they to be considered at risk of developing schizophrenia and thus in need of early intervention? We argue that this position is problematic. In The Netherlands, Marius Romme and Sandra Escher have made a detailed comparison of clinical and non-clinical voice hearers. Their work suggests that although some of these people are happy to accept medical interpretations of their experiences, many use a variety of explanatory frameworks, including psychodynamic, mystical and parapsychological (Romme & Escher 1993). Put simply, the question is this; what right do we have to impose on others explanations for their experiences that may conflict with their understanding? This question has ramifications into all levels of mental health care. It lies at the heart of individual encounters between psychiatrists and their patients. It should also colour our interpretation of frameworks and guidelines for mental health services. Its implications for the troubled encounter between Western psychiatry and non-Western cultures, locally and globally, are of even greater significance. Service Frameworks and Clinical Guidelines on Schizophrenia stress the importance of 'working in partnership' with service users, but as we shall see they are deeply rooted in modernism, and assume that we must adopt a bio-medical framework towards psychotic experience to the extent that this will be imposed upon individuals against their will. We must also remember in this context that the British government's proposals to reform the mental health leg-islation in England and Wales includes a broader definition of mental disorder than was the case in the 1983 Mental Health Act, thus potentially increasing the numbers of people who will fall under the gaze of psychiatry. Psychological interventions such as cognitive behavioural therapy are seen merely as treat-ment adjuncts to 'assist in the development of insight'. The real purpose of psy-chological interventions is to reinforce the idea that the person's experiences are to be understood in terms of schizophrenia for which medication is required (NICE 2002b: 16). Our position here is one that will continually resurface. We question the ethical and moral position of practice that is based upon sweeping assumptions about the interpretation of distress and psychosis, and imposes its own interpretation of distress upon individual patients, communities and cultures. Questions of ethics must come before questions of technological effectiveness. There are two further issues. The first concerns the nature of the technology that psychiatrists use to make a diagnosis. In other words, we are concerned here with phenomenology. This will be a major focus of the second section of this book. The second concerns the relationship between the technology of psychi-atry and local understandings of distress. Of course, the litmus test of this rela-tionship is how psychiatry relates to cultural difference. Our concern is that the profession, along with others who work in the community in mental health, simply see this in terms of 'cultural competence' (see, for example, Department of Health 1999: 47) rather than looking more deeply at this relationship. Our position, which will become clearer in the second and third sections of this book, is that it is the epistemological basis of psychiatry itself that is the prob-lem. This means that improving the outcomes and experiences of people from BME communities who use mental health services cannot be achieved simply by 'bolting on' modules in cultural competency in psychiatric or other profes-sional training. It is here that a critical philosophical perspective on psychiatric knowledge and practice is of greatest value.

Undermining local knowledge

At the beginning of this chapter, we described briefly the globalization of psychiatry. This is having an adverse effect on local belief systems and support structures for those who experience distress and psychosis. Higginbotham & Marsella (1988) have described how in the capital cities of Southeast Asia, psychiatric care varied little, in spite of large social, cultural and linguistic differences between the inhabitants of these cities. The mechanisms of international mental health education, consultation and collaboration created a form of psychiatric practice that looked to the West for its conceptual foundations and for ideas about innovation and progress. It was hoped that these developments would improve patient care, but in reality the care received by many people with mental health problems deteriorated. The authors stood back from the general approbation associated with the export of psychiatry and presented evidence for serious adverse ' *after-shocks*' within local cultural systems. They demonstrated how the diffusion of Western-based knowledge promoted professional élitism and institutionalized responses to distress, all of which undermined local healing systems and practices. We shall return to their work in Chapter 10.

The issue we are concerned with here is the globalization of a very narrow notion of psychology, normality, distress and healing, which replaces local understandings and indigenous frameworks. In turn, this weakens local ways of life. This is part of a global trend in which all the peoples of the planet are becoming incorporated into the international system of consumption and production.

Every day, more and more people in different parts of the world come to understand their lives, their needs and their relationships within the terms given to them by manufacturers of goods, services and entertainment. Our point here is that in the field of mental health, it is clinical neuroscience, mediated in large part by the interests of the pharmaceutical industry, that defines how we should think about our feelings and the terms we use to interpret our distress.

In our view, there is an exceptionally strong case to be made for help and support networks for people in distress that are primarily non-technical in low and high income countries alike. Kwame McKenzie and his colleagues point out that despite huge inequalities in resources, the rich countries of the world have something to learn from the poorer countries (McKenzie *et al.* 2004). They describe how traditional care in poor countries, such as structured community support for mothers following childbirth, or community-based rehabilitation services with workers drawn from local communities, can result in improvements in outcome and quality. This is not to idealize or romanticize local cultures, their understandings of distress and madness, and the support networks they contain. Neither is it to deny the importance of economic justice for the poor countries of the world. At the end of this book, we shall argue that the limitless expansion of Western technological approaches to distress and madness are simply unsustainable. There is a powerful case for restructuring mental health systems in the West in ways that diversify the workforce. This means building up infrastructure in local communities through community development. It has major implications for the structure of mental health teams, and for our roles as doctors working in mental health.

Implicit values of psychiatry

We tend to see psychiatric knowledge as simply the inevitable outcome of Western scientific thought, progress and innovation. Madness and distress are no longer to be understood in terms of religious, spiritual, cultural or political frameworks, but in terms of clinical neuroscience and cognitivism. The latter lie at the heart of contemporary psychiatry, and are assumed to be scientific, neutral, disinterested and acultural. Such a position marginalizes more than 20 years of historical, sociological, philosophical and anthropological research that challenge this self-understanding. These disciplines argue that psychiatric concepts and treatment, and the narrow medical framing of distress are far from neutral, but value-laden, and saturated with Western assumptions about the relationship between body and mind, mind and society. The prominent role of science and technology is apparent in the mhGAP initiative, which is based in 'scientific and technical evidence for what works' (World Health Organization 2002: 8), and the NSF and NICE guidelines. All these assume that Western science and technology are neutral, objective and universal truths that can be applied in any situation without regard for the context in which this knowledge came to be, or for the context in which it is to be used. Scientific evidence largely originates in research from high-income countries, but this is applied across a wide variety of cultural and socio-economic contexts, making it difficult to generalize the results. This is yet another facet of the troubled encounter between global psychiatry and local knowledge. Kleinman & Cohen (1997) point out that the preoccupation with clinical neuroscience is a peculiarly Western phenomenon, and that a myth has embedded itself in psychiatry:

> . . . that a knowledge base compiled almost exclusively from North American and European cases can be effectively applied to the 80% of the world's population that lives in Asia, Africa and South America as well as to the immigrant communities of North America and Europe. (Kleinman & Cohen 1997)

Thornley & Adams (1998) raise essentially the same issue, albeit from a different perspective. They observe that the majority (54%) of therapeutic trials in schizophrenia have taken place in North America, yet only 2% of the world's population live there. They make the following point:

> How applicable the findings of these trials are to the 43 million other patients in Africa, Australasia, and Europe is difficult to assess. Further problems with generalisability arise from the fact that most participants in trials were people in hospital, even in the 1990's. (Thornley & Adams 1998: 1183)

The mhGAP initiative, through its processes of consciousness raising and education with governments and public, is designed to create the demand for more psychiatric treatment and to ensure that the means are there to provide this. This devalues local understandings of, and responses to, psychosis in favour of Western modalities of treatment based in neuroscience and cognitivism. In the face of this, developing countries will continue to be seen as backward, second-best and dependent. The problem is that the value we attach to science and technology can blind us to their limitations and downsides. We must also remember that the scientific and technical evidence used to justify the claims made for the effectiveness of drug treatment in psychiatry is not without its weaknesses. For example, there are serious doubts about the quality of information from RCTs (Thornley & Adams 1998), and conflicting evidence on the advantages of atypical neuroleptics over conventional drugs (Geddes *et al.* 2000) advocated for by NICE. The issue is that like all clinical practice guidelines, the NICE guidelines are enormously influential. They are circulated to PCT Chief Executives, NHS Trust Chief Executives, GP Partners and all Consultant Psychiatrists in England and Wales, and health professionals are '. . . expected to take it fully into account when exercising their clinical judgement.' Our concern relates to the power and influence of clinical practice guidelines, and whose interests they really promote. We shall return to this theme in detail in Chapter 6.

Conflict, paradox, and the end of certainty

We do not deny the virtue of WHO initiatives and NSFs designed to improve the circumstances of those who experience mental health problems. Both represent a shift away from seeing hospitals and institutions as a solution to the problems of mental disorder. Both recognize the importance of responding to distress in primary care. Both appear committed to challenging the stigma associated with mental illness. Both make an plea for a new approach to mental health. But what does this really mean? For the WHO, it appears to mean that governments across the world must spend more money on psychiatry, with more mental health care practitioners identifying and treating more cases of mental disorder, presumably with more drugs. The main priority of the mhGAP programme is the global expansion of mental health services, and the exportation of models and understanding of psychosis and distress founded in modernism. Much the same can be said about the NSF. The emphasis in Standard 4 is on the management and containment of risk through technologies of care, especially medication. Only brief reference is made to the importance service users attach to the contexts of their difficulties and the issues that we know matter to service users from user-led research, such as good housing and income, as well as social contacts and ways of structuring time (p. 46), or their preferences for crisis houses and sanctuaries (p. 48).

We want to be quite clear that in looking critically at service frameworks and clinical guidelines, we are not denying that they have a valuable role to play in health care. The public expects doctors to be well informed about the effectiveness of different treatments, and there has to be some way of ensuring that this is the case. However, our concern is that evidence and the idea of evidence-based practice have become ends in themselves and are drawn into conflict with values. We are particularly concerned that service frameworks and guidelines have become important mediators of pharmaceutical company influence. Their purpose ostensibly is to enable doctors and patients to be aware of the best evidence for making decisions, but as we shall see in Chapter 6, there are serious doubts about the impartiality of this evidence. Haynes & Devereaux (2002) have pointed out that people make decisions, not evidence. This applies to the processes of negotiation between individual clinicians and patients, or those that operate when governments write guidelines and frameworks. Smith (2000) points out that evidence-based medicine is not simply the application of technology to clinical problem solving, but an ethical project:

> The evidence supports decision making, but the evidence can't make the decision. The values of the patient or the community must be a part of the decision. Effective interventions have risks. How can benefits be weighed against risks? (Smith 2000: 1364)

The processes of clinical decisions making are complex, and clinical guidelines, which apply to 'average' patients, must be flexible enough to take into account individual patient preferences and circumstances. This, as Geddes & Wessely (2000) point out, is primarily an ethical project. There are bound to be situations that arise from time to time where adherence to guidelines may do more harm than good. In addition, what happens if there is a lack of agreement between doctor and patient as to the nature of the patient's problems? Perkins (2001) points out that choices have to be made as to whose view of effectiveness counts. Most research in psychiatry defines effectiveness in terms of symptom resolution, but many service users reject notions of illness, or that their experiences are to be accounted for as symptoms. In other words, recovery means remission of symptoms; it means no longer hearing voices or having unusual beliefs. This view of recovery (and thus effectiveness) we will challenge in Chapter 8. Historically, service users have been excluded from having any voice in decisions as to what constitutes effectiveness, but as we shall see in the next chapter, user-led research is changing this (Faulkner & Thomas 2002). This represents an enormous political challenge to expert guidelines and evidence.

The democratic aspirations of the NHS Plan, its talk of citizens and partnerships, and of remedying social exclusion, constitute a serious challenge to the dominant position of the biomedical model in mental health services. Standard 1 of the NSF draws attention to the importance of cultural, social and political contexts and the effect these have on our emotional well-being. It challenges mental health practice that occurs in a vacuum, and treats people as individuals removed from human contexts. As this book progresses, we shall argue that a central theme of biomedical psychiatry is that its focus on the individual downplays the importance of human contexts. The NHS Plan with its commitment to tackling health inequality and seeing patients as citizens, not passive recipients of services, brings politics right into the heart of health care. It confronts us with an agenda that sits uncomfortably with the notion of health care professionals as experts, as neutral and disinterested scientists or technicians. It offers an opportunity for us to rethink the ways in which we understand illness and disease, and how we relate to those we serve—our patients and the public.

We agree that mental health services need to change, but a fundamental aspect of our analysis is that the tools of change, evidence-based medicine and clinical neuroscience, are couched in the idioms of modernity and progress. Progress is not to be made through science alone, which is incapable of tackling issues such as racism, disadvantage, poverty, lack of educational attainment, discrimination and social exclusion. This has implications for the way we work with people whose lives are blighted by such adversity. It also has implications for our understandings of madness and distress. In particular, how might we have to re-conceptualize madness and distress if we are to recognize the significance of the contextual factors that shape and colour the experiences of our patients? What sort of services might result from such an analysis? To start to answer these, we must next consider the experiences of service users. There is much to be learnt from facing up to and engaging with the disaffection and criticism expressed by service users about their experiences of mental health services. For us, this disaffection can no longer simply be dismissed as 'antipsychiatry'.

2 What counts as evidence?

Evidence, and the research upon which it is based, is not neutral. Investigators perform research and interpret evidence from a particular viewpoint or perspective. In doing so, they are driven by a variety of interests and concerns. Some of these may be understood in terms of scientific curiosity, some in terms of a commitment to extending knowledge in order to help others. Some may be less idealistic. In Chapter 6, we will describe how other interests shape and influence scientific knowledge. We will see that the pharmaceutical industry has created a grey area in which its interests are paraded around under the guise of science. In this chapter, we consider evidence that openly acknowledges the interests of service users. After Chapter 1, it is important that we clear a space for the voices of those who use mental health services. Then we will be in a better position to commence our critique of the philosophical underpinnings of psychiatry in the second section of this book. We have tried to access service user experience in two ways; through the many survivor narratives that have been written over the years, and through the growing corpus known as user-led research (ULR). There are a many personal testimonies and narratives in which we find authentic accounts of service user and survivor experience. The anthology *Speaking Our Minds* (Read & Reynolds 1996) is a reader for the Open University's course *Mental Health and Distress*, and consists of contributions by more than 50 people who have used mental health services. We have chosen to focus on this selection of personal narratives because the contributors include some of the leading survivors in England, including Peter Campbell, Louise Pembroke and David Crepaz-Keay, three founder members of Survivors Speak Out. Their voices have inspired countless other survivors, here and in other parts of the world. We consider some of these narratives in the first part of this chapter. They merit close inspection. They reflect a wide range of opinion and experience, from negative to positive.

ULR places service users' perspectives and interests in the foreground. ULR in mental health is unique. There is no equivalent in general medicine. It has developed out of frustration with the failure of professional-led research to engage with issues and outcomes that are important to service users. We draw on two main sources of information: research studies designed, implemented and disseminated by service users (i.e. ULR); and material published in the form of personal narratives that raise particular points about our work as psychiatrists. The first examine two examples of ULR. *Users' voices: the perspectives of mental health service users on community and hospital care*, deals with users' experiences of and satisfaction with community- and hospital-based mental health services. It examines user satisfaction with mainstream mental health services. The second, *Strategies for living*, examines users' experiences from a more personal perspective. It is concerned more with how users understand, cope with and recover from distress. Although these studies ask different questions, they reach broadly similar conclusions. We shall describe the design and implementation of these studies, and then outline the main findings. We have deliberately focused on those findings that are most relevant to the narratives presented in the first part of this chapter.

Survivor narratives

It is important to recognize that although many of these accounts describe negative experiences of psychiatry and mental health services, this is not exclusively so. We find diverse opinions about psychiatric treatment, both positive and negative. Leonard Taylor (1996) describes his experience of electro-convulsive therapy (ECT) as barbaric. On the other hand, Rachel Perkins (1996) chose to have ECT when she was depressed because she believed that it would help her to recover more rapidly. Richie B (1996) was given a diagnosis of schizophrenia, which for him did nothing other than to symbolize the abuse that he experienced as a child at the hands of his alcoholic father. He is enraged by psychiatry's failure to grapple with his life story and the early childhood experiences that he believed to be central in understanding why he heard voices. On the other hand, Richard Jameson (1996) found the diagnosis of schizophrenia to be real and meaningful. Accepting the diagnosis meant that he could get on with his life. Likewise, Christine McIntosh (1996) was angry that she had not been told earlier that she had a diagnosis of manic-depressive psychosis, but was then relieved when she found out. Knowing that her experiences could be accounted for through a diagnosis meant she was able to get on with her life.

The general tenor of these accounts is redolent of the results of earlier surveys of user experiences, such as that undertaken by Rogers *et al.* (1993). About a third of their 516 respondents said they had found psychiatric nurses to be the most helpful group. Only 12% found psychiatrists helpful. In fact, psychiatrists were reported to be the least helpful group by more than 21% of respondents. Nearly two-fifths reported their psychiatrists' attitudes to be either unhelpful or very unhelpful. They used adjectives such as '...reserved...', '...detached...', '...godly...' or '...condescending...', '...complacent benevolence...' to describe the attitudes of some psychiatrists. In fairness, others found their psychiatrists helpful. The point we want to make is that it is not possible to dismiss the accounts that follow on the grounds that they are unrepresentative. Time and time again service users report positive and negative experiences of psychiatrists and mental health services. In our view, all points of view must be acknowledged and taken seriously. It does not make sense to us to dismiss things that we may not like to hear as 'antipsychiatry', as often happens under these circumstances. For one thing, it betrays an ignorance about the true nature of antipsychiatry (see Chapter 3). We believe that there is much to be gained from a serious and open engagement with those who take up an oppositional stance.

There is another point to emerge from survivor narratives. When we examine them carefully, it is clear that people use many different ways of interpreting their experiences in their attempts to make sense of them. These range from traditional readings of the medical model to strong pleas for contextualized accounts of distress. *Speaking Our Minds* reveals the user and survivor movement in its complex diversity. Jim Read (1996) points out that the survivor movement, or at least those engaged in self-advocacy, has always had different opinions about how best to conceptualize emotional distress. Within the movement, there is debate and controversy as to whether mental illness exists, the role of drugs and whether compulsory detention is ever justifiable. These concerns are increasingly shared by growing numbers of psychiatrists and mental health professionals. However, there is broad agreement about the principles on which mental health services should operate. These resonate with the findings of ULR which we shall consider later in this chapter: information, choice, self-help and self-organization. In addition to this, our reading of these narratives reveals a number of themes that lie close to the heart of postpsychiatry; the importance of contexts and meaning in understanding distress, the ethical problems of psychiatry as a form of technology, and the role of power and control in mental health service.

Contexts and meaning

Several contributors describe the importance of understanding their experiences of distress within a variety of contexts. Some of the examples we cite here are all the more striking because they raise once more the baleful effects of racism in people's live, and the close relationship between racism and the experiences of psychosis. This increases the poignancy of David Bennett's story. Patricia Brunner (1996) describes how her psychosis became meaningful through her experiences as a Black woman, and those of her mother who also experienced psychosis after moving to this country. Her parents emigrated from Jamaica in the 1950s but returned to the island after her father retired. Back in Jamaica, her mother was quite different:

> When I see my mother in (Jamaica), doing her chores, ministering deftly and sympathetically to a sick relative, being hospitable to neighbours and old friends, I think of the woman she might have been, and of the appalling waste of a human being this signifies. All those years in England—all those years of grief, heartache and racism. Perhaps there had always been a rational person inside her struggling for assertion, but conventional methods of treatment failed to achieve much. Yet the simple act of returning to a society in

which she could be both accepting and acceptable has done more than the
years of shock treatments and drug therapy. (Brunner 1996: 17)

The links between her experience of psychosis and her mother are complex,
but what stands out is a contrast between her understanding of her psychosis,
and that of psychiatry, which locates psychosis in the disordered brain of the
individual. This identifies the solution in treatments that operate at the level of
the individual, and which purport to rectify disordered brain function. Patricia
Brunner, on the other hand, understands her psychosis partly through her
mother's experiences, and their situations as two Black women, mother and
daughter, within a predominantly White culture. Culture, conflicts about
cultural identity, and racism are also important in Veronica Dewan's (1996)
understanding of her experiences, especially in view of her mixed cultural
heritage (Indian and Irish Catholic). Thus the problems of living in a rejecting,
racist society lie at the heart of her psychosis, problems that were exacerbated
by her hospital admissions, and her encounters with mental health professionals.
She says:

My mental health, race and culture are inextricably linked. This link has been
ignored, denied, mocked, excluded, avoided, misunderstood, rejected by
institutions and individuals—and also by me in the many disorientated
moments of my life. (Dewan 1996: 27)

We find in her words pointers to the next theme, that of the ethics of
psychiatry as technology.

The ethics of psychiatry as a form of technology

We may think of psychiatry as a technology in the sense that it is a means
through which scientific knowledge acts in the human world. This raises many
questions. How is this knowledge used? What practices does it give rise to?
How are these practices experienced by those who are subjected to them?
What are the ethical contingencies of these practices? These issues emerge in
several stories in *Speaking Our Minds*. Mary O'Hagan's contribution is a vivid
example. She juxtaposes her account of her experiences of an admission with
the medical entries made at the same time by her psychiatrist. We find a stark
contrast between her intensely felt personal experiences of psychosis,
especially the agony and isolation she endured, and the detached and remote
attitude of her psychiatrist towards her. In the extract below, her account is in
italics and her psychiatrist's in non-italic font:

*Today I want to die. Everything was hurting. My body was screaming. I saw
the doctor. I said nothing. Now I feel terrible. Nothing seems good and
nothing seems possible.*

I am stuck in this twilight mood

where I go down

like the setting sun

into a lonely black hole

where there is room for only one.

Flat, lacking motivation, sleep and appetite good. Discussed aetiology. Cont LiCarb 250 mg qid. Levels next time. (O'Hagan 1996: 46)

This suggests that there is an unbridgeable gulf between Mary O'Hagan's suffering and the disinterested, objective stance of her psychiatrist, who uses clinical terms to describe her mental state and then refers to the aetiology of her distress and its treatment with lithium carbonate. It seems from this that he is unaware of the depths of her pain. There is no reference to it, and on occasions his words appear to minimize her distress ('Impression of over dramatisation' p. 46). The psychiatrist hopes that medication (chlorpromazine) 'will break the chain', but she refuses to take this because she is afraid that medication will dull her mind. '...and the meanings in there will escape for ever.'

In this account, there is a deep split between two humans beings, the patient and her psychiatrist. Mary is deeply distressed, grappling with profound issues about her existence as a human being. Her psychiatrist is there to help her recover. That is what doctors are supposed to do. But there seems to be no point of contact between the two. Although the psychiatrist is aware of his patient's distress at times, he appears to turn away from it. Kathleen Jones (1988) has suggested that the medical model has a protective or adaptive function for psychiatrists. As the care of patients has shifted into an increasingly hostile community, psychiatrists have rejected models that engage with painful social realities in favour of a narrow biomedical stance, so that they can see themselves as:

...experts in pharmacology rather than experts in human behaviour. Abnormal behaviour patterns could be controlled: they need not be understood. The psychiatrist could carry out his work as other doctors did—relieved of the burdens of attempting to follow the processes of disturbed minds, the strains and complexities of unfamiliar lifestyles, the pressures of unemployment, squalid housing conditions and poor nutrtition. There was no need to enter the jungle of human emotions—love, hatred, pain, grief. (Jones 1988: 83)

Seen in this light, the use in psychiatry of a particular form of phenomenology sometimes referred to as descriptive psychopathology, which strips away lived experience from its all too painful human contexts, serves the purpose of a coping strategy for the profession, which removes from psychiatrists the obligation to engage with their patients' experiences, other than for the purposes of making a diagnosis. But as Jones points out, this quest takes place in people whose lives are lived against a backdrop of poverty, disadvantage, stigma and oppression. In this sense, we can see that phenomenology in the guise of descriptive psychopathology offers a safe retreat into a world of expert knowledge which distances psychiatrists from their patients' suffering. We shall be returning to this issue in depth in Chapter 4.

Psychopathological interpretations of experience also exclude other ways of interpreting and understanding psychosis, for it marks out and excludes all superstitious and spiritual belief as irrational, as Louise Pembroke's account indicates. She provides a detailed description of her own explanatory framework, and then goes on to show how this was misinterpreted and ignored by psychiatry. This had ramifications into all areas of her life. She begins by pointing out that she had always been a spiritual person (Pembroke 1996). She recalls experiencing a spiritual presence at the age of 10, which waited outside her bedroom door trying to get in. She was afraid of what might happen if it did; she feared it would harm her. This continued every night for 7 years, until a spiritual healer suggested she speak to the presence. When she did, the presence went away immediately, but shortly after she awoke feeling as though her own spirit had died. She was terrified that her physical body would die, and at that point took her first overdose. When she had recovered from this, she discovered that another spirit had entered her body, replacing her own spirit. She felt contaminated, as if there was something rotten inside her, so she saw a priest who performed an exorcism. Again, the spirit left her only to return shortly afterwards through a hole in her aura. However, she discovered that by simply covering the hole with her hands, she could block the ingress of spiritual entities into her body.

Two years later, at the age of 19, the spirit told her that its name was Fred, and that it was the Devil's Advocate. It occasionally issued her with commands, but more typically it made critical and derogatory comments about her:

> ... and the single words would drop into my head. It was almost like my head was a cup and you could drop an object into it. That object would bang at the bottom. (Pembroke 1996: 169)

The voice could send forth snakes, which drove her 'catatonic' with fear. She describes hearing their heads thumping against the door, before entering the room. She would see them not:

> ... in a way that I can see this chair and this table. It's hard to explain how I could see them, because it's not that kind of literal vision. It was more like I know their dimension, their shape and their size. It is a different type of vision. (Pembroke 1996: 169)

Sometimes a snake would enter a drink, and she would swallow it without realizing. On other occasions she would see them moving over her body. These experiences were vivid. She could hear them hissing, and smell their burning flesh if they entered the fire. She felt helpless, paralysed with fear, unable to explain to others what was going on.

Most psychiatrists reading this would conclude that Louise was suffering from schizophrenia. In the language of psychopathology, she describes verbal auditory hallucinations in the second person, sometimes uttering imperatives, and what are almost certainly passivity experiences. The voice is also able to drop words into her head, suggestive of thought insertion. Finally, her observed behaviour would probably be described as catatonic. She describes being 'paralysed' with fear. Her first contact with psychiatry occurred at the age of 17, when she had problems eating and with vomiting. She was diagnosed as suffering from an eating disorder. Following this, she told her consultant (or to use her words, 'I made the mistake of telling my consultant') about Fred and the snakes. Her diagnosis was changed to schizophrenia, and she was given depot neuroleptics. This made her feel even more powerless. She felt that her own understanding of her experiences had been completely ignored, and she was left struggling to cope with profound uncertainties over her existence. She believed an evil spirit had replaced her spirit. It was as if she was dead. How could she possibly still be alive if her own spirit had been forced out of her body? Until this point, apart from the overdose, she had never deliberately harmed herself. The diagnosis of schizophrenia left her with more questions than answers, and left her feeling even more powerless. She started to cut herself, because of her anger and frustration. She found it impossible to express her distress by screaming, and at that point she started to hear the voice of a woman screaming. Louise describes this voice as a metaphor for her unvoiced distress:

> So I think I would hear my own screaming and I would cut myself instead of crying. Because when the blood ran away, it felt like tears. The injury was doing the crying for me. (Pembroke 1996: 170)

Louise Pembroke found psychiatry harmful and damaging. It offered her no opportunity to make sense of her experiences. It ignored her understanding of her experiences; indeed, it turned her understanding around and used it against her in order to re-create her as a schizophrenic. This strengthened her belief that she had no control over her life. In the end, she resisted. She refused to accept her neuroleptic medication, and escaped psychiatry. She established contact with other survivors with whom she could share her experiences, and became a founder member of Survivors Speak Out, one of the leading survivor organizations of the 1980s and 1990s. For her, this was the key to recovery.

The issues raised by Louise Pembroke and Mary O'Hagan are central to the arguments we shall be developing later in this book. Why is it that when we try to do what we sincerely believe is helpful for our patients we paradoxically impede recovery, or make things worse for them? We do not believe that this is intentional. We will try to show later in this book that it is to do either with the interpretation of psychosis that we use, or the way in which we use it. How should we respond to despair and psychosis? What are the ethical implications of failing to respond to (or worse, denying) the suffering of another? Do our theories shield us from the reality of our patients' suffering, and we turn to face them with a blank stare, as Kathleen Jones suggests?

Psychiatry challenged Louise Pembroke's understanding of what was happening to her. It also had the power to force medication on her. But her explanatory framework challenges widely accepted notions of reality and selfhood. It may seem to us that what she experiences, and her way of understanding this, is completely irrational, but if we are to be able to help Louise, and those like her, we have to suspend our judgements about the nature of reality and metaphysics. She found that if she pointed out the position of the snakes on her body to her friends, and they acted as though they were physically lifting the snakes off her skin, her distress was eased considerably. Thus the acceptance of the reality of her experience by her friends was a transforming experience:

> It helped that someone believed me. Somebody was taking me seriously and doing something. It did not necessarily help the snakes to disappear, but I didn't feel totally alone. *It does not help to tell me that they are not real, because they are. There is no point in denying what is happening to me.* (Pembroke 1996: 171)

The act of removing snakes that we cannot see, that are not physically there, places us in a curious moral dilemma. If we act in such a way, we may be accused of colluding with madness. This accusation is one of a number of factors that have prohibited mental health professionals from discussing patients' experiences. We shall examine the role played by phenomenology in this in Chapter 4. If we follow the logic of psychiatry and do not engage with that other reality, we keep madness in its proper place; it remains bound, alienated and isolated. A recent study of psychiatrists' interactions with their psychotic patients suggests that Louise Pembroke's experience is far from unusual. McCabe *et al.* (2002) investigated psychiatrists' engagement with their psychotic patients, using conversation analysis in routine out-patient consultations of 32 patients (diagnoses of schizophrenia or schizoaffective disorder) with seven psychiatrists. They found that patients actively tried to discuss the content of their psychotic experiences with their psychiatrists, asking direct questions and repeating the questions at the end of the consultation. The psychiatrists' responses were characterized by hesitancies, or replying with a question rather than an answer. Sometimes they smiled or laughed in responses, suggesting that they were embarrassed. They were either reluctant or unable to engage with their patients' concerns. The authors suggest that this reluctance may be institutional, that the professional view is that it is unhelpful to dwell on psychotic material.

The power of psychiatry

We have already glimpsed the devastating effects that our power can have in people's lives. It is the most difficult aspect of our work for us to face up to. It is also a theme that recurs in many survivor stories. Most of us enter the caring professions out of the deepest and most sincere intentions to help others, to care for them and help them through the most difficult times in their lives. We find it painfully difficult to acknowledge the fact that there are highly oppressive aspects to our work, but we have to acknowledge that our work draws us into a paradox between care and control. Peter Campbell (1996) talks explicitly about the power of psychiatry, and the influence and control this had in his life. His experiences as a survivor of mental health services led him to conclude that the psychiatric system does little to assist people in retaining control over their lives at times of intense emotional distress. In his view, the medical model is the key to understanding psychiatric power. He makes two points here. First, the medical model provides the dominant framework for the way in which society interprets psychosis, and this in turn gives rise to the dominant view in our culture, a negative one, of illness as a 'one-way street' from which recovery is not possible:

> The idea of illness, of illness that can never go away, is not a dynamic, liberating force. Illness creates victims. (Campbell 1996: 57)

His view of the power of psychiatry presages the type of critical analysis that we shall present in Chapter 3. It also lies at the heart of our analysis of recovery in Chapter 8. Another point concerns the role played by the judgement 'lack of insight' in disempowering service users:

> The concept of... lack of insight is one of the most powerful and insidious forces eroding our position as competent and creative individuals. (Campbell 1996: 57)

He points out that if we say that someone has no insight, we are not stating a fact, we are uttering an opinion. It is this judgement, made by psychiatrists, that confines him to a:

> ...category of persons whose experience is devalued, status diminished and rational evidence dismissed, simply because at a certain time or times I lost contact with the consensus view of reality agreed on by my peers... (Campbell 1996: 57)

This judgement, together with his diagnosis of manic-depression, strips him of his power as a person. It means that psychiatry and the mental health system are founded on inequality, symbolized by the power to detain and to treat. Compulsion and coercion are inescapable facts lurking beneath the surface of all encounters between mental health professionals and service users. Because of this, many users see their time in hospital as punishment. The move to the community may have shifted the focus of care away from institutions, but the legacy of compulsion and coercion remains. Biomedical psychiatry has not relinquished its power to interpret and control people's experiences simply by virtue of a change in scenery. This point is hotly debated as we write. The British Government intends to introduce a new legal framework that will enable compulsory treatment in the community for those mental health service users who persistently refuse to take medication, and have repeated admissions. Certain aspects of community care are seen by politicians, policy makers and some mental health professionals to be in need of higher levels of control and coercion. There is now even talk that the government is considering the introduction of a mental health version of the so-called Anti-Social Behaviour Order (ASBO) for offences such as stalking. This would result in a considerable broadening of the concept of mental disorder, and draws attention to the twilight zone between psychiatry and social control. As Peter Campbell observes, this controlling aspect of the work of psychiatrists has moved out of the asylum into the community:

> If we are made to feel victims and powerless by methods of dispensing care, if we are made to appear inferior by the systems supporting us, it is more than optimistic to expect that relocating the service-points will miraculously end our isolation. *It is what the psychiatric processes are doing to our status and self-image that is important, not where it is happening.* (Campbell 1996: 60; emphasis added)

In words that evoke Foucault, he sees psychiatry as a monologue about madness:

> Simply to keep repeating their (psychiatrists') sagacity in a loud voice does not mean that the experts are entering into a dialogue. (Campbell 1996: 60)

User-led research

It is clear that many service users find the experience of using mental health services and seeing psychiatrists as highly unsatisfactory. There will always be those psychiatrists and mental health professionals who will deny this. They will refuse to accept the authority of the voices that we have heard so far. They will question their legitimacy to speak for the great majority of those who use services. 'Whose interests do they represent?' they will ask; to which we would rejoin 'Whose interests do *you* represent?' This is one reason why service users and survivors from academic backgrounds have engaged on the project of establishing an evidence base that openly acknowledges the interests of service users. This project, better known as ULR, has grown out of frustration with the failure of professional-led research to engage with issues and outcomes that are important to service users. A great deal of ULR is modest and small scale. It takes place at a local level, bringing the benefit of ecological validity, that is to say the findings accurately reflect the concerns and experiences of a small group of service users within a specific context. However, this means that the findings may be difficult to generalize to a wider audience. There have been two large-scale ULR studies in England that have tried to overcome this limitation, and we describe these in some detail. The first, *Users' voices: the perspectives of mental health service users on community and hospital care*, deals with users' experiences of and satisfaction with community- and hospital-based mental health services. It deals with user satisfaction with mainstream mental health services. The second, *Strategies for living*, examines users' experiences from a more personal perspective. It is concerned more with how users understand, cope with and recover from distress. Although these studies ask different questions, they reach broadly similar conclusions. We shall describe the design and implementation of these studies, and then outline the main findings.

User-focused monitoring (UFM)

UFM is a method for evaluating and researching the experiences of mental health service users of community and hospital care, developed by Diana Rose at the Sainsbury Centre for Mental Health in London (Rose 2001). The main benefits claimed for UFM are that it empowers service users by providing them with real work as interviewers. It also claims to access the voices of the most disabled service users. UFM starts from the premise that who decides which questions are to be asked, and who asks them, is of paramount importance. For this reason, service users are closely involved in all aspects of UFM. They design questionnaires, coordinate the research, carry out interviews and conduct focus groups. Data are analysed from a service user perspective by the project coordinators. The research methods used are conventional social science methods of questionnaire design, interviewing and data analysis, but the study began with the involvement of service users at six sites across the country. This developmental work involved visits to day centres, work projects and drop-ins to explain the project to service users. UFM groups decided which areas were to be investigated. The questionnaires have their roots in a different epistemological tradition:

> UFM groups meet fortnightly or monthly, depending on the project timetable. The first three or four meetings are spent constructing a questionnaire, site visit workbook, or set of focus group questions. *These meetings are vital because they are the means of ensuring that the instruments are firmly rooted in users' experiences of community and hospital services.* This method of generating user-defined instruments distinguishes UFM as a method from research designed by professionals. (Rose 2001: 16; emphasis added)

The questions researched by UFM differ from those asked by professionals. Let us consider medication. Diana Rose argues that professionals frame questions about medication in terms of compliance, whereas UFM groups approach medication in terms of choice, dignity, respect and information about side effects. UFM questions about medication tend to be more open, making it possible for people to specify what it is they like or dislike about medication.

In terms of research design, the study used random sampling to gain a representative sample of views and opinions, and also to enable statistical analysis to be undertaken. Because they used random sampling, they only achieved a 30% response rate, raising the possibility of sample bias. There were no demographic differences between those interviewed and those not interviewed, suggesting that there was probably no systematic sampling bias. All interviewers were given rigorous training in the use of the questionnaire, although the report gives no analysis of inter-rater reliability. It does show that the questionnaire had satisfactory construct validity. The global rating of user satisfaction was statistically significantly correlated with a number of individual items on the questionnaire. UFM is methodologically robust, and is not to be dismissed as 'soft' research simply because it is undertaken by service users.

As far as the results are concerned, only about half of those who responded to the questionnaire believed they had sufficient information about the problems and side effects of medication, and a third said they felt overmedicated. Most of the questions dealing with satisfaction with information available about medication were significantly positively correlated with the general satisfaction scale. In other words, the availability of information about medication is an important measure of service quality. The study also examined care delivery and users' views of the CPA (care programme approach) process. Again, lack of information was an important aspect of people's experience. Most users did not know the purpose of the CPA process. Either it had not been explained to them, or they were unable to understand the explanation given. Most did not know who their care coordinator was, or the date of their next CPA review. This suggests a 'lack of transparency' in the CPA process, a serious problem in view of the importance attached to user involvement by government policy. The study paints a picture in which service users feel that things are done to them, rather than with them. This is reflected in the scepticism expressed by many service users towards user involvement in service planning.

Medication dominated the area of clinical issues. About two-fifths of respondents were on depot neuroleptics, and at the two London sites Black and minority ethnic (BME) service users were much more likely to be on medication than White service users. In general, service users expressed mixed views about medication. Most said they gained some benefit from it, but at the expense of unpleasant side effects. About a third said they felt overmedicated, and this was associated with lower levels of satisfaction. People whose doctors negotiated medication with them expressed higher levels of satisfaction with services.

> Discussing medication levels is one way of showing respect for a client. Ensuring that users do not feel overmedicated immeasurably increases their quality of life and ensures dignity. Overmedication can involve putting on a lot of weight, jerking, shuffling and dribbling. This is not dignified and it can lead to stigmatisation and social exclusion. Indeed, the visible effects of overmedication are a real problem for service users who know that these effects single them out as different. (Rose 2001: 97)

The study also examined satisfaction with different professional groups. In London, most users were neutral about their key workers and consultants. In

Table 2.1   Care standards

Service level standards

Community Mental Health Teams to hold full information on issues relating to community care.

Information on side effects of medication to be available at all sites that dispense medication.

The provision of alternatives to in-patient care, and improvement to the remaining in-patient units.

Individual standards

Needs assessments to take into account users' strengths and abilities.

Doctors to negotiate medication with service users.

Users never to feel overmedicated.

Users to be involve in care planning.

From Rose (2001).

general, community psychiatric nurses received the highest satisfaction ratings, with social workers close behind. The interview schedule also included a 10-point global satisfaction scale. The mean global satisfaction scores across the sites were on the positive side of neutral (range 5.3–7.7). This suggests that there was no evidence of the halo effect that gives unrealistically high levels of satisfaction in professional surveys. Based on a statistical analysis (the details of which are not presented in the text), the report sets out a set of care standards, three service level and four individual (Table 2.1).

UFM thus has a clear rationale for establishing service user standards, which complements evidence-based medicine and professional quality standards. It is designed to work alongside statutory frameworks. Even though there may be contradictions and tensions between different perspectives, UFM is essentially pragmatic, not idealistic. The study's main conclusion is that mental health services must change if they are to become more responsive to users' needs, and to respect their rights and responsibilities. This, it argues, can be achieved by moving from an illness- or problem-oriented approach, to a recovery or strengths model. It also requires service user involvement at all levels of care, from the individual to national planning.

Strategies for living

The Mental Health Foundation's Strategies for Living Project was a large systematic study of the experiences of service users in England. It began life as a questionnaire survey of service users, the results of which are described in the report *Knowing our own minds*. This was then followed by a depth interview study, *Strategies for living*, in which 71 service users identified through the questionnaire survey were interviewed by user-researchers. Again, service users were involved in the design, implementation, analysis and dissemination of the results. A steering group guided the project, with representatives drawn from a range of national service user organizations. The study was thus grounded in the concerns of service users and survivors. Unlike *Users' voices*, which examined service users' experiences of statutory mental health services, *Strategies for living* concentrated on service users' attempts to cope with and make sense of their experiences. *Knowing our own minds* and *Strategies for living* cover four main areas: explanatory frameworks; experiences of medication and physical treatments; coping strategies; and complementary and alternative therapies. Here we summarize the main findings in the first three areas.

The questionnaire survey (Mental Health Foundation 1997) drew 401 responses, mainly from London and the South East of England. There were roughly equal numbers of men and women, largely aged between 26 and 50 years. Despite the attempt to recruit subjects from ethnic communities, the sample poorly represented people of Asian origin (only 1% came from Indian backgrounds for example), although 15% of the sample came from African-Caribbean backgrounds, and 4% from Irish. About half the sample had been in contact with mental health services for >10 years, and >60% were still seeing a psychiatrist. The interview study (Faulkner & Layzell 2000) recruited five service users who were trained by consultants from the National Centre for Social Research to interview subjects about their experiences. All were employed on a sessional basis. The study used a purposive sampling strategy to identify a total of 76 potential interviewees, of whom 71 agreed to participate. The sampling strategy was meant to ensure that interviewees were representative of service users by gender, age, ethnicity and geographical region. Interviews were carried out using a topic guide that covered the main issues to be explored. The aim was to use subjects' own words as far as possible to describe their experiences.

Explanatory frameworks

The questionnaire asked respondents to state how they saw their mental health problems, rather than give their diagnosis. Most (70%) gave a diagnosis, although some chose to provide a personal description of their problems. Depression was the most common diagnosis, followed by manic depression, psychosis (schizophrenia and psychosis) and anxiety. However, almost as many people said they had been treated with neuroleptics as had received antidepressants, suggesting that there may have been under-reporting of terms such as 'schizophrenia'. A fifth of subjects chose their own way of expressing their problems, such as,

> Occasional feelings of being overwhelmed by events, people and bad memories. I prefer the term emotional distress to mental health problems, as it seems to be more accurate.

> I hear voices and I see things. I don't see it as an illness. (Mental Health Foundation 1997: 26)

The interview study (Faulkner & Layzell 2000) reveals more about the complex ways in which people frame their experiences. Many considered themselves ill only when they were unable to cope with their problems. Although some accepted the idea that their experiences could be accounted for by a diagnosis, others rejected diagnosis outright and used social concepts to describe their experiences. People were more likely to accept a diagnosis if this was consistent with their own explanatory framework. Some found a medical label a useful way of making sense of their experiences, but many had a complex, shifting relationship with the notion of diagnosis. A shift towards a medical interpretation of distress often occurred when the person found they could no longer cope alone:

> I got to the point where I knew I needed professional help, because I couldn't cope with it on my own. And something had to change. (Faulkner & Layzell 2000: 15)

and

> At the time I was horrified... but I've realised since that is actually true. But at the time I wasn't happy with it at all... but I've actually recognised that it is probably an accurate diagnosis. (Faulkner & Layzell 2000: 15)

This suggests that the individual's understanding is not fixed and static, but dynamic and evolving over time. This fluid, ambiguous relationship with diagnosis will surface again in Chapter 8. An important factor that influenced acceptance of a psychiatric diagnosis was the stigma associated with specific diagnoses. This woman had a diagnosis of bipolar affective disorder, and also had past experience of nursing people with severe mental health problems:

> Very, very frightened because the few people that I have seen on long term... were very severe... I was very frightened and I didn't see any particular hope and they didn't offer me any community support or support talking to other people. I felt totally alone and they didn't talk to my family. It was a horrible diagnosis. (Faulkner & Layzell 20007: 16)

Two diagnoses were particularly troublesome: schizophrenia and borderline personality disorder. Both were strongly linked to stigma in the eyes of those to whom the labels were attached. This was especially so for African-Caribbean men with a diagnosis of schizophrenia. This person linked the diagnosis and his blackness to the perception by others that he might be violent:

> People think I'm different and will kill them or whatever. (Faulkner & Layzell 2000: 18)

For women, the diagnosis of borderline personality disorder was particularly problematic. One interviewee rejected this diagnosis completely She believed that the reason she had been given the diagnosis had more to do with the nature of her relationship with her worker. When her psychiatrist changed, she was able to negotiate the diagnosis and get it changed.

Some people preferred to talk about their experiences from within a psychosocial framework, and others expressed anger and resentment at the imposition of a medical interpretation of their experiences. The following person was diagnosed schizophrenic. She disagreed:

> Just because I was shouting in the street, I don't really feel that makes me mentally ill, but I was homeless ... I had nowhere to live ... I felt, well, that the way that I was taken into hospital on that last occasion was a bit of a, it was a bit of a cheek to arrest somebody for shouting about God. (Faulkner & Layzell 2000: 17)

Another woman understood her problems in terms of her life history, not a biological disorder:

> I just don't think I've got a mental health problem. I've got problems, which, um, things, things that have affected me. Made me the way I am. But it's because of things that have happened, that have made me who I am, not because I've got a chemical imbalance in my brain. (Faulkner & Layzell 2000: 17)

Thus some people understood their distress in terms of their personal histories or the circumstances in which they found themselves. In other words, they contextualized their distress. This appeared to be the case in women from South Asian communities, many of whom understood their distress within the context of their family circumstances.

Medication and physical treatment

The questionnaire study contained a series of questions about medication (major and minor tranquilizers, antidepressants and mood stabilizers) and ECT. No distinction was made between atypical and typical neuroleptics. Over 90% of the sample had been prescribed psychiatric drugs at some point, most commonly antidepressants (67%) and neuroleptics (60%). People's views about the value of these drugs varied considerably, especially regarding neuroleptics. Many found them damaging, and their effects frightening, but some found them helpful. Others related distressing changes in their subjective awareness of self to medication:

> Although helpful, as stated, on the high dose it took away my psychic awareness which was quite disappointing and also deadened me emotionally leaving me very demotivated and I spent three years mostly sleeping and watching TV.
>
> They made me feel completely out of it, confused and lethargic. (Mental Health Foundation 1997: 26)

Such comments help us to understand why many find it so difficult to take long-term neuroleptics, and decide to discontinue. This indicates the importance of listening carefully to people's experiences of medication. In contrast, most people (two-thirds) found antidepressant medication helpful, although a small number (10%) said they were the most damaging drugs they had ever experienced.

The need to take medication evoked much ambivalence:

> I feel trapped by having said it was helpful. It is a drug and I **hate** it. It has not really helped me but right now I need to take it as there is no other alternative. (Mental Health Foundation 1997: 35; emphasis in the original)

Half the respondents had experienced forced treatment, most commonly in the context of taking neuroleptics. Many of the comments made here convey the lack of choice that accompanies coercion. If people are allowed to exercise choice over their treatment, they feel that they have been respected:

> I was forced to take major tranquillisers in order to regain custody of my seven week old baby, who was taken into foster care at just 5 days old. (Mental Health Foundation 1997: 37)

ECT evoked the most negative views. Over a quarter of respondents had experienced it, but only 30% found it helpful. Nearly half (47%) found it damaging or unhelpful, with most of the negative comments relating to memory loss.

For many people in the interview study, medication was associated with negative connotations of chronic illness, coupled with anxiety about potentially harmful long-term effects of drugs. On the other hand, some people gained benefit from medication, despite side effects. As with diagnosis, the most powerful theme to emerge here was that of ambivalence.

> I don't think it's fair on the tablets, because you've got to take them consistently. I didn't... and actually, taking medication was like acknowledging that I was ill. (Faulkner & Layzell 2000: 37)

This ambivalence was a complex phenomenon with several components. The potential benefits of medication were balanced against the disadvantages of short- and long-term side effects, and the way that medication, for some, symbolized illness. As the following extract reveals, part of this process included attempts to come off medication:

> I had made a conscious decision that I did not want to take medication any more, I got sick of it, and so I went to this conference and went very, very paranoid, and I just felt crap, really... it ruined everything really, because I just could not communicate with people, you see... I was so paranoid that I could not talk to anybody. (Faulkner & Layzell 2000: 37)

Many gained benefits from medication, such as feeling calmer, being able to sleep better, feeling more stable, feeling better able to cope with other people, and to function more effectively in life, for example by getting back to work. Medication also helped to reduce experiences such as voices, depression, or feeling too high, when these became too distressing. People were also very clear about the position of medication in their coping strategies. Nobody used it as their only coping strategy. References to medication were nearly always qualified through the use of expressions such as the 'right' medication, or 'appropriate' medication. In other words, people had very clear views about the ways in which medication was either beneficial or harmful. The difficulty for many people was that they felt they had been given insufficient information about the side effects of medication to make an informed decision about it. This can be seen in the following extract:

> I would prefer it if the doctor had told me, yes you will put on weight with these tablets but they never told me, so I just suddenly got fat and woke up one morning and could not get my clothes on—it was practically overnight it happened—so I wish the doctor had said... maybe I could have done something about it because... it is horrible to find out that you are fat, it took me ages to accept it because I would prefer being thin. (Faulkner & Layzell 2000: 41)

However, the real conflict to emerge from these interviews concerns power and control over medication. At issue here is not the obvious situation in which someone is forced to take medication under the Mental Health Act, but something more subtle. If psychiatrists prescribe medication for their patients strictly according to the medical model, then the most important element that determines the prescription is the psychiatrist's diagnosis. For example, if you hear voices, are distressed and show no evidence of mood disorder, you will probably be diagnosed as schizophrenic and given neuroleptic medication. The more rigidly the psychiatrist follows the medical model, the less likely it is that his or her opinion will be swayed by other considerations, such as what the patient finds helpful. Many people in the study had clear views about what was right or appropriate medication for their problems. Their views were often in conflict with what the psychiatrist considered to be appropriate. These judgements were highly subjective in nature, based on personal experiences of medication, balancing wanted against unwanted effects, the potential adverse symbolic function of medication (i.e. symbolic of illness), its possible positive and negative effects on distress, and whether the person felt a drug helped them to function more effectively. Thus decisions on whether or not to take medication were complex. It was here that conflict arose. Whose understanding influenced which drug will be offered, the psychiatrist's or the patient's? How does the psychiatrist interpret the patient's decisions; as a complex, rational choice or in terms of lack of insight and poor compliance? The quality of information provided by the psychiatrist about medication had an important influence on this conflict, in particular the extent to which people felt their psychiatrists engaged them as active partners in the decision-making process.

Coping strategies

One of the real benefits of ULR is its ability to draw attention to how people interpret, understand and cope with their experiences. The survey reveals how service users became experts in their own experience, through the development of coping strategies using different frameworks. Spiritual and religious beliefs were particularly important in helping people to make sense of and cope with their experiences. Just over half the respondents said that these beliefs were an important part of their lives, especially people from BME communities (78%) compared with White people (55%). For Christians, belief in God as a supportive figure was the most common theme to emerge. Faith brought meaning into people's lives, and a reason for suffering

> The knowledge that I am a part of a greater whole which is in the being of God's love, and that there is a far greater meaning to things than their surface appearance implies. (Faulkner & Layzell 2000: 74)

Personal spiritual beliefs unrelated to a particular religion also helped people to make sense of their suffering. This raises the importance of our common need to understand ourselves and find a purpose in suffering. In general, mental health services overlook the importance of this in people's lives.

The interview study helps us to see how different frameworks are integrated with coping strategies. People who regarded self-reliance as a virtue used positive self-affirmation strategies to achieve peace of mind. Peace of mind, or a sense of contentment within self, was often related to spiritual and religious beliefs. For example, this woman's firm belief that God loved her meant she could believe that she was a good person, making it easier for her to bear her illness:

> To know that I'm a good person and I try, and if the mental illness has come, then I'll just have to live with it, 'cause as long as I know I'm a good person... that makes me cope with my illness a lot better. (Faulkner & Layzell 2000: 74)

Religious faith brought a number of benefits into people's lives, including tranquility, the value of prayer and inner spirituality, support from others and sensing the presence of God. Prayer, or reading the Quran or the Bible, helped to establish peace of mind and self-acceptance:

> Now I think, when I want to pray or when I read simple books about Islam and the essence of Islam, I find them very very peaceful and it doesn't matter what crazy world I am in at the time, with stress around me, I just feel very at peace... (Faulkner & Layzell 2000: 86)

A sense of inner spirituality could also be identified with positive human or family relationships and human characteristics or nature quite independently of religious affiliation:

> My religious belief is that God is within yourself, there's nobody up in the sky looking on you. God is within yourself which is your spiritual within yourself, your honesty in everything. Now it's got to be taught to you from somewhere, but once it's within you, then you find it surrounds you. (Faulkner & Layzell 2000: 87)

For others, the friendship and companionship of others was an important aspect of coping. A sense of belonging, through companionship with others who have faced similar difficulties, brought a sense of meaning into people's lives. This was drawn from relationships with families or partners, or through identification with particular communities, such as the gay community, ethnic communities, or through a sense of solidarity with the wider service user community. It could be found in a self-help group, a day centre or through engagement in creative activities of physical exercise with others. In addition, caring about, or being cared for by others brought meaning into people's lives, and for some gave a significant reason for living. Having the opportunity for engagement in creative work and activities such as writing, poetry or painting was a particularly important aspect of coping for some.

Some general points

Both studies used a variety of methods to describe service users' opinions about services and their experiences of emotional distress. The important question is not which is the most suitable method or design, but who uses it. In both studies, service users are in control. This may account for the similarity of the results in common areas, and in turn this validates the findings. No matter what methodology or design is used, there is a consistency in what service users have to say about their experiences of mental health services. Common themes to emerge from these studies are the importance of adequate information, especially regarding medication, and the value of a negotiated approach to the use of medication, as opposed to coercion (power and control). *Users' voices* argues that the process of research is more important than the scientific methodology used. In this sense, URL has much in common with participatory action research (PAR) as a way of going about research. In PAR, researchers work explicitly with and for people, rather than undertaking research on them. According to Meyer (2000), it has three important elements: it is participatory; it is democratic; and it contributes both to social science and to social change. These elements are common to ULR and *Strategies for living*. Their participatory nature is clear. This means that the boundaries between researcher and researched are blurred. This serves an important epistemological purpose. It questions the distinction important in scientific research between the enquiring mind of the researcher and the phenomenon under investigation. In Chapters 4 and 5, we will explore the origins of this distinction in detail, and question its underlying philosophical assumptions.

The process of negotiation and engagement with service user concerns is an indication of their democratic impulse. As Meyer points out, the real value of this is that the research process becomes more meaningful and valid, because it is rooted in the reality of peoples' experiences of clinical practice. Finally, ULR not only contributes to social science, but is also an important vehicle of social change. The empowerment of service users lies at the heart of both studies. This approach forms the basis of an evaluation of a community development project in Bradford to be described in Chapter 9.

Conclusions

ULR, especially *Strategies for living*, places service users' reflections on their experiences in the foreground. What emerges from this is the great complexity of their understandings, and their emotional responses to the situations they encounter as users of services. There are several themes we want to take forward from this chapter. We have already described three important features of user experience that resonate strongly with postpsychiatry: the importance of contexts; ethics and technology; and care versus power and control. Two of the themes to emerge from the *Strategies for living*, explanatory frameworks and coping strategies, are particularly important, and relevant to our discussion of recovery in Chapter 8. In the second section of this book, we will explore in some detail specific features of psychiatric knowledge and understanding that we have drawn attention to in early chapters. The areas we are primarily concerned with here are the power of psychiatry to define our experiences, the failure of psychiatric understandings to engage with contexts and the problems of narrative in psychiatry.

The miracle drug

Zeal: an ardent feeling taking the form of love, wrath, righteous indignation.
Eager desire, longing (yes, for something much better). Ardour in the pursuit
of an end or cause (I really like that bit). Zealot: one who is carried away by
zeal; a fanatical enthusiast. That's what the Shorter English Dictionary *has to*
say about my favourite word. When did you last use it? When did you last
experience eager desire and ardour in the pursuit of an end or cause? Such
words discomfort us these days. They have religious connotations, albeit with-
out the mumbo-jumbo. They conjure images of an irrational past. Is our pre-
sent rational, I ask? We are slaves to progress, but good, old fashioned zeal
still burns deep in me, I tell you! God! An inferno kindled by the rubbing
together of grinding poverty with privilege and wealth. Now, if I just put
this . . . here, in the bottom corner of the window, they can't avoid seeing it
when they come.

> ## *Hands off Iraq!*

Poverty, hm! The streets I played in as a lad were cobbled streets that rattled
the rag and bone man's cart; streets laced with dog shit that stuck to my fore-
head when I headed the scuffed casey through Mrs McCormack's parlour win-
dow. Oi! You little buggers, look what you've done to my best carpet. Wait till
I tell your mam, Kevin Quinn! Poor Mrs McCormack. Mean narrow streets
that sat cheek by jowl with the quality. The quality! Up the brow and over the
bridge in Higher Broughton were wide leafy lanes with lace-windowed houses,
shiny Rileys and Rovers resting in the calm cool shade of old oak trees and
limes. And in those fancy mansions lived folk who went to hear Sir John at the
Free Trade Hall, without even wondering why it was called the Free Trade
Hall, folk who bought their clothes in arcades off St Anne's Square, and drove
to Buttermere with Wainwright laden knapsacks. I didn't hate them, these mill
managers and factory owners, shopkeepers and teachers. Nor did I envy them.
Once they were my kith and kin. They were ordinary folk who just happened
to prosper and better themselves. My uncle was one of them. No! It was the
system that was at fault, I hated the system. There was no way I would be tied
to it, driven by the flywheel of consumption. And that's the irony. Having spent
all my life fighting one system, rejecting it and all it stood for, I've found myself

tied down by another system, one that lives symbiotically alongside its big brother.

Of course, Rachel and Doctor-mind-my-Gucci-shoes-on-your-stinking-carpet-because-I-don't-want-to-contaminate-the-interior-of-my-BMW-with-your-ordure are tied to it. What will it be today, I wonder? Will it be the black silk suit, or the Rohan jacket? Does it matter? They sap my energy.

Going off again, that's what she said last week. Cheeky cow. Going off because I'm not taking my medication, that's what she said to my housing officer. What business is it of his? She has absolutely no right to discuss my circumstances, or my health if that's the way she sees it, with anyone else. I am up to here with nosey parkers sticking their fingers into my affairs. Is there no such thing as privacy these days? So this one should go well here I think.

> *End global tyranny now!*

Every way you look these days, there's someone laying down rules, telling what you can do and what you can't do, what you can think and what you can't think, what you can feel and what you can't feel, what you can do with your body and what you can't do with your body. I kid you not, and you may think that I am absolutely stark staring bonkers, right. You may think I've completely lost the plot, but I've even gone as far as crapping in the garden at night because for all I know Blair's state has stuck a minicam down the pan to spy on my turds. Seriously? 'Hmm. I see Mr Quinn's out of order again today, six grade three floaters. That's the fifth time this week. Can't have that. Take a note Miss Williams! To Whom It May Concern; Kevin Quinn needs more roughage and less fat. See to it that his diet is amended immediately. He'll have a heart attack if he sticks to that diet. And we know that an eighty per cent hit rate on grade three floaters is associated with a two point seven per cent increased risk of colonic cancer in the next 5 years. God knows what that will cost the NHS. Ask Radio Five Live to put it out immediately' I ask you! Of course I daren't tell them that. They wouldn't recognize hyperbole, even if it was the size of Mount Everest covered in green fur.

It was the same when I was a lad. There was always some nosey parker from the welfare, some oversized overscrubbed girl guide from the Town Hall, Our Lady Bountiful of the Black Shirt. We've had a letter from the school, Mr Quinn. It is our duty to inspect the sanitary conditions of this house. So what if there was a bit of a reek? Those la-di-da buggers couldn't stomach the smell of honest working class sweat and toil. What do you expect if you herded nearly 2000 folk together in those narrow streets? You tell me how much space is there at the back of Salford Royal, between Silk Street and the Irwell. I'm guessing; 20 mills, 10 foundries, 5 chemical works, 500 two up two downs? Our house, number 17, was due for demolition. Outside privy, no hot water, but inside there was no time for carbolic, Lanry Bleach, donkey stones or dolly blue. Because the only thing we had time for in our family was talk, conversation, argument, putting the world to rights, talk of heroes and martyrs, of passion and struggle. We lived it, talk all day, and talk all night. From my dad, we understood the history of the working class movement, and revolution. From my mam, we heard tell of the poor soil of County Clare in 1849 and families shattered by famine.

But in this house of parley something else began to crystallize in my mind. Dad worked in a factory. He would smuggle little jars of chemicals home to show us simple experiments. I loved the colours; the intense violet dust of potassium permanganate, sky blue copper sulphate crystals like little sapphires that melted on your fingers, the rushing fizz of granulated zinc and hydrochloric acid, and the whooping explosion of hydrogen when he stuck a match in the mouth of the test tube. Uncle Joe from Sedgeley Park bought me a chemistry set for my 11th birthday. What joy! A magic world of changes and metamorphoses, and all in a litany you could understand; 'Take five cubic centimetres of the light blue copper sulphate solution and carefully pour in the solution of caustic soda. Note the soft, flocculent precipitate of copper hydroxide thrown out of solution.' Chemicals were predictable. Although they had their own passions and affinities for each other, sometimes with explosive consequences, these followed set patterns.

In the Chapel of Ease, I asked Mother Bernadette if I would be able to study chemistry at secondary school. She was only off the ferry 3 months and wept each night for Westport. She told me that I'd only study chemistry if I passed the 11 plus and went to De La Salle, adding that that was not for the likes of me. It was the Holy Sisters' responsibility to ensure that those who went to De La Salle were fit and deserving. I wasn't in that august company because of my Dad, a communist, a Godless man, she said, with his head full of dangerous ideas. She demanded to know what heathen thoughts he had instilled in my head. This one goes in the back door window.

> *Smash capitalism!*

Looking back I'm glad things worked out the way they did. People change in unpredictable ways. Fuck knows what would have happened if I'd gone to De La Salle. You see it all the time. Folk get educated, leave their roots behind, think they know better than their parents, and before they know it they get sucked in to buying a house, a bigger car, holidays abroad; spend, spend, spend, and for whose benefit? No, people change; but chemicals don't. Again, you may think I'm crazy to say this, but there's something wonderfully pure about chemicals. You always know how they will behave. You know that if you add exactly 1.95 grams of A to 3.90 grams of B, you'll always get 2.26 grams of C and 3.59 grams of D. Do you see what I'm getting at? There's no messing about with chemicals. They tell the truth. They have their own laws. No, that's not quite the right word, it's more like a set of higher ideals. Fidelity and incorruptibility. They will always yield to truth; they know no other way. They are impassive and austere, beyond influence by man's tawdry interests. Theirs is a serene beauty. In a way you might even say that they too are zealots. They are utterly committed to fulfilling without question their own natural laws. There is inevitability about them, the sort of inevitability you find in a Bach fugue. It could only possibly fit together one way. Once you know their rules, you become a witness to their beauty, their passion and their ardour.

I am convinced that Man is the problem. First he realized there were rules, then he discovered them, and having discovered them put them to work for his own ends, even to turn them back on nature, to pervert nature for his own ends. That's scandalous. You want profit? No problem, we can rape and wrench out of nature what we want for our own greed, or to control, and manipulate others, to hold them in bondage, to ruin the environment. How it drives me mad. Those beautiful, austere, serene rules debased by our lust for power and control. Will they ever get the message? This is my favourite, over here in the middle of the window.

> *Buck Fush*

It's the way she wrinkles her nose and purses her lips when she comes in. I have to laugh. She can't stand the stench of poverty; she can't allow it into her body; it's an affront to her sensibilities. Like I said, last week she was going on and on about my health, about how much weight I'd lost, about the state of the house, and the smell. Of course I can't live off what I get, but I didn't tell her I was sharing my benefit with the bloke next door. You think I'm hard up? He gets fuck all. He hopes his wife and kids are still in Afghanistan. He hasn't spoken to them for 2 years. He doesn't even know if they are alive. The next day she came with Doctor-mind-my-Gucci-shoes-on-your-stinking-carpet-because-I-don't-want-to-contaminate-the-interior-of-my-BMW-with-your-ordure. He had this spiel about this new medication; what was it he called it, a clean drug? What bollocks! Anyway, I caught him eying my books and of course he noticed it and picked it up. He ran his finger up and down the spine and asked me if it was mine.

    K. Quinn
    1978
    Doctor of Philosophy
    University of Salford

He read the title page; Pauli's Exclusion Principle and Magnetic Quantum States of Neon. *And do you know what he said, this arrogant man in Gucci shoes and a BMW, shall I tell you what his response was? He asked me how could someone of my intelligence not realize that I was ill and in need of medication. For only the second time in my life I was lost for words. What can you do? What can you possibly say in the face of such blind arrogance? Do you know, I have never in my life hit anyone, but I swear that I was so close that day, I shall never know how I managed to restrain myself.*

Do you have a PhD, doctor? You shouldn't call yourself 'doctor' unless you have a PhD, doctor. You can't be a real doctor, doctor, without a PhD, doctor. Doctors who don't have doctorates, doctor, aren't fucking doctored doctors doctor so fuck you Doctor doctor. No doctorate? No doctor, doctor.

He said something to her about dys, dysmorphia or something or another like that, oh and thought disorder of course. That old favourite, thought disorder. Then he asked if I had any interesting new ideas. And I said, yes. Oh yes! I told him about it. I gave it to him straight. It's the big one, I said, the one that will change the world for ever, the one that I've been working on since I was a lad, the miracle the world has been praying for . . . the drug to cure the world of capitalism.

3 The battle for acceptance

Defining the relationship between medicine and the world of madness and distress

Mad Pride and the power to define reality

One of the most active user organizations in the UK in recent years has been the group Mad Pride. Tragically, one of its founders, Pete Shaughnesy, died at the end of 2002. Pete was very clear: his writing and activism were dedicated to establishing Mad Pride alongside other groups that celebrated difference while campaigning for human rights. Mad Pride has never been concerned with attempts to find a cure for madness. It has never argued for more or better psychiatric research. Mad Pride has been about embracing madness as a fundamental feature of human life: a feature that is sometimes painful and terrifying but also something that can be the source of creative and spiritual insight and renewal. This movement regards madness as an aspect of our humanity; sometimes we can explore it positively. It rejects the medical framing of such states of mind and regards psychiatry's attempts to do this as often oppressive and dehumanizing. References to Gay Rights feature prominently in the writings of Mad Pride activists.

One of the first moves of the Gay Rights movement involved challenging the idea that homosexuality was an illness. The fight against discrimination and oppression combined with a positive campaign in which gay people struggled to 'define' themselves and develop their own agendas for the future. Alongside arguments against the medical framing of homosexuality as some sort of disease was a move to celebrate gay culture.

As we enter the 21st century, we have government ministers who are openly gay and TV programmes made by gay people for gay people. Progress has been made, but only when this process is complete will gay people feel that they are accepted fully as citizens. The proponents of Mad Pride argue for substantial similarities between the social position of gay people 30 years ago and the position of those who experience states of madness and distress today. They regard their struggle as one of the last great battles for emancipation. For Mad Pride, real improvements in the quality of life of those who experience states of madness will not come about through the development of new drugs, new therapies or even new services, but through social and cultural change.

As with gay people, mental health service users will know that things are better when they feel accepted as full citizens of the country in which they live.

We are broadly in agreement with the arguments of Mad Pride and groups such as the Hearing Voices Network. We have worked and campaigned with both organizations for a number of years. While at the radical end of the service user movement, we believe that they express with great clarity the central importance of power in the world of mental health.

This connects directly with the first theme of postpsychiatry: the need to move away from a dynamic of social exclusion and towards a positive framework invoking the concept of citizenship. As we saw in the last chapter, this theme emerges directly from the individual testimonies of service users. It also echoes the findings of research that has sought to grasp users' priorities for change. We agree with Mad Pride, the Hearing Voices Network and others that full citizenship involves more than the absence of discrimination against a particular group. It also involves a more positive move through which the group in question realizes the power to define itself and to set its own agendas. In this, the contribution of that group to the wider society also comes to be recognized and valued.

While real change will be social and cultural, we recognize that mental health professionals can assist this process or can work to hinder it. In the next part of this chapter, we shall first define what we mean by citizenship. We shall then examine what a loss of citizenship has meant for service users. In the third, we shall look at the relationship between psychiatry and the social exclusion of madness and argue that current campaigns against stigma, while well intentioned, are in some ways serving to continue the status quo; possibly working to undermine real social change. In the fourth part, we turn to the more positive aspects of the citizenship agenda. We argue for a need to redefine the relationship between medicine and the phenomena of madness and distress. This will require a look at the nature of power in modern societies and, in particular, the connection between power and knowledge. Our argument is that for psychiatry to really help service users achieve full citizenship it will need to move beyond the modernist framing of its relationships with service users. We believe that this will have benefits in both directions.

Citizenship and its loss

The *Oxford English Dictionary* says that the word citizen refers to 'an inhabitant of a city or town, especially one possessing civic rights, as a freeman'. We use the word to refer to someone who is allowed to, and feels able to, participate fully in the society of which he/she is a member; someone who benefits from the rights and carries the responsibilities available to other members of that society. The citizen only forfeits his/her rights if he/she contravenes the laws of that society. However, the level of responsibility expected of any individual varies throughout the life cycle and particularly in relation to episodes of illness.

We also use the term to indicate something beyond these legalistic connotations. Our analysis is close to that of the writer Michael Ignatieff who says that:

> Citizenship has its active modes (running for political office, voting, political organizing) and its passive modes (entitlement to rights and welfare). (Ignatieff 1989: 63)

Ignatieff makes the point that both these modes of citizenship go together and cannot be separated. Conservative political voices have often tried to assert the former over the latter. Thus:

> Conservatives want citizens to be free, but cannot refrain from fastidious distaste towards what most people do with their freedom. Moreover, conservatives believe the polity exists to maximize private freedom but do not believe the polity should provide the means to enable all citizens to be free.

> There is nothing wrong with enterprise, personal responsibility or even the lawful pursuit of private profit. What is incoherent is believing these goals can be achieved without a citizenship of entitlement, without the shared foundation that alone makes freedom possible at all. (Ignatieff 1989: 74)

Citizenship is about much more that holding a passport or being on the electoral role of a particular country. To us, being a citizen is about being regarded as a full human being, entitled to expect the same from life and the society in which one finds oneself as everyone else. On a basic level, it involves being free of discrimination, exclusion and oppression. On a more positive note, it means being able to define one's own identity and to celebrate this identity in different ways.

Some people are born into situations where their citizenship is curtailed. Such things as one's ethnic background, religious group, social class, physical or mental disability can all mean that one is denied the same rights as others. Even the simple circumstances of one's birth, such as being born out of wedlock, can also have the same effect. (This was certainly the case in Ireland in the years up to the 1980s. Many children born to unmarried parents were placed in 'industrial schools' run by religious orders where they were made to suffer for their parents 'sins' and were generally regarded by the people who ran these institutions and the wider society as in many ways 'second class', see Raftery & O'Sullivan 1999.)

Other people lose their citizenship as they move through life. This can happen for diverse reasons depending on the prevailing culture. Asylum seekers are perhaps the best example of a group of people who have lost their social position and their citizenship (see below).

Not being a full citizen of one's society means that essentially one has a 'life less worthy' than others. The implications of this are extremely serious and pervasive, and no list of the effects of loss of citizenship will ever be complete. However, the following are important:

(1) Loss of life: inmates of mental hospitals were sent to the gas chambers by the Nazis alongside others who became 'non-citizens' such as Jewish people and homosexuals. At least 250 000 people with mental or physical impairments were killed in this way (United States Holocaust Memorial Museum 1996).

(2) Violence: being regarded as 'mentally ill' can lead to violence and physical abuse. Read & Baker (1996) found that of 778 service users who responded to a survey 47% said that they had been physically attacked at some point. This violence included having eggs thrown at them while being called a 'nutter' and having dog faeces or lit paper pushed through their letterbox.

(3) Restriction on parenting rights: this ranges from forced sterilization programmes to unwarranted questioning of parental skills. The former took place in the USA and in a number of European countries (Sweden, Norway, Denmark, Finland, Estonia and Germany) in the first half of the 20th century in an effort to reduce the number of the 'feeble minded' in society (Lombardo 1983; Sayce 2000). The latter is still very prevalent today. Mental health service users can make good, bad or indifferent parents. There is no consistent or convincing body of evidence that people with a mental illness diagnosis are necessarily poor parents (Mowbray *et al.* 1995). In spite of this, parents with a psychiatric diagnosis lose custody for reasons that would rarely lead to the same outcome with 'normal' parents such as 'bad attitude or sexual promiscuity'. (Stefan 1989).

(4) Restriction on migration: a history of 'mental disorder' in itself can debar an individual from entry to the USA. Liz Sayce quotes from the visa waiver form that entrants to the USA are given. The entrant is asked if any of the following apply to him/her: 'moral turpitude, prior engagement in espionage, terrorist activities, genocide—or mental disorder' (Sayce 2000: 56).

(5) Discrimination and exclusion in different areas of social and economic life: there is evidence that people with a history of 'serious mental illness' move down the social ladder and often end up living in poverty (Pilgrim & Rogers 1999). This is usually understood in terms of the 'social drift' hypothesis according to which 'schizophrenia', in itself, undermines the individual's ability to work productively. However, there is also evidence that poverty, social exclusion and isolation result from discrimination in areas such as employment (Read & Baker 1996) and housing (Page 1977).

Huxley & Thornicroft (2003) point out that in the UK in recent years, 'the employment level of psychiatric patient populations rarely reaches more than 10% and when working they work fewer hours and earn only two-thirds of the national average hourly rate' (p. 289).

(6) Poor physical health care: standardized mortality rates for people with a history of mental illness are much higher that the population average. Medical personnel sometimes do not take the medical complaints of mental health service users seriously. As a result, diagnosis of cancer and other serious illnesses can be delayed (Sayce & Measey 1999).

(7) Complaints to criminal justice agencies not taken seriously: having a history of mental health problems or psychiatric service involvement can mean that complaints to the police and other agencies are not taken as seriously as they warrant. Individuals in this situation may be thought of as being an 'unreliable witness' (Home Office 1998). There is mounting evidence that rape has been commonplace in psychiatric hospitals and yet few prosecutions have been successful.

(8) Exclusion from society: some politicians and organizations continue to campaign for the social exclusion of people with mental health problems. Thus we heard from a recent UK Minister of Health that 'care in the community has failed'. The implications of this statement are extremely serious; essentially it is an assertion that such individuals have no right to be 'in the community'. One study found that two-thirds of mental health service providers surveyed (both statutory and voluntary sector) had experienced 'nimby'[1] opposition to planned service changes between 1992 and 1997 (Repper *et al.* 1997).

How does 'mental illness' lead to a loss of citizenship?

There are a number of different ways in which mental illness and loss of citizenship are related. Some of these work in both directions. Thus being socially excluded for non-mental health reasons can lead to marginalization and loneliness and through these states to depression, anxiety and sometimes paranoia. A good example in Britain at the moment involves the position of asylum seekers. By definition, such people are 'lacking citizenship'. One Labour MP in the Midlands refused to see asylum seekers at his clinic because they were not on the 'electoral roll' (*Guardian* 2003). They are maginalized, poor and vulnerable and subject to a very negative campaign in the media. Their mental health problems often stem from these realities.

It is also clear that individuals and groups who are not necessarily 'at the margins' can also be subject to social inequality and that this can result in distress, despair, confusion and dislocation (Williams 1999). This is particularly

---

[1]'Not in my back yard'.

well documented in the case of gender (Williams & Watson 1996), ethnicity (Fernando 1991) and class (Pilgrim & Rogers 1999).

In the other direction, being a psychiatric service user can also lead to marginalization, exclusion and sometimes isolation. Huxley and Thornicroft point out that:

> Both the inherent nature of mental health problems and discriminatory responses to them have deleterious effects on interpersonal relationships, leading to reduced social contacts. Patients are four times more likely than the average not to have one close friend, and more than one-third of patients say that they have no one to turn to for help. (Huxley & Thornicroft 2003: 290)

Poverty is very often the common factor that links mental illness with marginalization. We noted above the low levels of employment achieved by people who use psychiatric services. About 50% of people in contact with a community mental health service in England were not receiving their full benefit entitlements (McCrone & Thornicroft 1997). Low income can exclude people from leisure activities and social occasions.

A fear of difference and 'otherness' is often given particular force by the coverage of mental health issues in the media. Traditional negative images of people with mental health problems are presented on a daily basis in many newspapers, TV and radio programmes, and in popular novels and films. Mental illness is connected strongly with ideas of violence and dangerousness. If mental illness is only mentioned when a user or ex-user of services commits a crime, a very distorted view of users is being presented to the public. As Scheff comments:

> Even if the coverage of these acts of violence was highly accurate, it would still give the reader a misleading impression because negative information is seldom offset by positive reports. An item like the following is almost inconceivable: Mrs Ralph Jones, an ex-mental patient, was elected president of the Fairview Home and Garden Society at their meeting on Thursday. (Scheff 1966: 72)

This media onslaught against service users (and by connection often their carers and professionals as well) goes back a long way; Scheff was writing in the 1960s. It also appears to be widespread even though some British commentators have argued that it is particularly bad in their country (Sayce 2000). Perhaps some forms of madness and distress have always been stigmatized. We shall return to historical questions below. What is clear is that in our society, to be a psychiatric service user is to be regarded as a sort of 'second class citizen'. We take this as a given based on the evidence presented above. In this section, we want to ask the questions: why does this happen? What is the role of psychiatry? Are current anti-stigma approaches to discrimination and citizenship adequate?

Traditional psychiatry and 'anti-stigma'

Traditional psychiatry has argued that the loss of citizenship associated with being a service user has been essentially due to two processes: first it has to do with the impact of mental illness on the individual's social functioning, and secondly it has to do with ignorance amongst the public with regard to the true nature of mental illness. Furthermore, psychiatry has been clear about how best to respond to these processes. On the one hand, downwards social 'drift' caused by the person's illness is to be combated by more aggressive treatment. Roth and Kroll write:

> Job loss, family disruption, economic hardship, loss of educational opportunities, and social drift downwards are all frequent consequences, rather than causes, of serious mental illness. A significant part of this suffering and loss can be prevented with readily available pharmacological and psychological treatments. (Roth & Kroll 1986: 2–3)

On the other hand, stigma is to be challenged by education campaigns aimed at the public and attempts to change the representation of mental illness in the media. The Royal College of Psychiatrists has recently run an anti-stigma campaign along these lines (Royal College of Psychiatrists, Changing Minds, see RCPsych website).

While this approach has a certain amount of validity, we believe that it fails to engage with the 'full story' about stigma. We agree that some people who are withdrawn, paranoid or confused do have difficulties maintaining a meaningful role in society because of their mental problems. We also accept that stigma and discrimination are a daily reality for very many service users. We accept as well that the phenomenon of 'downward drift' has been supported by the findings of studies in some countries at least (e.g. Goldberg & Morrison 1963).

However, the real questions relate to why this process takes place. We believe that the illness effect is only part of the picture. Given the evidence above about the way in which being a psychiatric patient involves a loss of citizenship, it is likely that a great deal of the downward social mobility associated with mental illness is due to social exclusion and, in particular, to lack of access to proper employment opportunities[2]. Also, understanding rejection and exclusion in terms of 'stigma', 'ignorance' and the solution in terms of 'education' effectively lets professionals (particularly psychiatrists) 'off the hook'. It ignores the possibility that psychiatry itself may be part of the problem and allows psychiatrists and others to assume a position of moral superiority over an ignorant public and over equally ignorant fellow professionals.

---

[2]For an excellent overview of these issues see the report 'Mental Health and Social Exclusion' prepared by the UK government's Social Exclusion Unit on http://www.socialexclusion.gov.uk

There is a historical dimension to this. Introductory chapters in psychiatric textbooks and the writing of a number of historians sympathetic to the project of psychiatry present the story of the discipline in terms of ever-increasing scientific knowledge of madness. This perspective is presented forcefully by Roth and Kroll in their defence of medical psychiatry:

> ... having regard to the successes of the medical models in recent decades, we can reasonably expect that clinical practice and the public health approaches to the problems of mental health will acquire a more and more solid foundation and thus become more precise and effective. This is because medical models pose clear questions that can be refuted or upheld by scientific investigation (Roth & Kroll 1986: 66)

No talk here about the politics of social exclusion, about progress, democracy and citizenship: medical science holds the answers and we (users and professionals) will simply have to wait for 'scientific investigation' to come up with 'more precise and effective' interventions. This account involves a gradual move from superstition, cruelty and exclusion in the pre-Enlightenment era towards scientific psychiatry, humane treatment and social inclusion in the modern period. We shall return to the question of stigma below, but first we need to look at somewhat different perspectives on the relationship between psychiatry and exclusion.

The anti-psychiatry perspective

A counter-discourse to the traditional understanding of this relationship has gathered strength in recent years. Those who challenge the self-image of psychiatry and its legitimacy do so from many different perspectives. We shall encounter some of these at various points in this book. The term 'anti-psychiatry' was first used in the late 1960s to describe the views of a range of psychiatrists, psychologists and sociologists who argued that psychiatry was essentially an instrument of oppression. Although from diverse backgrounds, these writers were united by a belief that medical psychiatry had the effect of crushing the individuality and subjectivity of its patients. Its treatments were seen as repressive and its diagnoses as limiting. One of the most powerful advocates of an anti-psychiatry perspective was the Scottish psychiatrist R.D. Laing.

However, the counter-discourse to traditional psychiatry has taken paths other than the arguments put forward by Laing. Perhaps of greatest irrelevance to our argument is a substantial body of historical opinion that casts the relationship between psychiatry, stigma and social exclusion in a very different light from the story of linear progress traditionally favoured by psychiatry itself. We touched on this issue in the Introduction. Historians such as Roy Porter, Michel Foucault, Klaus Doerner and Andrew Scull have argued that, in reality, psychiatry itself was the *product* of social exclusion. Their accounts of psychiatry's history vary greatly, but they are united by an attempt to get away from (what they would see as) a simplistic linear and progressive view of this story. Doerner (1981) writes about the 'sequestration of Unreason' during the European Enlightenment:

> The genesis of psychiatry as a modern science must be seen against the background of a movement that radically changed the social landscape of seventeenth-century Europe. The Age of Reason, mercantilism, and enlightened absolutism coincided with a new and rigorous spatial orientation. It put all forms of unreason, which in the Middle Ages had been part of a divine world and in the Renaissance a secularising world, the civil world of commerce, morality, and work, in short—beyond the pale of the rational world—under lock and key. (Doerner 1981: 14–15)

This process took place across Europe but took different forms in different countries. Various buildings (workhouses, prisons, penitentiaries, hôpital général and orphanages) were used. Doerner emphasizes the economic changes taking place in Europe in the wake of the industrial revolution and the rise of a powerful bourgeoise with a world-view based on reason and order. Roy Porter is in broad agreement, and writes that, for a number of reasons, at the time of the European Enlightenment there was a cultural focus on the power and benefits of reason and rationality. This prizing of rationality developed from:

> The growing importance of science and technology, the development of bureaucracy, the formalization of the law, the flourishing of the market economy, the spread of literacy and education…(Porter 1987: 15)

In this context, there was a move to exclude 'unreasonable' elements from the midst of society. Foucault stresses the idea that the emergence of the institutions in which 'unreasonable' people were housed was not in itself a 'progressive', or medical, venture. It was simply, and crudely, an act of social exclusion. His term for Doerner's 'sequestration of Unreason' is the 'The Great Confinement' (Foucault 1971). Like Doerner, Foucault stresses the economic background to this Europe-wide phenomenon and argues that confinement had more to do with a shifting perspective on labour than with any concern with health. He says:

> Before having the medical meaning we give it, or that at least we like to suppose it has, confinement was required by something quite different from any concern with curing the sick. What made it necessary was an imperative of labor. Our philanthropy prefers to recognize the signs of a benevolence toward sickness where there is only a condemnation of idleness. (Foucault 1971: 46)

Furthermore, he argues that it was only when such people had been both excluded and brought together that they became subject to the 'gaze' of medicine. According to Foucault, doctors were originally involved in these institutions in order to treat physical illness and to offer moral guidance. They were not there as experts in disorders of the mind. As time went on, the medical profession came to dominate in these institutions and doctors began to order and classify the inmates in more systematic ways.

Medical superintendents of asylums gradually became psychiatrists, but they did not start out as such. Alongside the increasing hegemony of psychiatrists, the concept of mental illness became accepted. In other words, in this account, the profession of psychiatry and its associated technologies of diagnosis and treatment only became possible in the institutional arena opened up by an original act of social rejection.

This has obvious importance for how we understand the relationships between stigma, exclusion and psychiatry. In these accounts, psychiatry is very much a part of the problem, being the product of a social movement that was essentially repressive in nature. Its origins are very different from the origins of medicine itself which draws on an ancient quest to ease pain and cure illness. Instead, psychiatry is seen as a relatively recent phenomenon; brought into being to legitimize the exclusion of those who did not have a role in modern society.

In this light, psychiatry shows up a controlling force: it 'confines', it 'excludes'; more an arm of the modern state than anything else. While Foucault and Doerner focus their attention on the very early origins of psychiatry, Andrew Scull writes about the later history of the discipline. However, his account resonates in several aspects with theirs. In particular, he links the movement towards the use of asylums in Britain to economic developments. He says that the segregation of mad people from the rest of society:

> can...be asserted to lie in the effects of the advent of a mature capitalist market economy and the associated ever more thoroughgoing commercialization of existence. (Scull 1979: 30)

Scull argues that psychiatry represents just one of the many modern apparatuses of social control. In 'mature' capitalist economies, the control of deviance becomes one of the central functions of the state. In such economies, a regulated, healthy and consuming workforce is a necessity. In these circumstances, the state turns to certain groups, often professionals, to operate this regulation. Scull agrees with the accounts of Foucault, Doerner and Porter that historically this has taken shape through an initial segregation of a broad group of deviants from the surrounding community. When this has happened, there is then a differentiation of various subgroups of deviance. He writes:

> From this perspective, the differentiation of the insane, the rise of a state-supported asylum system, and the emergence of the psychiatric profession can be seen to represent no more than a particular, though very important, example of this much more general series of changes in the social organization of deviance. (Scull 1979: 17)

He describes how psychiatrists fought to secure and extend their control over the care of mentally ill people in the face of many challenges.

Psychiatry, stigma, and exclusion

While the work of Porter, Doerner, Foucault and Scull is historical, it raises serious questions about how we should understand the problems of exclusion, stigma and mental illness in our own time. If, historically, psychiatry emerged to label those who had already been rejected, it is not surprising perhaps that its diagnoses quickly became symbols of rejection in themselves. While a number of psychiatrists and historians have questioned various aspects of Foucault's account and it has become increasingly clear that the story of psychiatry has varied greatly from country to country (Foucault's focus was upon developments in France), nevertheless there is a general acceptance that his rejection of a simple 'progressivist' version of psychiatry's development is justified (Gordon 1990).

The essential move in most anti-stigma work is to assert that mental illness 'is just the same as physical illness' which is not so heavily stigmatized. Being depressed is said to interfere with one's functioning in ways similar to the effects of having a broken leg. The difference being that the mental illness is 'inside' and invisible. This might be plausible if there was no controversy about the medical framing of states of madness and distress. This is not the case, and there is clearly a great deal of dispute about the benefits and risks of such a framing.

While a medical diagnosis can be useful in the short term in getting help and support and time off work, in the long term it can be counter-productive. It can lead the individual and his/her carers to adopt a passive position in relation to 'the illness'. This can be very dis-empowering. The individual's experiences are turned into symptoms. These are understood to be the result of some form of pathology and something to be got rid of. Eventually, the individual can begin to think about his/her life as being racked by 'symptoms'. This approach tends to rob such events of meaning and strips them from the background context (social, cultural and personal) from which they may have arisen. The effects of this are many. It can lead to a lessening of a search for meaning by the user, his/her family and the professionals. Explaining the phenomenon of 'hearing voices' as being simply a symptom of schizophrenia means that there is no point in further efforts after understanding. It is a full stop. But many people who hear voices have been helped by framing this experience as being the result of such things as life events or spiritual crises. Perhaps most importantly, a narrow medical framing can lead to a situation where the user starts to think of him/herself as someone who has a 'mind' or a 'life' that is of less value to others. Once one starts to think of one's thoughts, emotions and behaviours as 'diseased', it is a short journey to this conclusion. This can also be confirmed when one's reports of things such as sexual assaults or medical symptoms are not taken seriously by others. For many service users, frameworks involving a mixture of spiritual, political, social and biological factors are more meaningful and helpful.

It is also the case that in the public imagination, being mentally 'sick' is actually morally worse than being simply 'evil'. We hear the term 'sick' being used to express utter disgust and revulsion. Diagnostic labels such as 'personality disorder' 'borderline' 'schizophrenic' and 'neurotic' are sometimes used as terms of abuse.

From this, it can be seen that while the medical framing of states of madness and distress initially appears straightforward and value-neutral, in reality the situation is a lot more complicated. If this analysis is correct, then anti-stigma campaigns that argue for the similarity between mental illness and physical illness might actually be counter-productive. This is certainly the long-held view of Thomas Szasz. He has argued for many years that the very concept of 'mental illness' is dubious at best and oppressive at worst. Szasz writes from a philosophical and 'logical' perspective and argues that the concept of 'mental illness' should only be used as a metaphor. Because psychiatry refuses to acknowledge this metaphorical nature of the term, it has caused a great deal of confusion in the public imagination. As a result, we have the 'myth' that mental illness is, in reality, a real form of illness. Under the guise of this 'mythology,' psychiatry functions to confine, subdue and control people who are not really ill. Szasz says that this amounts to 'the greatest scandal of our scientific age' (Szasz 1976).

However, we are also unhappy with the anti-psychiatry response in so far as it simply understands psychiatry as some sort of repressive force. This is a limited understanding and, in our opinion, fails to do justice to the complex reality of contemporary mental health care. In the next section, we tackle directly the question of power and how it operates to shape this reality.

Power, psychiatry, and the creation of subjects

In their 1986 book, *The Power of Psychiatry*, Peter Miller and Nikolas Rose brought together a number of voices all broadly critical of psychiatry but also seeking to move beyond a traditional understanding of how power operates in this field. In his chapter, Peter Miller made the important point that by the late 20th century psychiatry was no longer simply about people being locked away against their will or having physical treatments forced upon them. Instead:

> ... psychiatry is no one thing, but a loosely assembled set of practices that extends from the 'hard' core represented by the asylum and electro-shock, passes through the recent and emergent community mental-health moves, and extends to the 'soft' end that takes the form of various psychotherapies. The history of psychiatry is a history of reorganizations and transformations of this 'system'. (Miller 1986: 15)

Miller goes on to chart the development of critiques of psychiatry in the 19th and 20th centuries. He argues that these critiques have largely directed their attention at the 'hard core' institutional structures of psychiatry. He suggests that this position is too limited and has failed to engage with the contemporary reality of the mental health system. Indeed, his argument is that many of these critiques have actually helped extend the authority of psychiatric discourses to other parts of our lives. Anti-psychiatry of the 1960 and 1970s emerged in the midst of a wider cultural concern with personal autonomy and subjectivity. Miller argues that the various elements of what we call anti-psychiatry were united by a core belief that psychiatry was in essence about the domination of subjectivity:

> In the work of Goffman this took the form of a preoccupation with the degradations and profanations of the self that asylum psychiatry wrought. Laing's concern was with the existential experience of mental illness. And Szasz attacked institutional psychiatry for its harmful effects on the individual and its insufficiently contractual basis. In these different ways anti-psychiatry was based on an a priori philosophical position that elevated to maximum importance the category of subjectivity. (Miller 1986: 28–29)

Miller's point is that this elevation of subjectivity fails to grapple with the way in which power in our modern and postmodern worlds actually functions. Traditional anti-psychiatry does not help in our understanding of 'those forms of power that operate by seeking to invest the individual with subjectivity rather than to crush' (p. 29).

Miller, like other contributors to *The Power of Psychiatry* book, draws heavily on the ides of Michel Foucault. We have already encountered Foucault's history of insanity above and opened our book with a line from the quotation below. We have noted his phrase the 'great confinement' and his argument that psychiatry was the direct product of a massive European move towards the social exclusion of 'unreason'. In this work, Foucault was still operating with a 'negative' understanding of power. Like the anti-psychiatrists, he presented psychiatry as being about the domination of madness. At first, the mad were confined along with the poor, the unemployed, the chronically sick and general criminals. Subsequently, because of their inability to engage in 'rehabilitative' labour, they were confined separately in asylums. As discussed above, by and large, these institutions were run by doctors, and the inmates were understood to be suffering various forms of mental illness. This historical move meant that the voice of madness, which had been heard in different ways during the Middle Ages and the Renaissance, was now silenced:

> ... the constitution of madness at the end of the eighteenth century, affords the evidence of a broken dialogue, posits the separation as already effected, and thrusts into oblivion all those stammered, imperfect words without fixed syntax in which the exchange between madness and reason was made. The language of psychiatry, which is a monologue of reason about madness, has been established only on the basis of such a silence. (Foucault 1971: xii–xiii)

By the 1970s, Foucault had moved away from an understanding of power as something negative. In numerous articles and interviews and in the books *Discipline and Punish* and *The History of Sexuality* (Vol. 1), he developed an account of power as something productive. In particular, he made the point that power is productive of knowledge. This position challenged the Marxist and liberal idea that knowledge could be separated from ideology. This relationship between power and knowledge is so pervasive that we should really speak about 'power/knowledge' as a single entity. In *Discipline and Punish* he writes:

> power produces knowledge (and not simply by encouraging it because it serves power or by applying it because it is useful); that power and knowledge directly imply one another; that there is no power relation without the correlative constitution of a field of knowledge, nor any knowledge that does not presuppose and constitute at the same time power relations. (Foucault 1977a: 27)

In this book, Foucault charts the emergence of modern ways of thinking about crime and punishment. He argues that a type of 'disciplinary' power came into being in the modern period. This involved a shift in focus: away from the criminal act itself and onto the offender him/herself. In this focus upon the individual offender, Foucault argues that a new figure, a new subject of knowledge and power, came into being: the delinquent. This shift in focus from the criminal act onto the life of the criminal that was to be 'normalized' through various types of intervention coincided with an increasing preoccupation with the collection of biographical details about the identity of the offender, independent of the crime itself. The delinquent had to be analysed through the examination of instincts, drives, tendencies and character. In this setting, the conditions for the emergence of the discourse of criminology were set. In the modern prison, it was possible to compare one individual with another and by this process to exercise a 'normalizing' judgement. However, disciplinary power and normalizing judgements and interventions were not confined to the prison. Foucault speaks about a 'carceral network'. Throughout modern society, we find such forms of power at work. 'Cases' of different sorts are identified in different settings. These are both objects of knowledge and sites of power. In this situation, the individual is both an object who can be described, judged, measured and compared with others, and also someone to be trained or corrected, classified, normalized or excluded. He writes:

> The judges of normality are present everywhere. We are in the society of the teacher-judge, the doctor-judge, the educator-judge, the social worker-judge; it is on them that the universal reign of the normative is based . . . The carceral network, in its compact or disseminated forms, with its systems of insertion, distribution, surveillance, observation, has been the greatest support, in modern society, of the normalizing power . . . This policy required the involvement

of definite relations of knowledge in relations of power; it called for a technique of over lapping subjection and objectification; it brought with it new procedures of individualization. (Foucault 1977*a*: 304–305)

According to Foucault, in modern societies, power is exercised most often through 'regimes of truth': expert discourses through which we understand ourselves and our motives, our desires and our behaviours. Furthermore, such discourses have their experts who act as commentators, advisors and judges. We come to live our lives through these discourses and think about our priorities and values in the terms that are given to us. Because they are 'regimes of truth' they provide the backdrop to our ethical debates and through them it becomes possible to utter the 'truth'. In fact, what is to be regarded as true or false is set by these discourses.

Psychiatry is a clear example of what Foucault had in mind when he wrote about disciplinary power operating outside the prison. In the 20th century, psychiatry became something much bigger than simply the governing power of the asylum. With the advent of psychoanalysis, behavioural and cognitive therapies, community mental health workers and psychiatric rehabilitation, it has become something much more extensive, pervasive and influential. While debates take place between medical models and psychological models, these take place against a certain set of assumptions about the nature of human beings and their relationships with the social body. These assumptions are shared across the different arms of what is broadly regarded as the mental health field. In their encounters with this system, individuals may never be detained or even admitted to a psychiatric hospital. They may never receive electro-convulsive therapy (ECT) or even drug treatments, but they are still bringing their lives into a system invested with the sort of power/knowledge that Foucault describes. Individuals are not just given a diagnostic label but a way of understanding themselves. Their encounters with madness and distress are formulated in terms which draw on discourses produced by the system.

In his book, *Governing the Soul*, the sociologist Nikolas Rose writes about how 'the management of the self' has become a key element of political governance in modern societies. While the self and questions of identity have always had a political aspect, Rose argues that in modern and postmodern times, this has mushroomed. Rose situates the rise and expansion of psychiatry and allied professions in this context. He writes about an emergent 'expertise of subjectivity':

A whole family of new professional groups has propagated itself, each asserting its virtuosity in respect of the self, in classifying and measuring the psyche, in predicting its vicissitudes, in diagnosing the causes of its troubles and prescribing remedies.

The multiplying powers of these 'engineers of the human soul' seem to manifest something profoundly novel in the relations of authority over the self. (Rose 1989: 2–3)

The power of psychiatry and allied disciplines can no longer be thought of in terms of the silencing of deviance. Something very different is now underway. Instead of repression, psychiatric power is now operating to produce an enhanced notion of subjectivity, an expanded sense of selfhood. This has happened in different ways, but most importantly through the production of new discourses of the self. We now think and talk ceaselessly about ourselves, our childhoods, our desires and our relationships. We have new words and idioms through which to conceive and debate our problems and our states of distress and alienation:

> The new languages for construing, understanding and evaluating ourselves and others have transformed the ways in which we interact with our bosses, employees, workmates, husbands, wives, lovers, mothers, fathers, children and friends. Our thought worlds have been reconstructed, our ways of thinking about our personal feelings, our secret hopes, our ambitions and disappointments. Out techniques for managing our emotions have been reshaped. Our very sense of ourselves has been revolutionized. We have become intensely subjective beings. (Rose 1989: 3)

In this framework, psychiatry has moved beyond the physical and intellectual constraints of the institution. Psychiatry, psychology and psychotherapy now make up a 'psy complex' which extends into many new aspects of our lives. An approach to this complex that sees it as simply repressive is inadequate.

However, not everyone agrees that this has been as profound a shift as claimed by Miller, Rose and others. In their book, *Mental Health Policy in Britain*, Anne Rogers and David Pilgrim argue that the demise of institutional psychiatry has been greatly overstated. They point to the focus on risk and safety issues in recent British mental health policy, arguing that this underscores a mental health agenda that remains centred on control and exclusion. They maintain that little has altered in this regard during the past 100 years. The locations in which this agenda has taken shape may have changed, little else. Medical psychiatry is still in control of this agenda, and other professional groups such as nurses, psychologists and therapists continue in a handmaiden role.

At the end of the 19th century, the asylum, as total institution, provided care, control and accommodation. These functions are now delivered through a network of smaller psychiatric units, community teams and housing agencies. This network is connected through a range of legal arrangements, policies and government directives. Rogers and Pilgrim quote Department of Health figures for the operations of the 1983 Mental Health Act:

> formal admissions under the 1983 Mental Health Act rose more than 60 per cent from 16 000 in the year 1988–89 to 27 000 in 1998–99. (Rogers & Pilgrim 2001: 179)

They also argue that the late 20th century has witnessed a reassertion of biological approaches within psychiatry. This has happened in spite of the rise of the user movement and 'its demand for more talking treatments'. They contend that in-patient care is still at the heart of psychiatry, that this is dominated by biological approaches with little attention to social or psychological issues in the patient's life and that coercion continues to be a primary focus of the whole system. In other words:

> in many ways recent mental health policy does not reflect the post-modern agenda about voluntary relationships, 'minor' mental health problems and the production rather than the repression of selfhood. Instead, it continues to place centre-stage responses to the threat which embodied irrationality (unintelligible conduct) poses to a social, economic and moral order. (Rogers & Pilgrim 2001: 177)

There is a great deal of truth in these observations. Anne Rogers and David Pilgrim are two of the most astute and respected observers of the mental health scene in Britain. However, there is a danger that we fall back on an 'all or nothing' position when it comes to our understanding of mental health politics. In the conclusion to this chapter, we will outline our thoughts on how both these perspectives are not necessarily mutually exclusive.

The postpsychiatry position

While we agree with Rogers and Pilgrim's analysis of the current policy situation in Britain, we believe that their presentation of this as some sort of rebuttal of a Foucauldian perspective is mistaken. We do not read Foucault as maintaining that all power is productive in modern and postmodern societies. Nor do we believe that his thought leads to the conclusion that the politics of discourse should replace a political understanding centred on the question of coercion.

Our understanding of postmodern thought is that it represents an addition to, rather than a rejection of, previous critical positions. This may sound like a fudge. It isn't! For us, postmodernism is centred on the belief that no single analytic frame will explain the world and all its contradictions. Postmodernism is suspicious of meta-narratives. While we are sympathetic to Marxist, liberal and other political perspectives that seek to challenge institutions of social control, we refuse the demand that we should endorse any one position as being inherently superior to others. This is not a flight to mindless relativism but simply a recognition that different situations and events will require different forms of analysis. Postmodern thought represents a struggle to free ourselves from the idea that there is only one path to the truth, one way of using reason, one form that science and serious reflection should take. This echoes Foucault's demand that we should get beyond the 'blackmail' of 'being for or against the Enlightenment' (Foucault 1984: 45).

We believe that as we enter the 21st century, power is exercised in many different ways around our planet. For example, the globalization of market capitalism has been achieved through different methods. At the time of writing, the USA and Britain have deposed the government of Saddam Hussein in Iraq and are now involved in the process of shaping the Iraqi economy in a way that suits the interests of major international corporations (*Guardian* 2004). The war was short-lived and served to demonstrate to the world at large the military might of the USA. It also showed that the USA is quite prepared to use this military power to shape political and economic structures in different regions of the world. This represents globalization 'through the barrel of a gun'. At the same time, globalization moves forward through the increasing involvement of the global economy in local worlds. There are many facets to this process, but the insertion of new discourses of the self into these local worlds is of great importance. International capitalism can only continue to survive and prosper as more people around the planet come to see themselves (and feel themselves) as consumers. Michael Hardt and Antonio Negri write that:

> The great industrial and financial powers thus produce not only commodities but also subjectivities. They produce agentic subjectivities within the biopolitical context: they produce needs, social relations, bodies, and minds. (Hardt & Negri 2000: 32)

Every day, more and more people in different parts of the world come to understand their lives, their needs, their relationships within the terms given to them by manufacturers of goods, services and entertainment. So, globalization proceeds through naked military force and coercion and also through the production of subjectivities. Power is exercised in negative and positive forms.

This also resonates with our understanding of the increasing turn towards drug treatments in psychiatry. We agree with Rogers and Pilgrim that there has been a substantial turn towards biological theories and interventions within psychiatry in the past 20 years. We noted the dominance of reductionism in the Introduction. In fact, the ruling ideology of psychiatry in recent years has been biological reductionism. However, this is not simply a return to the past or even a sign of 'professional inertia' as they put it (Rogers & Pilgrim 2001: 180). In many ways, it represents psychiatry's attempt to come to terms with postmodern cultural developments. In the past 20 years, 'man' and human nature have not disappeared, as Foucault predicted at the end of *The Order of Things* when he wrote that the normative ideal of 'man' might soon be 'erased, like a face drawn in sand at the edge of the sea' (Foucault 1970: 387). That this face has changed and become more blurred is not in doubt, but effaced? No. Instead, new narratives of human nature and new discourses of the self have emerged. The resurgence of biological models of human suffering has to be understood in this light.

In an article entitled 'From vastation to Prozac nation', Alice Bullard considers two revolutions in our recent conceptualization of depression. The first is the modern revolution in the late 19th century that involved a shift from a religious to a psychological outlook; the second is what she calls the 'postmodern revolution' in which there has been a turn to biochemical narratives. Bullard discusses how in the idiom of psychoanalysis and related forms of psychotherapy, depression shows up as meaningful. Therapy is targeted at unwinding the intricate knots of emotional pain and hurtful relationships. If successful, individuals emerge with a deeper understanding of themselves and indeed of the human condition in general. The self is a site of struggle; deeply layered, complexly textured. Depression emerges from the wounds inflicted over years on this self by the vicissitudes of personal relationships. It crucially involves our contact with 'the other'. This clearly echoes the sort of analysis presented by Nikolas Rose, discussed above.

Bullard contrasts the self that emerges in the psychoanalytic narrative (deep, layered, meaningful) with the self that emerges in narratives of biochemical depression:

> Under the influence of Prozac it becomes possible and most probably advisable to constitute the self not through remembering, but through forgetting, through systematic omission of the void, the abyss, the darkness of depression's shadow. (Bullard 2002: 277–278)

In the culture of postmodernity, the self that we are offered is able to choose its moods, to switch off its past. Narratives are no longer deep and complicated. Our stories of ourselves and our suffering are short. Our identities are increasingly the stuff of 'lifestyle' choices instead of personal struggle. Bullard writes:

> All those hours in analysis now appear like time spent inventing fairy tales. All those mornings lying in bed enthralled to visions of doom and pondering the whys and wherefores of this peculiar persecution; the early relationship with one's mother, the older brother who beat you, or a God who has abandoned you, faith that has been eclipsed by evil, every possible element has been drawn into a drama motivated by chemical instability. One feels poorly because one's chemicals are out of wack, that's all, end of story. (Bullard 2002: 283)

We are neither 'for nor against' the emergence of postmodernity[3] and its new narratives of the self. There is nothing inherently better (in an ethical sense) about psychological and psychoanalytic accounts of depression when compared with more recent biological versions. In different ways, these seemingly diverse ways of understanding ourselves both reflect background

---

[3]Perhaps it is important to point out that there is a difference between postmodern *thought* and postmodern *culture*. The former is a way of understanding and is thus something we can choose or reject. The latter refers to a contemporary social, cultural and political *condition*, something we simply find ourselves living through. In this sense, our postmodern culture is not something we *choose*. Rather it is something we have to come to terms with for good or bad, see Bracken (2003) and Lewis (2000).

socio-economic developments. They underscore the various ways in which the projects of our lives and the ways in which we deal with sadness and loss are bound up with our position as individuals trying to survive in the midst of consumer capitalism. While Bullard describes a transformation that has taken place since Nikolas Rose's *Governing the Soul* was first published in 1989, both authors describe a self shaped by issues of choice, autonomy and identity. Rose ends his book with the lines:

> . . . modern selves have become attached to the project of freedom, have come to live it in terms of identity, and to search for the means to enhance that autonomy through the application of expertise. In this matrix of power and knowledge the modern self has been born; to grasp its workings is to go some way towards understanding the sort of human beings we are. (Rose 1989: 258)

We believe that this analysis still rings true, but capitalism never sleeps, and the last 10 years have seen the massive expansion of the pharmaceutical industry and the advent of brand-based consumerism (Klein 2001). The psy complex has changed accordingly and is less focused on the 'codes and vocabularies of psychotherapeutics' (Rose 1989: 254) and more on the technologies of diagnosis and 'cosmetic psychopharmacology'[4]. Bullard writes:

> The biochemical revolution cuts the self free from depression's narratives. This radical freedom opens onto uncharted terrain for the elaboration of selfhood. (Bullard 2002: 269)

The point is that if we are to understand the massive consumption of psychotropic drugs in our culture, we require the sort of Foucauldian understanding of the self developed by Rose and others. However, we also need the insights of more traditional forms of critical discourse centred on the role of the economy. The writers Herb Kutchins and Stuart Kirk, in the book *Making Us Crazy. DSM: The Psychiatric Bible and the Creation of Mental Disorders*, make the point that the pharmaceutical industry has played a substantial role in shaping the agenda of psychiatry in the past 20 years. It funds a large number of researchers and has directly contributed to the development of the Diagnostic and Statistical Manual (DSM). They write:

> the companies have a direct financial interest in expanding the number of people who can be defined as having a mental health disorder and who then might be treated with their chemical products. For this reason, drug companies are disturbed by the findings of many surveys that have found that a majority of people whom DSM would label neither define their own problems as mental illness nor seek psychiatric help for them. For drug companies, these unlabelled masses are a vast untapped market, the virgin Alaskan oil fields of mental disorder. (Kutchins & Kirk 1999: 13)

---

[4]In many ways, 'cosmetic psychopharmacology' involves a coming together of the modernist reductionist impulse at the heart of psychiatry (discussed in the Introduction) with the shifting nature of the postmodern self.

As well as expanding the number of psychiatric labels through which individuals might come to frame their problems, the drug companies have also been at pains to extend the range of indications for their use in conditions such as schizophrenia. Thus, in recent years, there has been a major focus on the idea of 'early intervention'. The concept of 'duration of untreated illness' (DUP) has been introduced. This is said to be related to outcome and thus there is a logic for aggressive early treatment with new antipsychotic drugs.

Conclusion

This chapter has looked at the first theme of postpsychiatry: the relationship between psychiatry, exclusion and coercion. We have argued that these links were forged in the Age of Reason, but have been developed in different ways through the course of the past two centuries. We agree with Anne Rogers and David Pilgrim that they remain at the heart of government policy and psychiatric practice. However, we have argued that we need an analysis of psychiatric power that serves to highlight its more productive aspects. We have turned to Foucault for this. Psychiatry and its allied disciplines control deviance through their interventions and treatments, but they also provide us with the narratives through which we understand ourselves and our problems. There is really no contradiction here. We started the chapter with Mad Pride. They campaign against discrimination but also, more positively, for the right to be heard in their own words. Foucault spoke about the thrusting 'into oblivion (of) all those stammered, imperfect words without fixed syntax in which the exchange between madness and reason was made' (Foucault 1971: xii). Organizations such as Mad Pride, Mad Women, the Hearing Voices Network and the Self-Harm Network are demanding a return to dialogue; a move away from monologue. As we enter the 21st century, their words are far from stammered, but articulate and powerful.

We put forward the idea of citizenship as something that can hold a number of agendas at the same time. It represents both a campaign against exclusion and coercion and a demand that users be allowed to articulate their own voice and develop their own vision of how the world of mental health could develop. We believe that the concept could also serve to provide a unitary focus for users, carers and professionals in their struggle to improve the lot of those who endure states of madness, alienation or distress. Groups such as Mad Pride are clear that they are not in the business of changing services but changing society. Increasingly the wider user movement is beginning to shift in this direction. Peter Campbell (2001) writes:

> The great irony about service user action in the past 15 years is that, while the position of service users within services has undoubtedly improved, the position of service users in society has deteriorated. As a result, it is at least arguable that the focus of service user involvement needs adjustment. Service

users and providers should accept that the quality of life of people with a mental illness diagnosis in society, indeed their proper inclusion as citizens, depends on education and campaigning. (Campbell 2001: 88).

'Education and campaigning' are activities that can bring the different stakeholders together, but only if the full meaning of the concept of citizenship is understood by all sides. Psychiatry has argued that its medical framing of madness is a major step forward and understands stigma as being due to 'ignorance'. As a result, it puts great score on the notion of public 'education'. The argument is that if the public came to see schizophrenia as being in the same league as measles or diabetes, the associated stigma would disappear. In this chapter, we have argued that 'education' needs to be thought of as something more than arguments in favour of the medical model being presented to a sceptical public.

The ring

Dr Ian Cooke
The Surgery, Quarry Cliff

Dear Dr. Cooke

Re: William Murphy

Many thanks for referring this 22-year-old single man who came to see me in the clinic this afternoon. He was accompanied by his mother.

His problems started 3 weeks ago just as he was about to return to university for the final year of his psychology degree. Earlier this year, his father died unexpectedly of a heart attack. He attended the funeral, had some time off his studies, but from his mother's account during the last few weeks of his second year, he became increasingly withdrawn, stopped going to lectures, and didn't sit his end of year exams. A month ago, a friend was killed in an accident, following which he became very preoccupied. He felt that things were specially arranged; he said 'These things just do not happen this way.' He felt God's presence, and thoughts from God entered his head. He believed that God could control his thoughts and actions, for example he told me that God could make him cry. He believed the Masons were spying on him, but wasn't able to explain why. He also describes hearing voices addressing him in the second person, but he was reluctant to discuss the details with me.

His mother corroborated this story. She told me that she was very concerned about her son because he was so preoccupied and withdrawn. He had started to neglect himself, letting his appearance go, and often missing meals. He spends much of his time in his bedroom reading the Bible.

William lives at home with his mother and younger sister. His early life and development appear unremarkable, although he does appear to have been a somewhat sensitive child. His mother said that he had always been a bit shy, and he refused to go to school at the age of 11, when he moved to secondary school. Despite this, he excelled, academically, and after a year out travelling, went to university. His physical health is excellent, and he has never before seen a psychiatrist. He is on no medication and, apart from moderate cannabis use (2 or 3 times a week), there is no history of serious drug misuse. He has never had any close relationships.

At interview he presented as a tall, slim young man with moderately severe acne. He was dressed in a dirty old t-shirt and jeans. His hair was unkempt; he was unshaven and unwashed. His attention and concentration were poor. His speech frequently tailed off in mid-sentence and he found it impossible to pick up the thread of what he was saying (thought block). He kept repeating 'Why is this happening?' His affect was blunted, and he displayed clear evidence of first rank symptoms of schizophrenia (delusions of control and thought block), and on several occasions I thought he was experiencing verbal hallucinations (whispering to himself), although he denied this on questioning. He was fully orientated in three spheres.

Opinion and recommendations

I have no doubt this young man is suffering from acute paranoid schizophrenia. Although recent life events may have triggered this, his pre-morbid personality is such that he will not have a good prognosis. I have started him on risperidone tablets, increasing to 2 mg b.d. over the next week, and I have also referred him urgently to our new early intervention service that specializes in treating first onset schizophrenia. I am sure they will be in touch with you in due course.

Yours sincerely
Denise Menas MPhil., M.D., FRCPsych

Consultant Psychiatrist

In her office, my mouth swung to attention but silence streamed out in all its beauty. I was trapped. She was polite, efficient, coldly decorous and but her little white pill, guidelined with such precision, melted on my tongue and froze my brain. My gushing thoughts ground to a halt—I couldn't think anymore. I tried it for a few days but couldn't sit still; I was on edge all the time; no energy. So I stopped it yesterday, and they're coming tomorrow.

It is important that I try to explain this. I say 'this' because I still don't know what to call it, or how to understand it. It isn't a thing to be dismissed so readily with a name. It must have started in January. We had been walking the dog down by the river. The blizzard had blown itself out. When we got back, he grabbed his chest, made this strange noise in his throat, and fell down. It happened so suddenly. I didn't know what to do. I froze as my dad coughed his life away.

Yes, that's when it started. Back at college, things were sort of okay for a while, but the week before I was due to sit exams, my granny died. She was a very religious lady. At the funeral, the minister kept repeating our dear departed sister, safe and away in the arms of Jesus, bathed in the blood of the lamb. I was really close to my gran. She used to look after me and my sister when we were small. Afterwards, I kept getting these images of a lamb drowning in a sea of blood, struggling for its life, being dragged down and down, choking and gasping for breath. I couldn't shake them off. Night after night I would lie in bed staring at the ceiling, watching this over and over again.

I didn't get back to college to sit my exams. I stayed at home, numb with no feelings or thoughts, nothing. I'd try to read or watch telly. I'd sit for hours staring at blank pages that stared back, mocking me, telling me that I'd lost the plot, so I gave it up. Then my best friend Chris returned from university and tried to get me out for a pint, but that was no good. I felt on edge, especially in the local. We live in a small village, the sort of place where everyone knows everyone else's business. They all knew my dad, and they'd say they were sorry about your dad, and what a good man he was. But that only made things worse. I believed that I had let my dad down, watching him die, not knowing what the hell to do to help. I felt useless and guilty because it was my fault that he died. I loved him, and all these people in the pub knew him, and respected him, reminding me of him. Chris tried to reason with me, saying I wasn't to blame, and I could have done nothing to save him. In the end, I stopped going out, and stayed in. Chris kept phoning to see if I was okay, but I didn't want to speak to him or for anyone else to see me in such a state.

A few weeks later my mum had to go into hospital for an operation, nothing serious but something she had to have done. The day before, it was my birthday, and she gave me a ring that belonged to my dad. Originally it was her father's, but he gave it to my dad the night before they married. I don't know why she gave it to me; perhaps she believed that if I had something special that belonged to my dad it would help me to get over his death. I don't know. Anyway, I opened this tiny black box inside which was the most amazing gold ring. My granddad was a Mason, and the ring had the sun and an eye with rays coming out against a turquoise background. I've always been vaguely interested in the Masons because of the ritual and secrecy. When she gave it to me, she kissed me on the forehead. This is to watch over you and guard you and keep you, she said. He looks down on you across space and over the centuries. The next day she went in for her operation, and that night Chris was killed in a car accident.

Then it hit me, the losses, my dad, my gran, and Chris. It didn't make sense. Things like that just don't happen, do they? There must be a reason for them, some sort of logic. Chance, random events? Losing those you love the most as though through the throw of a dice. There had to be some purpose in it. All this flooded my mind, and I was alone. My mum was recovering from her operation, my dad and gran dead and buried. I was lost and utterly alone.

That evening I found myself walking down by the river where I went with my dad the day he died. It had been really hot for several days but now the weather was breaking. It was heavy and sultry. Everything was still and quiet. The trees and bushes were lifeless. No birds flew. The world was waiting for something. It started raining; the first heavy drops were like great tears falling from heaven. I wanted to cry too, but couldn't. As the earth's thirst was slaked, its sweet sharp fragrance broke out. The sun appeared from behind a great tower of black clouds throwing its rays across the river. Flaming clouds of gold and vermilion drew across the east against a turquoise sky. The rain came heavier, drenching me, not now the sky's tears but my own. God was there; I was no longer alone. God was with me and I stood there for what seemed like ages. As the silence deepened, I could see everything with the greatest clarity; my senses connected with the world in the most intimate way, making everything emerge with the most intense clarity. Its beauty was astoundingly painful, as I was drawn into creation with a sense of duty. I realized I was seeing the world through God's eyes. I became that sun and those clouds, that river and those trees, that sky, rain and earth; all these beautiful things alive in me, fused with me. And I heard God saying 'You are being watched.'

A moment, an aeon in a microsecond, passed. God has not returned but they are, tomorrow, with the consultant. I am being watched over. I'm still in a state of shock. Dr Menas says she wants me in hospital. In the last few months, I have changed. My life will never be the same, but it doesn't make sense. They say I need medication. I don't believe in God. I'm not religious. I don't go to church or anything like that. But now I read the Bible and the Koran. They say they'll have to get me in to force me to take it. I don't know what the answer is, perhaps there isn't one. Perhaps the answer isn't important, but the search for one is. They want me to stop searching. They say it's illness. How can they say that? They weren't with me by the river. They didn't see what I saw, hear what I heard. How can they say that? How can they?

4   Foregrounding contexts

What kinds of understanding are appropriate in the world of mental illness?

Introduction

In Chapter 3, we looked at the relationship between psychiatry and the world of madness and distress. We noted how for much of its history that relationship was predicated upon a concern with control. While coercion has been central to the way in which control has been exercised by psychiatry, this is far from the full story. The professional models we create and defend so vigorously are the means through which we structure the experiences of service users. These are powerful tools, and are often experienced as destructive and controlling by recipients. Through these models, we see power being exercised 'positively'; power as shaping reality through discourses, not simply as repressive and silencing. The way in which we have come to discuss our states of distress and alienation through a language of psychology, psychiatry and therapy is not neutral but based on certain values, assumptions and priorities. In other words, it carries a strong element of control. In previous centuries, the formulation of such states through a religious idiom served to bind individuals to the institutions of the church and invested power in priests and other officials. The 19th and 20th centuries witnessed a decline in the authority of the Christian religion in Western countries. With this decline came a corresponding increase in the power and influence of what Nikolas Rose has termed the 'psychological complex' (Rose 1985).

In this chapter, we turn away from a direct engagement with questions of power, control and coercion and look instead at a related matter: the issue of what sort of understanding is brought to bear when an individual comes into contact with the mental health system. We shall look particularly at the process of assessment and diagnosis. Although a great deal of the discussion in this chapter will be philosophical, issues of power and control are never far from the surface.

As a medical discipline, psychiatry argues that diagnosis is a fundamental part of its practice. In general medicine, the making of a diagnosis plays a pivotal role. History taking, examination, investigations all lead towards the generation of a diagnosis. It gives whole departments (bacteriology, pathology, biochemistry and radiology) their raison d'étre. Medical and surgical interventions are guided by diagnosis. In short, modern medicine could not be practised without the use of diagnosis. A medical diagnosis puts a name on the patient's condition. However, it does more. It brings to bear an explanatory framework through which the emergence of the symptoms and signs of the illness makes sense. It is true that different individuals may suffer from the same disease in different ways and with different levels of severity. However, this does not negate the idea that a medical diagnosis delineates the essential 'truth' of the patient's condition. We shall encounter the way in which philosophers, psychologists and others have used a contrast between the *form* and the *content* of various phenomena later in the chapter. Here, let us simply point to the way in which the named disease (the diagnosis) represents the form of the illness, while the illness as experienced in particular patients corresponds to the notion of 'content'. The form of the disease is universal, i.e. is the same in everyone who suffers it regardless of context. The actual symptoms and signs, 'the content', can vary from individual to individual. For example, these will vary depending on the age, nutritional status and psychological state of the patient. The role of the doctor has to do with outlining the form; in practice, this means finding the right diagnosis. While the patient will be concerned to learn about the diagnosis (form), their central concern, on a day-to-day basis, is more likely to be the content, i.e. the actual symptoms and signs experienced.

Not surprisingly, psychiatry has followed medicine in its focus on diagnosis. In its efforts to establish itself as a *bona fide* medical enterprise, psychiatry has invested considerable effort in attempts to establish diagnostic systems that are valid and reliable. This has gathered even more urgency in the USA since the introduction of managed care. In this system, doctors do not get paid unless they generate a diagnosis for the patient. This fact, alongside other factors such as the decline of psychoanalysis, created the conditions in which the production of DSM III and its successors has been so important (Kutchins and Kirk 1999).

Diagnosis has traditionally been the preserve of medically trained psychiatrists. While nursing staff, psychologists and others can perform most other clinical tasks (such as psychotherapy) as well as, if not better than, psychiatrists, diagnosis has always been the job of the doctor. Thus, assessment and diagnosis lie at the heart of psychiatric theory and practice.

In the era of DSM, psychiatric textbooks continue to assert that diagnostic assessments are based upon an understanding of the 'phenomenology' of 'psychopathology'. Writing in the *Comprehensive Textbook of Psychiatry* in 1995, Mezzich states:

> The manifestations of mental disorder constitute the focus of the so-called phenomenological description of psychopathology

and notes that the DSM III is

> characterized by a phenomenological emphasis in the conceptualisation and
> organization of mental disorders...' (Mezzich 1995: 692 and 700)

So, psychiatry maintains that *phenomenology* is the tool through which it is able to conceptualize and make apparent the nature of psychiatric 'symptoms'. It is also the means through which 'symptoms' are classified.

In this chapter, we ask: what sort of understanding lies behind the issue of diagnosis in psychiatry? What assumptions are involved? What is the nature of the phenomenology used by psychiatrists? Are there other ways of encountering and understanding states of madness and distress? Are there different ways that we can think about the notion of diagnosis? Are there other forms of phenomenology that might be helpful in this regard?

At the core of this chapter is a discussion about where the focus of our understanding should be when it comes to grappling with madness and distress. Our argument is not that psychiatric assessments are 'false' but that they are limited by the conceptual assumptions currently underpinning psychiatric practice. Behind this lies a particular understanding of phenomenology. We shall argue that psychiatry needs to grapple more with issues of context if it is to progress in its understanding of patients' experiences. A key element of what we call postpsychiatry is the view that modernist psychiatry has been built on what some commentators have called 'methodological individualism', the assumption that different psychological states can be examined in isolation from the world around them. Postpsychiatry seeks to overcome this orientation by bringing contextual issues centre stage. By contextual issues, we are referring to the fact that human psychology is always embodied (wrapped up in the complex biology of a human body), encultured (involved in the linguistic, cultural and political reality of the society in which it exists) and temporal (never fixed, but constantly in flux and always involved in a journey from past to future).

Our argument is that these dimensions of human reality have somehow been pushed back to the edges of our understanding of mental states, in particular states of distress. Not completely dismissed but usually of marginal interest only; external 'factors' impinging on an individual mind which is understood as something apart from the world around it. Traditional psychiatry and different forms of psychotherapy have theorizied on the basis that there is some basic core of human psychology that is universal, not context bound. We disagree. We believe that the 'mind' is social through and through, cannot be understood apart from 'its' body, and never static. In this chapter, we outline the theoretical aspects of this debate; in later chapters, we shall spell out our position in the context of case examples and make reference to a substantial (and growing) literature from different discourses that supports this position.

Phenomenology in contemporary psychiatry

In his foreword to the English translation of Karl Jaspers' *General Psychopathology*, Anderson writes that '. . . the phenomenological approach involves painstaking, detailed and laborious study of facts observed in the individual patient at the conscious level' (Anderson 1963: vi). Anderson was keen to differentiate this approach from that of psychoanalysis with its focus on unconscious processes and conflicts. This understanding of phenomenology has guided mainstream psychiatric thinking about assessment and diagnosis throughout the latter half of the 20th century. One British psychiatrist defines phenomenology simply as 'the precise description of psychopathology' (Mortimer 1992: 293). In contrast to the vague speculation of psychoanalysis, the phenomenological approach is held up as being more clear-cut and precise; ultimately more scientific. Most contemporary psychiatrists would argue that their assessments involve a detached, factual listing of the patient's symptoms accompanied by a clear analysis of the person's mental state. This is what is meant by the term phenomenology in contemporary psychiatric practice.

In this process, the experiences that trouble the patient (or an interested third party in some situations) are taken out of the patient's own language and reformulated in psychiatric terminology. In medical practice, 'a pain in the tummy' becomes 'left-sides hypogastric pain' in the words of the doctor. In psychiatry, a person might complain of feeling 'empty', 'without direction' 'fed up' or simply 'miserable'. These feelings are often bound up with such things as unhappy relationships, difficult work situations or physical ill health. In the psychiatrist's formulation, these feelings become 'dysphoric mood' or 'symptoms of depression'. Painful thoughts about the possibility of ending one's life, with all the cultural, religious, personal and family implications and nuances that such thoughts invariably bring to the fore, become simply 'suicidal ideation'. Voices that discuss and comment upon the actions of the individual become 'third party auditory hallucinations'. This process is carried out in an attempt to render psychiatric practice more scientific, the idea being that if we are to have a science of psychopathology, we need a clearly defined language through which a scientific discourse can proceed. Without this, we are 'limited' to a level of interpretation that is based only on personal narrative and locally defined meanings. A science of psychopathology demands concepts that are universally valid and reliable. In other words, it demands a concern with the 'forms' of psychopathology.

Psychiatry has never really doubted the idea that a science of psychopathology is needed or even possible. The assumption has been that without a specifically scientific approach to the framing of troubling thoughts, emotions and behaviours, psychiatry itself would never progress. It has never been in doubt that there *are* forms, diagnostic entities 'out there' awaiting identification and clarification.

However, whatever the demands of a scientific psychopathology, in the actual lived lives of individuals, painful thoughts, feelings and experiences are always woven in with other psychological, cultural and practical realities. In the course of the person's day-to-day life, such thoughts and feelings relate to particular situations and circumstances; they are often associated with longer-term worries and conflicts. They reach back to the past and look forward to the future. They also take place in the context of an embodied reality, a reality that wakes and sleeps and is subject to the rhythms of a personal physiology. The point is that the experiences brought to psychiatry are rarely, if ever, singular isolated events. They are most often varied and muddled. Forcefully present at one moment, less intense at a later time, and absent altogether in a different social setting. They emerge from within the tapestry that is the person's life.

The initial words used by the patient, the family and wider social group are given by the language and culture through which these events take shape. As such, they are intrinsically bound up in webs of meaning. These meanings may not be immediately obvious, they may be contradictory and far from clear-cut, sometimes they are actively resisted by the individual involved, but they are always present. But webs of meaning are always that: complicated inter-dependent networks of references. The philosopher Wittgenstein famously pointed this out in relation to our use of language. Words relating to concepts do not denote sharply defined concepts but instead refer to a set of family resemblances between the things labelled with the word. Furthermore, language only works on the basis of a shared practical world; a shared culture. As Hubert Dreyfus says:

> ... linguistic communication is possible only on the background of a shared world and ... what one communicates about is an aspect of that shared world. In communication something is explicitly shared on the background of an already shared affectedness and understanding. (Dreyfus 1993: 221)

Meaning involves relationships and interconnections; a background context against which things show up in different ways. The expression 'I feel like killing myself' may mean very different things depending on the context in which it is uttered, from a joking throw away remark to a serious expression of suicidal intent. The world of psychiatry, involving emotions, thoughts, beliefs and behaviours, is a world of meaning and thus of context. Indeed, it is the centrality of these twin issues of meaning and context that separates the world of the 'mental' from the rest of medicine. This world is somewhat different from the 'non-meaningful' world of physical processes that are the core territory of the various branches of physical medicine. A number of researchers in the area of artificial intelligence (AI) are beginning to realize this. These researchers have spent many years attempting to develop physical models of human thought. One prominent American AI researcher, Terry Winograd writes:

> The results of human reasoning are *context dependent*, the structure of memory includes not only the long-term storage organization (what do I know?) but also a current context (what is in focus at the moment?). We believe that

this is an important feature of human thought, not an inconvenient limitation.
(quoted in Dreyfus 1993: 118)

It goes without saying that there is a psychological element present in all of medicine. But psychiatry is precisely delineated by the fact that its *central* focus is the 'mental world' of its patients. Meaning and context are thus essential elements of the world of mental health and simply cannot be regarded as 'inconvenient limitations', issues that can be ignored or wished away.

In spite of this, just as the physician reformulates the patient's description of his/her feelings of sickness in a medical language that is sometimes opaque to the patient, so too the psychiatrist abstracts an account of individual psychiatric symptoms from the patient's own descriptions. Just as the physician is initially only concerned to describe in medical words in order that a diagnosis might be produced, leaving words such as 'misery', 'struggle' and 'suffering' to one side, so too the psychiatrist is trained to observe and describe in the technical language of psychiatric 'symptomatology'. Questions of meaning, relevance, connection to the past and the future, and social context might well be brought to bear later on, but they are deliberately excluded from the initial psychiatric act of assessment and diagnosis.

In current psychiatric practice, phenomenology simply means the description and ordering of the patient's symptoms. There is a fundamental assumption involved here. This is the belief that our lived psychological realities *can* be described and ordered in the very same way that our physical symptoms and bodily processes can. In other words, a belief that psychopathology is essentially no different from physical bodily pathology. Detached scientific observation, analysis and ordering are held to be equally relevant in both areas. Stemming from this is a secondary assumption: that psychological events can be reliably and accurately described in *isolation* from the meaningful context in which they emerge and have significance. Just as the physician can, through the processes of history taking, physical examination and investigations, come to a position where he/she is able to group my medical problems together and explain them by invoking causal processes operating in my body, outside my awareness, so too it is generally assumed that the psychiatrist can perform a detached assessment of my mental state and then order my psychological reality accordingly. The bodily processes explored by the physician are not 'meaningful' as such. They are not intimately linked to linguistic, cultural or social realities in the way that thoughts, feelings and behaviours are. Psychiatrists are aware of the importance of meaning, but if the psychiatrist who is assessing me seeks an understanding of how my particular psychological reality came about, this is seen as something different from phenomenology, which is simply about description and ordering.

While there is an on-going debate within psychiatry about the validity and reliability of different ways of classifying psychiatric symptoms (Kendell & Jablensky 2003), there is little worry about the above assumptions concerning the nature of phenomenology and psychopathology. A fundamental aspect of psychiatry's quest to establish its medical identity is the assertion that it has a scientific way of encountering the world of distress and madness. What we have called modernist psychiatry demands that we conceptualize phenomenology as a scientific process. Phenomenology has to be seen as something that allows the psychiatrist a neutral, scientific view of the subjective world of the patient. As we shall see below, this was a task that exercised Jaspers a great deal. However, before turning to Jaspers and his presentation of a 'scientific' version of psychopathological phenomenology, it is worth a brief discussion of how the authors of the DSM understand the meaning of phenomenology.

Increasingly, the DSM is the accepted classificatory system internationally, used by psychiatrists everywhere to frame the problems of their patients and to provide the diagnoses that are used to name these problems. The authors of the DSM argue that it is 'atheoretical' in its approach. They also claim that it is based on a phenomenological approach. The DSM Training Guide contains a statement to the effect that the DSM is: 'phenomenologically descriptive' (quoted in Mishra 1994: 130). This has been challenged by a number of writers who believe that this claim involves a misrepresentation of what phenomenology (as least in its Jasperian form) involves. For example, Gupta & Kay (2003) argue that the approach to assessment embodied in the DSM is not in keeping with the phenomenology of Jaspers. Instead they suggest that:

> this use of phenomenology is a particular, clinical deployment connoting the elicitation of characteristic signs and symptoms of a particular mental disorder. This usage has little connection to phenomenology as it is understood within philosophy or even as compared to the great variety of meanings that evolved as psychiatrists applied phenomenology to psychiatric practice and research. (Gupta & Kay 2003: 83)

Mishara (1994) argues that modern psychiatry, and the DSM approach in particular, has failed to grapple adequately with the importance of subjectivity. While phenomenology is often invoked, in reality psychiatric assessment is informed by a central focus on observable behaviour. Mishara laments the covert behaviourism of current DSM-centred psychiatry and contrasts this with the real possibilities of a phenomenological approach:

> By selecting a descriptive approach based on behaviorist assumptions in which behaviors are described and classified as clinical features of disorders, DSM-III-R inadvertently compromises not only the preconceptual aspects of the clinician's diagnosis, but also the future research into the causes of mental disorder. A phenomenological approach ameliorates this problem by providing categories for the description and conceptualisation of the genesis of the subjective structure of experiential meaning. (Mishra 1994: 132)

Thus, although phenomenology is still invoked by contemporary psychiatry, and even by the authors of the DSM, as providing access to the subject life of patients, there is serious doubt that what is actually meant by phenomenology in this context is anything like what was proposed by Jaspers in the early part of the last century. These writers, and many others, argue that what Jaspers offered was a much richer approach to the understanding of subjectivity. They argue for a 'return to Jaspers'. Our position is that Jaspers is very much a part of the problem, not a solution. Therefore, in the next section, we shall examine what was at stake in Jaspers' phenomenology. This is the central section of this chapter. In it we describe at some length the guiding assumptions, the philosophical orientation, of Jaspers' work. We believe that this is important because Jaspers' work, even if not followed precisely by contemporary psychiatry, continues to shape the fundamental approach to assessment. It provides the concepts, the assumptions and the attitudes that continue to inform psychiatric practice. Therefore, it is important to be clear about what Jaspers was doing. In the following section, we go on to argue that the form of phenomenology available to Jaspers when he was writing on psychopathology was limited. We make the case that the hermeneutic turn taken by continental phenomenology in later decades offers a much richer grounding for psychological theory. In this, the role played by meaning and context in structuring human reality is no longer an 'inconvenience' but instead becomes the central focus.

Before looking at the nature of Jaspers' phenomenology, it is important here to say something about the philosophy of Descartes and Husserl. One of the central arguments of postpsychiatry is the idea that modernist psychiatry has been locked in the embrace of Cartesianism throughout the 20th century. This has resulted in a neglect of contextual issues. We believe that the version of phenomenology bequeathed to psychiatry by Jaspers is largely responsible for this, together with the enormous influence of cognitivism within psychology over the last 50 years. Together, these two have resulted in psychiatry and psychology moving ever further away from recognizing the importance of contexts in human experience. While mainstream psychiatry has changed the meaning of the word 'phenomenology' and, as we have seen above, some psychiatrists believe that a 'return' to Jaspers would solve some major problems, we are not convinced. We believe that Jaspers' approach is fundamentally Cartesian in nature. There can be little doubt that Jaspers' orientation was modelled on the approach of Husserl. The hermeneutic phenomenology examined in the next section offers the possibility of getting beyond Cartesianism and holds out the possibility of a different sort of understanding of mental health problems.

Karl Jaspers' approach to phenomenology and meaning

Most psychiatrists who trained in the 20th century have looked to the *General Psychopathology* for their understanding of phenomenology. Even those who have never read the original have been introduced to this major figure in the introductory chapters of psychiatric texts or in the many shorter works focused on psychopathology.

Philosophical background to Jaspers' work: the Cartesian understanding of human reality

Let us first be clear about what we mean by Cartesianism. We are of course aware that there are different interpretations of Descartes. Our use of the term 'Cartesianism' and the 'Cartesian legacy' is indebted to Hubert Dreyfus' discussion in his *Being-in-the-World. A Commentary on Heidegger's Being and Time, Division 1* (Dreyfus 1991). There are two central themes at the heart of Cartesianism.

Knowledge and certainty: towards a scientific approach to subjectivity

Like other Enlightenment philosophers, Descartes was concerned with questions of knowledge and certainty. Can we be sure that our internal mental representations give us an accurate account of the external world? How can we explore the subjective world in a rational scientific fashion? He was impressed with the truths of mathematics. We can be certain of these. How can we produce a knowledge of the subjective realm and the outside world that is as certain as mathematics? His solution was to propose a method of systematic reflection upon the contents of the mind, and through this to separate what was clear and obviously accurate from what was uncertain and vague. In his *Meditations on First Philosophy*, he argued that by way of systematically doubting everything that was unclear, we could eventually reach a situation of certainty with regard to our own existence, the existence of God and the existence and nature of the external world.

His reasoning was as follows: even though I can doubt many things, there is one idea that I know always to be true: the fact that I am thinking. I simply cannot be mistaken when I think that I am thinking. To think that I am not thinking would be to logically contradict myself. This truth is certain and indubitable, of equal standing with any of the truths of mathematics. In fact, I know that I exist because I know that I am thinking. This insight has become known as the Cartesian 'cogito'; *cogito ergo sum*: I think therefore I am.

On the basis of this insight, Descartes goes on to argue that by examining our beliefs carefully, we can also be certain that other thoughts are true. While we can be deceived at times by our senses, if we accept that God is good, and 'on our side', there is, according to Descartes, no reason to postulate that he would have set the world up so that we would be *systematically* deceived by our senses. Thus, if we confine ourselves to thoughts and beliefs that are 'clear and distinct' (like the concepts of mathematics) we can work to avoid error.

For Descartes, our reason is a gift from God and as long as we use it properly we can use it to avoid mistakes. This is the essence of rationalism. While a 'non-deceiving' God was the ultimate guarantor of truth and certainty, his presence was not essential to his confidence in our ability to clarify our thinking and to separate the clear and distinct thoughts from others. Importantly, even if we remove God from the picture, there is reason to believe that systematic reflection on our thoughts and beliefs can lead to an accurate understanding of how the world works.

A central tenet of Cartesianism is therefore a belief in the possibility of, and importance of, reflexive clarity and the value of defining and mapping the ways in which internal representations are ordered and related. Serious exploration of the subjective was going to be scientific after Descartes. This view has been immensely influential and lies at the heart of Husserlian phenomenology; we shall see later that it is also to be found at the heart of cognitivism, and dominant approaches to ethics.

Cartesian dualism: metaphysical and epistemological

In addition, Cartesianism operates on a fundamental distinction between the 'inner' world of the mind and the 'outer' world with which it is in contact. This separation of the inner and the outer is predicated upon Descartes' metaphysical (or ontological) separation of the world into two kinds of substance. This is usually called 'Cartesian dualism'.

The term substance is the philosophical equivalent of the ordinary word 'thing' (*res*). Descartes separated out the soul from the material body in which it resided. The latter he characterized as follows:

> ...By body, I understand all that can be terminated by some figure; that can be contained in some place and fill a space in such a way that any other body is excluded from it. (Descartes 1968: 104)

In other words, the body is characterized by the fact that it possesses 'extension'; it occupies space. It is thus *res extensa*. In contrast to this, the soul is characterized by thought:

> ...I am therefore, precisely speaking, only a thing which thinks, that is to say, a mind, understanding, or reason, terms whose significance was hitherto unknown to me. I am, however, a real thing, and really existing; but what thing? I have already said it: a thing which thinks. (Descartes 1968: 105)

The soul, or the self, is thus 'a thing which thinks', a *res cogitans*. While it does not occupy space, Descartes still maintained that it was a substance, a *res*, a thing.

This application of the concept of thing or substance to the self has had major implications. In our reckoning, the most important result of Descartes' dualism is not the metaphysical notion of two separate substances existing in the world. This separation has underpinned an extensive and on-going debate about the relationship between the *mind and the body*. Important as this debate is for medicine and psychiatry, it is not the central focus of our discussion for the time being, although we shall return to this in Chapter 5. Our concern is the separation of *mind from outside world* that follows in the wake of Descartes' metaphysical dualism. We might call this his 'epistemological dualism'.

This arises as follows. The term substance is usually applied to familiar objects such as trees or chairs. In pre-Enlightenment, scholastic philosophy, a distinction was made between the attributes of a thing and that within which such attributes resided. This was in an era before atoms and molecules were identified. The understanding of 'things' was very much driven by philosophical speculation. It was clear, for example, that two chairs could have the same features (colour, size and shape), but they were still separate chairs. The features were known as attributes and what they resided in was called the *substantia*, that which 'stands beneath' the attributes. The substance, as that in which the attributes or properties of a thing inhere, cannot be readily perceived or described. Nevertheless, it is what gives the thing its existence as a singular entity. In the concept of substance used by Descartes, this contrast between the plurality of the attributes and the singleness of that in which they reside is fundamental. However, Descartes used this term to describe, not things in the outside world, but the nature of the self or the soul, that which thinks. When moved to the self, to the *res cogitans*, this contrast (between attributes and substance) is maintained, but operates in a somewhat different way. The attributes are not now size, shape, colour, etc., but instead our thoughts and beliefs (our representations). Frederick Olafson notes that:

> To the attributes of the standard substance or thing, there now correspond the representations or ideas of the things that the self perceives or otherwise thinks about; and to the mysterious nucleus in which those properties were supposed to inhere, there corresponds that in which these representations are contained. It is as though substance in the picture we ordinarily form of it had been turned inside out or, better still, outside in. Indeed, this is not a bad way of understanding the change that has taken place, since to the attribute that a thing like an apple displays to general view, there now corresponds a representation *within* the new kind of substance, but with this difference, that the representation is accessible only to the view from within and cannot be perceived from without at all. (Olafson 1987: 7)

Thus, thoughts, perceptions, beliefs, desires and other mental phenomena are the attributes, or properties, which inhere *within* the mind. Thought becomes the inner functioning of a substance, which we call a subject (*subjectum*). This subject is in contact with an outside world and has knowledge of it through sensation and through the representations it has of it. The point is that in this Cartesian view, the mind becomes something 'self-contained'. It stands outside the world and has a relationship to it. Mind (or 'subjectivity') becomes something conceivable apart from and separate from this relationship. It knows the world from the outside. Thus, there is an epistemological separation of mind from world.

It is this epistemological separation, based ultimately, as we have seen, on Descartes' metaphysical dualism, which provides the basis for what is known as the representational theory of mind and thought, concerned as it is with the relationship between inner states of mind and outer states of the world. We shall return to this later on, when we examine the influence of cognitivism in theories of psychosis. But first, we shall consider the Cartesian heritage of Husserl.

A brief introduction to Husserl's phenomenology[1]

For the most part, Husserl's orientation towards the Cartesian project was overtly positive. His fundamental method of enquiry, which he called 'phenomenological reduction' in works after the *Logical Investigations* (Husserl 1970), involved setting aside, or 'bracketing', the existence of an outside world in order to focus in a clear and unbiased way upon the phenomena of consciousness and experience. His aim was to reach what he called the 'transcendental standpoint'. This was to be achieved by a series of 'reductions' which, in turn, were operations performed upon everyday experience with the purpose of isolating the 'pure' consciousness which is obscured as long as it is not separated from the natural world. Like Descartes, Husserl was attempting to elaborate a method of investigation into the experiential world, which was solid and foundational. He also sought a science of the subjective realm.

Thus, while Husserl's views on phenomenology changed throughout his life, in most of his writings he saw himself as engaged directly with the legacy of Descartes. In his 1931 book *Cartesian Meditations*, he described his own phenomenology as a 'neo-Cartesianism' (quoted in Walker 1994*b*: 254). This is not a topic that we can deal with in any great detail here. We have neither the space nor the expertise to present an analysis of Husserl's complicated approach to phenomenology. We simply wish to point out the Cartesian orientation of Husserl's phenomenology. We believe that this orientation was passed on to Jaspers. In relation to this, we believe that it is safe to make the following claims about Husserl:

(1) In a large part of his work, Husserl was attempting to establish an indubitable basis for our knowledge claims. Like Descartes, Husserl was interested in mathematics and impressed by the fact that we can be certain about the truth of many mathematical statements. He wanted to establish a similar degree of certainty in other areas of knowledge. Following Descartes, he did this through an intense examination of the nature of human subjectivity. Dermot Moran writes that:

> More and more, he [Husserl] articulated his methodology in terms of the radical foundationalist project of Descartes's *Meditations*, understood as the grounding of objectivity in subjectivity. (Moran 2000: 138).

---

[1] Our account of Husserl is indepted to Dermot Moran's account in his *Introduction to Phenomenology* (2000).

Husserl was a philosopher. He hoped that his phenomenology would establish philosophy as a precise and ultimately scientific enterprise. As such, his work was very much a continuation of the Enlightenment project. Like Descartes and Kant before him, he was seeking to establish the ultimate grounds upon which we can have certain knowledge. His was a search for *a priori* truths.

(2) Also echoing Descartes, Husserl sought to engage with subjectivity as though it was something outside but related to the world around it. In the years after the publication of his *Logical Investigations*, Husserl wanted to establish phenomenology as a transcendental discipline. He rejected his own, earlier, account of phenomenology as 'descriptive psychology'. While he denied Descartes' presentation of the *res cogitio* as a separate substance, a 'thinking thing', he followed Descartes in presenting the 'inner' world as something apart from the world in which it exists. In other words, he endorses Descartes' epistemological separation of mind from world. In his book *Cartesian Meditations*, he uses the term 'monad' to describe human reality. He actually speaks of the self as a 'monad with windows' (Moran 2000: 174).

Thus, while Husserl was working some centuries after Descartes, his philosophy was very much influenced by a Cartesian understanding of human subjectivity.

Jaspers' philosophical assumptions in the *General Phenomenology*

In this huge work, first published in 1913, Jaspers brought together previous descriptions of psychiatric phenomena and provided psychiatry with a comprehensive account of psychopathology. Jaspers is quite clear in this work that phenomenology represents only one aspect of psychopathology. It is very much a subdiscipline. Most of the *General Psychopathology* is actually focused on other aspects of the field. But for Jaspers, phenomenology is essential. It provides an accurate description of, and a precise definition of, the symptoms and signs of mental illness. In the following discussion, we aim to demonstrate the Cartesian nature of Jaspers' phenomenology.

Jaspers is clear from the start:

> A textbook of psychopathology ... must be scientific and is valuable only for this reason, so that we are deliberately confining ourselves in this book to what can be understood in scientific terms. (Jaspers 1963: 2).

Not having the benefit of an encounter with philosophers of science such as Thomas Kuhn, who came later in the 20th century, Jaspers maintains that science is not concerned with value judgements. In fact, on page 1, he insists that a properly scientific psychopathology must proceed by separating off issues of value:

> Ethical, aesthetic and metaphysical values are established independently from psychopathological assessment and analysis. (Jaspers 1963: 1)

The 'field of values' he continues, 'has nothing to do with psychiatry' (p. 2).

While some of the other subdisciplines of psychopathology (such as the contribution of physiology) are un-problematically rendered in the logic of science, Jaspers recognizes that the psychopathologist is faced with a major difficulty when it comes to the development of an adequate methodology through which the scientific study of subjective life can take place. This is a problem at the heart of psychiatry's difficulties. While the scientific study of biology has underpinned the development of modern medicine, in many ways psychiatry still appears stuck on the 'starting line'. How can we begin to study and measure such things as thoughts and feelings? How can we render the 'inner' world accessible to the detached gaze of science? Psychologists of the behaviourist school have reacted to this problem by saying that there simply cannot be a science of subjective life. Subjective reports of thoughts and feelings are just too vague to be the subject matter of a proper scientific discipline. They then proceed as if subjective experience just does not occur. For its part, psychoanalysis has directly engaged with subjective life. However, alongside many others, Jaspers was unimpressed by the contribution of psychoanalysis. He regarded it as 'a confusing mixture of psychological theories' (Jaspers 1963: 359–360).

Husserl's influence on Jaspers

Aware of the many practical difficulties in the world of psychology and the major philosophical problems lurking behind, Jaspers turned to Husserl who, as we have seen above, was developing phenomenology as a method through which the nature of subjective human reality could be revealed in an exact and precise fashion.

In the philosophy of psychiatry literature, there has been a recent debate about the background influences on Jaspers' approach to phenomenology. A central question has been the extent to which Jaspers' thought *was* actually influenced by Husserl. Until this recent debate, the consensus had been that Husserl had a substantial influence on Jaspers, at least with regard to his understanding of phenomenology. This position was associated with the views of prominent figures such as the psychiatrist Shepherd (1983) and the historian of phenomenology, Spiegelberg (1972). Their views were supported by a number of statements made by Jaspers himself. For example, this is how he described the relationship in an autobiographical essay:

> After being confined to medicine for a long time I came in 1909 to know Husserl through reading him. His phenomenology provided a productive

method which I applied in understanding the experiences of the mentally ill. What was essential for me was to see how extraordinarily disciplined Husserl's thinking was ... Above all I appreciated his unceasing demand to clarify unnoticed presuppositions. In Husserl I found confirmed what was already working within me: the drive to press to the things themselves. And at that time-in a world full of prejudices, schematisms, and conventions-this was like a liberation. (Jaspers 1951; quoted in Wiggins & Schwartz 1997: 17; their translation).

More recently, German Berrios (e.g. 1993) and Chris Walker (e.g. 1988) have challenged Jaspers' account of his own debt to Husserl. They make the case that Jasper's use of phenomenology took him far away from what Husserl had been trying to develop. Chris Walker makes the case that Jaspers was more influenced by other philosophers such as Kant, Weber and Dilthey. In turn, Osborne Wiggins and Michael Schwartz (e.g. 1997) have disputed the Berrios and Walker readings of Jaspers. Michael Langenbach (1995) has also argued for a strong Husserlian influence on Jaspers.

For our part, we believe that there is truth in both sides of this argument. Thus we agree with Walker and Berrios that Jaspers diverged in a substantial way from Husserl. First, there were obvious differences in the subject matter that concerned them. Jaspers was primarily interested in exploring the symptoms of patients. His phenomenology was a sort of medical tool and not really philosophical at all. Husserl was a philosopher and his phenomenology was purely a philosophical enterprise. Secondly, for Jaspers, phenomenology was an *empirical project*, part of the empirical science of psychopathology. Husserlian phenomenology was *transcendental*, reaching beyond the empirical 'surface' of things to define instead 'pure essences'. Thirdly, for Jaspers, while phenomenology was an element of scientific psychopathology, philosophy was something very different. Philosophy could never be scientific. For Husserl, philosophy *was* science, in fact he wanted it to be a 'rigorous science'.

This last point is important. Chris Walker presents good evidence that Jaspers himself saw a clear gap between his position and that of Husserl on this issue. In fact, Jaspers wrote later that in his presentation of philosophy as a science, in the book *Philosophy as Rigorous Science*, Husserl had 'committed the most naïve and pretentious betrayal (Verrat) of philosophy' (Jaspers; quoted in Walker 1994*a*: 120). Jaspers did not accept the idea from Descartes and adopted by Husserl that philosophy should be a search for indubitable truth. In a monograph first published in 1937 on Descartes, Jaspers is explicitly critical of this position. He tackles the Cartesian *cogito* and states that while its truth is certain, it is, contrary to Descartes' view, neither clear nor distinct. He says that it does not tell us what 'thought is, what the I is and what the being of this I is' (Jaspers 1964; quoted in Walker 1994*b*: 254). Walker, quoting Jaspers, writes that:

> Both Descartes and Husserl claimed that their philosophy was scientific. For Jaspers, this 'confuses human knowledge [science] with the form of knowledge

peculiar to the angels [both certain and informative].' 'The knowledge of the angels is intuitive, innate and independent of things'. In contrast, science is 'not intuitive but dependent on logical inferences, not innate but dependent on experience and not independent but dependent on objects.' (Walker 1994*b*: 255)

Jaspers' Cartesian phenomenology

In spite of these clear differences, we believe that Jaspers *was* correct in his own estimation of the intellectual debt he owed to Husserl. In turn, we believe, through Husserl, there are strong Cartesian underpinnings to Jaspers' approach.

First of all, Jaspers had no doubt that a science of the mind was both possible and desirable. Like Descartes and Husserl, he wanted a method whereby subjectivity could be explored scientifically. The difference between them related to what *kind* of science was being developed. For Descartes and Husserl, this was to be some sort of eidetic or transcendental discipline; for Jaspers, it was to be empirical. There can be no doubt that Jaspers was attracted to Husserl's account of phenomenology because it appeared to hold out the possibility of a clear, accurate, precise account of human subjectivity. Furthermore, Husserl was convinced that phenomenology, if carried out properly, offered not just descriptions of individual subjectivities but rather a universally valid account of how we, as human beings, experience the world we live in. For Jaspers, like most others writing at the beginning of the 20th century, science was about the obtaining of knowledge that was universal and beyond dispute. If psychiatry and psychology were to aspire to scientific status, then they had to acquire clinical and research methods that gave them such knowledge about subjectivity. This was the central reason behind Jaspers' attempt to apply Husserl's approach to phenomenology in the world of psychiatry. He and Husserl were at one in their search for a scientific underpinning of psychology and psychopathology, even if they differed in their characterization of the relationship between philosophy and science.

In the following long quotation from the introduction to the *General Psychopathology*, Jaspers states very clearly what 'job' he wants phenomenology to perform:

> The first step towards a scientific knowledge of the psyche is the selection, delimitation, differentiation and description of particular *phenomena of experience* which then, through the use of the allotted term, become defined and capable of identification time and again. Thus we shall presently describe the different kinds of hallucinations, delusions, compulsive phenomena and the different modes of personal awareness, drives etc. So far there is no concern with the sources of such phenomena nor with the emergence of one psychic phenomenon from another, nor yet with any theories about underlying causes. The only concern is with the actual experience. This representation of the psychic experiences and psychic states, this delimitation and definition of them, so that we can be sure the same term means the same thing, is the express function of *phenomenology*. (Jaspers 1963: 25–26)

Secondly, Jaspers wants a phenomenology that engages with the subjective world of the patient as something separate. Phenomenology is to act like a scientific instrument through which the psychiatrist can examine the 'interior world'. The subjective world is encountered as something distinct from both the meaningful world around it and from the body in which it is located. This is reflected in the structure of the book.

There are six parts in all. The first part is devoted to a detailed account of 'individual psychic phenomena'. This part of the work is purely descriptive. He covers the objective manifestations of mental disturbance: motor problems and speech disorders for example. Phenomenology is presented as the way of exploring the subjective dimension. Subsequent parts of the book deal with the different ways in which the phenomena of psychopathology emerge. Jaspers deals separately with the 'meaningful connections' associated with 'morbid' experiences and their 'causal connections' (exogenous and endogenous). He also discusses a number of other issues in some depth including historical and social aspects of psychiatric conditions.

The structure of the book is important because through it Jaspers is making a clear distinction between the descriptive aspect of psychopathology and the search to understand the particular circumstances of the person involved. Most important for our discussion is the separation Jaspers makes between the task of describing the subjective world of the patient (phenomenology) and the search to understand the meaning of the patient's experiences. Jaspers is quite clear about this:

> Phenomenology presents us with a series of isolated fragments broken out from a person's total psychic experience. (Jaspers 1963: 27).

It is not the job of phenomenology to look outside the 'interior' to seek meaning, understanding or explanation. Phenomenology presents us with a 'static' picture of the person's psychological state. The search after meaning involves a 'genetic' approach:

> Genetic understanding (the perception of psychic connection) enlarges the 'hermeneutical round'; we have to understand the whole from the particular facts and this whole in turn preconditions our understanding of the facts. (Jaspers 1963: 29).

So Jaspers separates phenomenology from hermeneutics (interpretation). Of course, Jaspers is very much aware of the importance of meaning and context. But, for him, phenomenology is not about meaning. It concerns an effort to present a picture of the patient's mental state as described in the technical language of psychopathology. Phenomenology is concerned with the 'form' of psychiatric symptoms, not with their meaningful content:

> It is true that in describing concrete psychic events, we take into account the particular contents of the individual psyche, but from the phenomenological point of view it is only the form that interests us. According to whether we

> have the content or the form of the phenomenon in mind, we can disregard
> for the time being the one or the other—the phenomenological investigation
> or the examination of content. (Jaspers 1963: 59)

Phenomenology for Jaspers involves a particular sort of gaze into the patient's mind. This gaze does not seek to interpret or even to understand, but to identify and describe. The mind it engages is a separate realm, something that can be described apart from the world around it. The gaze is rational, scientific. It works to order, to define and analyse. For Jaspers, phenomenology is a technology: a particular way of framing and ordering the world of distress, madness, confusion and alienation. Phenomenology is different from hermeneutics, which seeks meaning and connections. This echoes a further assumption in Jaspers' approach: the separation of scientific psychopathology from cultural anthropology. Culture is something superficial. It only influences the content (not the form) of an individual's symptoms. The forms of psychopathology are universal:

> As far as we know today we find the same psychopathological phenomena in
> all the three great cultures of East Asia, India and the Occident. Content
> changes with the prevailing opinions. The phenomena are identical even in
> the individual neurotic deviations. (Jaspers 1963: 740)

Like the dominant tendency within psychiatry, Jaspers presents phenomenology as a search for the universal forms of psychiatric symptoms. The phenomenological part of psychopathology does not engage with the question of content. This is something local and variant.

We believe that the Cartesianism we have identified above in the work of Husserl is also manifest in that of Jaspers. As noted before, there are two important aspects to this. First, Jaspers endorses the idea of a specifically 'scientific' form of phenomenology. His is a phenomenology that separates off questions of meaning, narrative and ethics. The subjective world of the patient shows up as something to be analysed, categorized and described. Jaspers' assumption that this is both a possibility and a necessity is essentially Cartesian. Secondly, Jaspers separates the subjective realm both from the meaningful world around it and from the body in which it is held to reside. The phenomenologist is tasked with encountering the mental world of the patient in isolation from the rest of his/her lived reality. This is a necessary first step in the development of a scientific understanding of psychiatric problems.

These twin themes are not independent. Rather they represent two aspects of something more fundamental: the idea that phenomenology is about having knowledge of the other's mind. Like its rival, psychoanalysis, Jasperian phenomenology is about a science of 'the other'. It is ultimately about the doctor having a language, a framework, a knowledge about the patient that the patient does not possess. As we have seen in the last chapter, this is essentially a political issue. This was not apparent to Jaspers.

Phenomenology in a different key

We believe that there are serious difficulties with Jaspers' approach to phenomenology and the current form of psychiatric assessment that takes inspiration from it.

The assumptions that our psychological reality can be rendered accurately in a 'static' way and that this is best done through the technical language of psychopathology needs interrogation. Many service users find the process of psychiatric assessment painful and sometimes oppressive. Many react against a psychiatry that is based on this type of phenomenology, a modernist psychiatry involved in a search for knowledge about 'the other'. For in this form of psychiatry, the patient is always 'the other', is always 'outside', always inferior.

To be interviewed by a doctor who is seeking not primarily to understand but instead to classify can be disturbing. Of course, many psychiatrists fail to adopt the phenomenological (as described by Jaspers and the DSM) position and do indeed seek, in their assessment interviews with patients, to understand the meaning and context of what is happening. But in doing so, they move beyond the 'static' assessment position and engage in something else.

Our argument is that Jaspers' attempt to separate phenomenology from hermeneutics is problematic. Following Heidegger, we believe that any attempt to grasp human reality (and its problems) that neglects either:

(1) the way in which this reality is bound up with issues of social context,

(2) the way in which human reality is always an embodied reality and

(3) the question of temporality

will always be partial and potentially destructive. In other words, we do not believe that phenomenology can be separated from hermeneutics. Jaspers' 'static' phenomenology is false to the lived world of patients, doctors and the society in which they live.

In the next subsection, we shall argue that Heidegger developed an approach to phenomenology that moved substantially beyond the sort of Cartesian assumptions defined above. We shall argue that his phenomenology is something different from the 'scientific' encounter proposed by Husserl and adopted in a different way by Jaspers, i.e. as an empirical science. We shall also argue that Heidegger made substantial headway in his attempt to get beyond the sort of 'mind–world' split endorsed by Husserl and also used implicitly by Jaspers. In the following subsection, we shall discuss how such an approach to phenomenology helps to shape a positive postpsychiatry way of thinking about mental health issues.

Heidegger's approach to phenomenology

Heidegger worked closely with Husserl during the last years in which Husserl held his chair in Freiburg. Indeed, Heidegger was appointed to the same position when Husserl retired. Heidegger edited a series of Husserl's lectures, and his own work in phenomenology was initially guided by the older man. Heidegger's most famous book *Being and Time* was dedicated to 'Edmund Husserl, in friendship and admiration' (Heidegger 1962). One might suppose, therefore, that there was a lot in common between the sorts of philosophy developed by the two men. Not so. Although Heidegger did begin by follow-ing in the footsteps of Husserl, *Being and Time* actually represents a radical departure from the sort of Cartesian-inspired phenomenology of Husserl. As Hubert Dreyfus points out, the sort of philosophy developed by Heidegger was very much outside the tradition that linked Descartes with Husserl:

> Heidegger rejects the methodological individualism that extends from Descartes to Husserl to existentialists such as the pre-Marxist Sartre and many contemporary American social philosophers. In his emphasis on the social context as the ultimate foundation of intelligibility, Heidegger is similar to that other twentieth-century critic of the philosophical tradition, Ludwig Wittgenstein. (Dreyfus 1991: 7)

While in his later works [after his so-called *Kehre* (turning)] Heidegger is at pains to distinguish philosophy (what he then referred to as 'thinking') from science, in *Being and Time*, following Husserl, he uses the term 'science' in relation to his phenomenology. In spite of this, as Theodore Kisiel writes:

> ... *Being and Time* is manifestly a philosophy of being and existence and not a philosophy of science. (Kisiel; quoted in Hoeller 1988: 148)

Heidegger's aim in *Being and Time* was to examine the question of being, the central preoccupation of traditional Western metaphysics, in a completely new light. Dreyfus argues that:

> what Heidegger has in mind when he talks about being is the intelligibility correlative with our everyday background practices. (Dreyfus 1991: 10)

In other words:

> to raise the question of being (is) to make sense of our ability to make sense of things. (Dreyfus 1991: 10)

Heidegger's concern is about how the world 'shows up' for us; how there *is* a world in which we exist; how this world appears to 'hold together' in some way. The question of being is not about the nature of things in the world such as objects and thoughts; it is the question of how the world makes sense for us, of how it is meaningful. Things in the world (rocks, cows, paintings, concerts, religions, ideas, relationships) show up as meaningful for us only against a background context. A good relationship only exists because we know about bad relationships. A delusion (a false belief) is only a delusion because we know about 'correct or true beliefs'. The point is that we experience the things of our world as related or as contrasted, but always as 'holding together' in some way. But this background cannot be described comprehensively through a listing of things. It appears to resist lists and categorization. While things within the world are amenable to analysis in themselves or in relation to other things in the world, the background to everything, the simple fact that everything 'is' in some way, cannot be grasped in this way.

Heidegger distinguishes two areas of inquiry, which he labels 'ontological' and 'ontic'. Ontological inquiry refers to the question of being (the background 'holding together'), while ontic enquiry refers to a concern with entities and facts about them (Heidegger 1962: 31). Ontological inquiry has to be undertaken in a way different from any type of ontic enquiry. Being has to be 'exhibited in a way of its own'. Thus, for Heidegger, the question of meaning cannot, and should not, be framed as a scientific issue (Hoeller 1988). The meaning of being is simply not 'some*thing*' that can be grasped through a causal framework. In fact, it is not a 'thing' at all and it requires a very different type of understanding from that provided by science. For Heidegger, in *Being and Time*, the path to understanding the meaning of being was through an analysis of the only entity for which this question arose: human being. Heidegger's approach to understanding the nature of human reality takes him far from the sort of phenomenology put forward by Jaspers. In turn, this understanding opens up a very different sort of encounter with the suffering patient.

For Jaspers, the 'mind of the patient' is something to be encountered through the gaze of an empirical science. This science (psychopathology) seeks to analyse, categorize and label the contents of this entity. Phenomenology is essentially the technology through which this encounter takes place. Training in psychopathology is about the young psychiatrist learning this technology and incorporating its perspective, its assumptions, its outlook, its vocabulary. It involves the trainee psychiatrist positioning him/herself in a particular way in relation to the 'mind of the patient'. It involves a certain sort of gaze. He likens the psychiatrist to a histologist looking down a microscope:

> Just as the histologist describes particular morphological elements in detail only so that others can *see* them more easily, and just as the histologist must presuppose or induce this seeing-for-oneself in people who are really to understand him, so also the phenomenologist specifies features and distinctions and warns against confusions in order to describe qualitatively peculiar mental data. He must, however, count on others not *merely thinking* along with him but rather, in their interaction and conversation with patients and through their own making present (*Vergegenwärtigung*), *seeing* along with him (Jaspers 1968; quoted in Wiggins & Schwartz 1997: 30).

Heidegger argues that human reality resists analysis through the gaze of empirical science. He starts from the idea that human beings are not 'in' the world in the same way that these CDs are in their boxes or that there are hard drives 'in' the computer[2]. These things are passively situated one inside the other. But for a human being to be 'in' the world actually involves a sort of bringing that world into being. In some ways, we are responsible for allowing a world to be in the first place. And this world must be different for us as humans from that of other animal species. The way in which human bodies are made anatomically and physiologically means that a certain type of world 'opens up' for us. Humans have a certain way of hearing, seeing and smelling the world, a certain way of experiencing space and time. We bring colour and sound to the world. It is difficult for us to imagine what sort of world 'opens up' to a fruit fly, a fish or a bat. We are simply not 'in' a world that is separate from ourselves. Rather, we allow a world to be by our very presence. Heidegger uses the composite term 'being-in-the-world' in an attempt to describe the complexity of our involvement with our worlds. Traditional ways of thinking about ourselves as minds existing alongside an outside world and 'containing' representations of an outside world fail to grasp the complexity of this involvement. There simply is no world incorporating sights and sounds, waiting 'outside' to be represented. Heidegger seeks a very different vocabulary to describe our reality.

Alongside the fact that the worlds in which we live are brought into being through our physiological make-up, it is also the case that our involvement in a society, a culture, a historical period also plays a part in this process. This involvement provides the words, concepts, assumptions and attitudes that all contribute to the shaping of the world we encounter on a daily basis. The words of our languages do not simply name separately existing things in a world outside but rather structure that world in specific ways. Heidegger talks about human reality being a sort of clearing (*Lichtung*). The word *Lichtung* usually refers to a clearing in the woods (according to Macquarrie and Robinson, the translators of *Being and Time*). The noun *Licht* also means light. These words convey a sense of a world being disclosed through our presence 'in' it. We are the illumination that brings a world to light[3]. As pointed out above, the world that is disclosed through us is (presumably) very different

---

[2]Of course, our bodies are in the world in that sense, and can be spoken of in the same way that we may speak of other physical objects in the world. But the point is that 'human *being*' is an active phenomenon. It is not a physical entity, and it is wrong to think of it as one, and to treat is as such. We will return to this error in Chapter 5 when we consider Wittgenstein's later philosophy and its implications for metaphysical and epistemological dualism.

[3]It is worth noting here that there are close affinities between Heidegger's ideas, and those of Maurice Merleau-Ponty, who compares *Lichtung* with the light in a room. We may not be able to detect its source, but its presence makes objects in the room stand out for us. Merleau-Ponty also attaches great importance to the fact that we are embodied beings, indeed it is central to Merleau-Ponty's understanding of being-in-the-world. It is only by virtue of our physical bodies that it is possible for us to be subjects in the world. We are, to use Merleau-Ponty's expression, body-subjects. Langer (1989) comments that classical psychology's commitment to the standpoint of an impartial observer means that it fails to appreciate the fundamental difference between the body and other objects in the world. We cannot detach ourselves from our bodies and inspect them in space as we can other objects. It is because we have bodies that we can perceive the world in the first place and act meaningfully in it. It is through our bodies that the myriad objects in the world

from that which is available to other creatures. While this is an act of individual humans, it is never this alone. As Dreyfus puts it:

> We can thus distinguish *clearing* as an activity from *the clearing* that results from that activity. Think of a group of people all working together to clear a field in a forest. There is a plurality of activities of clearing, but all this activity results in only one cleared field. (Dreyfus 1991: 165)

When we open our eyes and ears, we see and hear a world around us. As Heidegger maintains, this act of perception is never passive: it is also an act of creation. We 'bring into being' the colours, shapes and sounds of the world. Furthermore, we experience the world, not as a collection of discrete items, but as a totality, something that 'holds together'. We experience it as meaningful. But we do this as a social group, not as a collection of individuals. Thus, any individual act of perception has a social dimension. It is dependent on our human physiology but also on our social embeddedness: our involvement in a world socially ordered through human practice, language and culture.

For Heidegger, human reality is always embodied reality and encultured reality. The Cartesian approach which positions our mental worlds as some-how outside and separate from our bodies and our social contexts is simply

---

act on us and become meaningful to us. We are not 'pure consciousness', but embodied beings. We have eyes and ears to see and hear with; our limbs provide us with the motility to move around the world and to become active in it. Our nervous systems are essential to our consciousness, but it does not follow as some suggest, that our consciousness, our personhood *is* the brain.

Having a body locates us in time and space. It positions us in culture and history, providing us with a perspective from which we move in to and out of the world. But the world stretches out in front of us endlessly ('inexhaustible' is the way Merleau-Ponty puts it), infinite in its variety and possibilities. We are positioned but never fixed. So being-in-the-world brings with it our attempts to 'exhaust' the world, to grasp it, encounter it, engage with it, understand and make sense of it. The point is that human experience cannot be dualistic. Our bodies, as the physical substrate of being and experience, provide an organic physiological background to experience. Matthews (2002) in describing embodiment draws an analogy with a stone. A stone is an inanimate object, 'in the world', but fixed and passive. It has its place in time and space, but is only acted on by other objects, Humans, as embodied subjects, have the capacity to engage actively with the world, to move around in it and to explore it intentionally.

The fact is that we do not experience the world in two ways: a mindful or mental way and a bodily way. In reality, we are unified entities. Using the term 'embodiment' instead of 'mind and body' helps us to move away from Cartesian ways of describing experience. Thus 'embodiment' offers a valuable way of dealing with body mind dualism, but it also helps us to think our way around epistemological dualism (mind/society dualism). Being a body-subject, as Merleau-Ponty suggests, also means that our being-in-the-world is just as much located in historic and cultural worlds as it is in the physical world. Our bodies inhabit the physical spaces of our houses, build-ings, streets, towns or country, and nations. These physical spaces, which we have created, are pregnant with cultural meaning and significance for us. They also represent an infinite variety of cultural institutions, family, home, school, mosque, temple, hospital, prison, theatre, and so on. Our lives are acted out in and shaped by these cultural physical spaces; they place us in unique relationships with each other; they signify meaningful social, spiritual, aesthetic and political realities. But it is always our bodies that bear us forward into these spaces of meaning. For Merleau-Ponty, cultural, social and political activities are not optional extras that just happen to come along with having a body. They are a vital, integral part of being-in-the-world.

false to the actual way we exist as human beings. However, there is a third essential element to our human way of being, our way of 'clearing' a world in which to live. This involves the fact that we are temporal creatures: we exist 'in' and through time. We shall not deal with this issue in any great depth. However, Heidegger's understanding of temporality also undermines Jaspers' notion of a 'static phenomenology' so it is important to mention this at least.

Just as I am not 'in the world' in the same way that my car is 'in the garage' or my brain is in my 'skull' so too I am not 'in time' is some sort of passive or merely observing way. Instead, just as I bring colour and meaning to the world via my physiology and culture, so too, I bring a particular sense of time and its passing into being. As far as we are aware at present, human beings are the only creatures who have an awareness of death and thus of finitude. This knowledge structures our engagement with the world in a profound way.

Time is usually understood to be a series of moments, a series of 'nows', each essentially disconnected from each other. While Aristotle conceived the 'now' as having a certain 'thickness', modern thought has sought to model the 'now' in atomistic terms. It is only from outside the series of nows that what is past, present and future can be established. Furthermore, the necessity of a possible atemporal position is also required to explain how any individual has a sense of his/her own position in time. In the model of linear time, the person who is 'in time' knows the past through representations. But there is a difficulty here as these representations are always *present*. Thus, it is not clear how the person can reach out of the present and establish certain representations as being of the past and then relate to them as such. Why is it that all representations do not simply collapse into the present? This is only avoided by postulating an atemporal position from which it is evident which representations are in the present and which are from the past. In some way it is understood that the person who is in time has access to the atemporal viewpoint. This model is obviously problematic and has caused a number of difficulties for philosophy. However, the postulation of an atemporal position is often an implicit rather than explicit element of the model, and so the problematic usually does not come to light. Modern commonsense and psychology simply assume a clear distinction between what is present and what is past.

The notion of an atemporal vantage point is deeply entwined with the positivist notion of causality which is closely allied to Cartesianism. Causal laws are understood to exist as 'hard and fast' unchanging connections between things. Such laws, by definition, do not change with time but work at different times and in different situations. As the psychologists Faulconer and Williams assert:

> The positivist notion of causality...relies on the assumption that static, atemporal entities are the fundamental kind of existing things and that other things exist only to the degree that they can be reduced to these static entities and their atemporal characteristics. Causal explanation is explanation in terms of these atemporal entities. In this sense causality *is* atemporality; the causal account is the atemporal one, and it is the only account by which

human being is intelligible according to the positivist point of view.
(Faulconer & Williams 1985: 1182)

Heidegger contradicts this by pointing out that time is at the essence of human being. To be human is to be temporal, involved in possibility and change. Without the presence of possibility, no *human* event can really occur. Heidegger maintains that human being, the clearing described above, is inherently temporal and simply cannot be grasped in terms of atemporal, static causality.

Heidegger argues that we have to stop thinking about time as a self-contained independent moment, existing as logically distinct from the past or the future. His move is to point to the internal complexity of time as it is actually experienced. For human beings, the 'now' is not simply a point in a series but rather it holds, or frames, time in such a way as to set up contrasts within itself between the past, present and future. Olafson says

> Another way of putting this is to say that, in the Now, time is stretched (*erstreckt*) in such a way that it holds on to what has been and awaits something that is to come. The former is thus taken as that which is no longer, the latter as what is not yet; and what is now the case is present in the strong Heideggerian sense of that term as what once was not and later will (or may) no longer be the case. If what is now the case were simply replaced in the next moment by something else, then in each of these moments what is the case would be a Now without a contrasting Then, a present without a past or a future. But there is a future only if what is not yet the case is something other than just a state of the world that is located, for some transcendental and nontemporal observer, further along the time dimension. (Olfason 1987: 85)

The essential point being made is that the present is not and cannot be something that is fixed and separate from the past and the future. The three are involved inextricably with one another. This is seen clearly if we attempt to imagine a person existing in the present tense alone, without access to a past or future. It is simply impossible to imagine such a state. Our worlds are always already configured for us and this configuration implies a past. It makes no sense to think of a present moment in which the world is not configured in some way. Likewise it makes no sense to think of a present without a future. It is akin to attempting to think of night without a concept of day, or vice versa. By speaking about a present at all, we are implying the existence of something else, we are implying a movement onwards[4].

We believe that Heidegger provides an account of human being that is closer to the reality of lived experience than those of Descartes, Husserl and Jaspers. The twin assumptions that run through the work of these philosophers (that the

---

[4]The great complexity of our human experiences of time is conveyed beautifully by Prince Myshkin in Dostyevky's novel *The Idiot*. In the following extract, the Prince is describing an encounter he had with a man he had met the year before, who was due to be executed for having committed a political crime. He had been taken to the place of execution along with some other prisoners, where the sentence of death was read out. Twenty minutes later, his reprieve was

mind has some sort of existence outside the world and that the contents of this mind can be described and analysed scientifically with little or no reference made to bodily, social or temporal context) are shown by Heidegger to be exactly that: assumptions. In their place he begins with human reality as we experience it in our everyday lives. This reality is *always* deeply shaped by context. To use a metaphor: for Descartes, Husserl and Jaspers human psychology is built like an avocado: at its heart is the stone of universal, context-independent processes. A scientific psychology or psychopathology seeks to grasp the nature of this solid object. It seeks to cut through and remove the flesh. This gets in the way of the true scientific gaze. In this picture, the flesh of the avocado represents the surrounding world in which the individual psychology is situated. In the hermeneutic phenomenology of Heidegger, human psychology is better likened to an onion. Here, there is no separate central, solid core. Just as the onion simply *is* its layers, there is no human psychology that is not bound up with context. In addition, at the heart of our reality as human beings lies movement, potential, constant change and open-ness. In some very profound way, our reality refuses capture by the fixing gaze of empirical science even if this is called phenomenology, as it is by Jaspers.

Towards a hermeneutics of distress

We have seen above that for Jaspers, phenomenology is concerned with the form of psychopathology. The assumption is that this can be separated from

---

announced. The Prince recalls his recollection of the 15 or so minutes between the two sentences as follows:

'He remembered everything with the most extraordinary distinctness, and he used to say that he would never forget anything he had been through during those minutes. Three posts were dug into the ground about twenty paces from the scaffold, which was surrounded by a crowd of people and soldiers, for there were several criminals. The first three were led to the posts and tied to them; the death vestments (long, white smocks) were put on them, and white caps were drawn over their eyes so that they should not see the rifles; next a company of several soldiers was drawn up against each post. My friend was the eighth on the list and his would therefore be the third turn to be marched to the posts. The priest went to each of them with the cross. It seemed to him then that he only had five minutes to live. He told me that those five minutes were like an eter-nity to him, riches beyond the dreams of avarice; he felt that during those five minutes he would live through so many lives that it was quite unnecessary for him to think of the last moments, so that he had plenty of time to make all sorts of arrangements: he calculated the exact time he needed to take leave of his comrades, and decided that he could do that in two minutes, then he would spend another two minutes in thinking of himself for the last time, and, finally, one minute for a last look around...Then after he had bidden farewell to his comrades, came the two minutes he had set aside for think-ing of himself; he knew beforehand what he would think about: he just wanted to imag-ine, as vividly and as quickly as possible, how it could be that now, at this moment, he was there and alive and in three minutes he would merely be *something*—someone or something—but what? And where? All that he thought he would be able to decide in those two minutes!' (Dostoyevsky 1955: 82–83) the content. With this distinction in mind, it becomes possible to think of two different discourses: the one concerned with form, the other with content. This appears to be how Jaspers understood it. For him, phenomenology was an empirical science, concerned with identifying and defining the forms of psychopathology. Interpretation, hermeneutics, was something different, concerned with the content. Thus there was a clear difference between the two. In Heidegger, we find a concern to engage with human reality in a unified way. Nowadays, this would be referred to as a 'holistic' approach.

We believe that Heidegger's critique of the Cartesian tradition holds for Jaspers' phenomenology as well. Heidegger does not have all the answers but his work helps to free us from the idea that knowledge is always about grasping the essential form of something[5]. In particular, he shows that when it comes to understanding human reality, the idea that this can be grasped through an idiom of static, causal elements is fraught with dangers.

The psychiatrist and psychotherapist Medard Boss, who was a friend and associate of Heidegger, attempted to bring the insights of hermeneutic phenomenology to bear on mental health issues some years ago. Like us, Boss argued that the traditional psychiatric approach to understanding psychiatric problems began from the wrong direction. When it comes to the fact of our embodiment, he argues that it is only through an understanding of what having a physical body allows us to do within the context of a meaningful social world that we can begin to appreciate the implications of what a loss of some bodily function or other will mean.

If we were not beings for whom communication is a part of our very make-up, then there would be no human illnesses characterized by a loss, or break-down, of communication[6]. Building up from the material facts of our bodies does not help us understand anything about loss of function. Boss uses the word 'bodyhood' to indicate the fact of our embodiment. He says:

> By positing the human body as some self-contained material thing, natural science disregards everything that is specifically human about human bodyhood. The natural scientific research method treats the body as it might treat works of art. Given a collection of Picasso paintings, for instance, this method would see only material objects whose length and breadth could be measured, whose weight could be determined, and whose substance could be analyzed chemically. All the resulting data lumped together would tell us nothing about what makes these paintings what they are; their character as works of art is not even touched by this approach. (Boss 1979: 100)

---

[5]The philosopher John McCumber argues that at the heart of many problems of Western philosophy and culture is the quest to establish fixed systems of truth. He identifies this with the Greek word *ousia* which refers to something similar to what is meant by the English words 'structure' and 'form'. McCumber finds in Heidegger's philosophy the greatest challenge to this tendency (McCumber 1999).

[6]There are strong resonances between this approach to the notion of illness and that developed (from within a different philosophical tradition) by Fulford in his *Moral Theory and Medical Practice* (1989).

We can only build up a picture of bodily function and impairment from a prior understanding of what meaningful human reality is like. We cannot move in the other direction. Let us think of one of the paintings by Picasso, and imagine that it has been damaged in a move from one gallery to another. Pigment has been scraped from some part of the canvass. The impact of the damage can only be judged by way of reference to the meaning of the painting as a whole. Loss of a certain amount of material from one corner of the painting might not render the painting as damaged as a loss from some other point on the canvas. The damage is *defined* by how the painting works as a meaningful whole.

Boss uses the example of colour blindness. He makes the point that this condition is supposed to be clearly and primarily 'hereditary-organic'. However:

> If we want to understand what it really is, we will have to find out from the afflicted person exactly how his ability to relate himself through perception to what reveals itself to him in his world has been impaired. We will discover that he cannot respond to the meanings 'red' and 'green'. Yet the potentiality in understanding 'red' for what it is cannot be understood on the basis of any molecular structure. Like color blindness, all of the other so-called primarily organic-hereditary illnesses are by nature nothing more than deficiencies in the ability to carry out potential ways of being which are usually there for people. (Boss 1979: 201)[7]

This leads to a concern with meaning and significance. We experience our world as, first and foremost, a world involving relationships of significance. We produce a scientific (in terms of physics and chemistry) account of that world only by stripping it of these relationships. The positivist and reductionist approach to the human world tries to move in the reverse direction, claiming along the way that the scientific world-view is actually primary. When it comes to the world of medicine, traditional approaches attempt to explain illness by 'working up' to 'subjective' human reality from the 'objective' descriptions of physics, chemistry, biology and (more recently) computer science. The 'hermeneutic phenomenological' account of illness, developed by Heidegger and Boss, attempts to reverse the direction of understanding, moving from lived human 'bodyhood' and being-in-the-world to an understanding of how certain phenomena limit the potential of this world.

---

[7]The example of colour blindness given by Boss also opens out the issue of values in human life. In societies that have cars and traffic lights, our ability to distinguish between red and green is clearly of great significance. Equally, we can conceive of a society or culture that has no traffic lights or cars, and where such distinctions are unimportant. The fact that traffic lights operate on the distinction between red and green is simply a convention. If our understanding of the significance of traffic lights operated on the basis of some other distinction (say between blue and yellow, which is uncommon), then people with red–green colour blindness would not be placed at a disadvantage. We can apply similar arguments to other types of human difference based on real (or imagined) biological differences, such as epilepsy, or a propensity to hear voices.

Conclusion

A hermeneutic phenomenology involves an understanding of knowledge as something that is not centrally concerned with the identification of forms. It is an approach to knowledge that is tentative and based on negotiation. In our opinion, it is potentially more democratic. In this conclusion, we summarize our approach to knowledge. These ideas are not put forward as some sort of hard and fast rules. At this stage, we are simply seeking directions, not destinations.

(1) A postpsychiatry perspective sees context first. From this comes the understanding of an individual reality. This is to reverse the Jasperian approach and the approach adopted by mainstream psychiatry. These seek to identify symptoms first and then to explain or understand them later. A postpsychiatry point of view sees an understanding of the context: social, cultural, temporal and bodily as the first step. From this emerges a sense of what the problems are. Understanding starts from a different point on the hermeneutic circle[8].

(2) While postpsychiatry does not rule out causal explanations of what is happening for the individual patient, it argues that a hermeneutic exploration of (i) meaning; (ii) significance; and (iii) value should always precede the move to causal explanation. More so than any other branch of medicine, psychiatry is *primarily* concerned with the meaningful reality of the patient's distress. We propose that an attempt to grapple with the meaning of an episode of low mood should precede attempts to dissect out any biological causes. These may well be present (infectious or endocrine illness for example), and with them the need for the causal logic of pathophysiology will come into operation. But we believe that it is a mistake to start with an assumption that the biology of the patient's condition is always primary or central.

(3) In the postpsychiatry approach, diagnosis becomes something other that the doctor defining the patient's world from the point of view of a detached expertise that arrives with its definitions and demarcations already in place. Instead, diagnosis becomes a process of exploration pursued by professional and patient together. It becomes an attempt to develop a framework of understanding and explanation that calls on different sorts of knowledge. A doctor may well bring a knowledge of genetics, medicine and pharmacology to bear on this process, but in a

---

[8]The phrase 'hermeneutic circle' refers to the circle of interpretation necessarily involved when understanding a work of art, literature or a social or psychological phenomenon. It is not possible to really understand any one part of a work/phenomenon until you understand the whole, but it also is not possible to understand the whole without also understanding all of the parts. One gains in understanding as one moves through the circle.

postpsychiatry approach this type of knowledge is not privileged over others. The patient's own understanding of his/her world moves centre-stage. While sometimes this will be challenged, the aim is not to silence this understanding but to attempt an opening up to other perspectives. Knowledge from other sources such as spiritual and religious may also be important.

(4) We have touched on the issue of temporality above. We believe that Jaspers' notion of a 'static phenomenology' is deeply flawed. In our experience, the psychological worlds of suffering patients are most often deeply structured through past experiences and future possibilities. They are rarely 'static' in any sense of the word. Attempting a framing of the person's experiences that is fixed in some way is often to do the shifting reality of the patient an injustice. A postpsychiatry understanding comes with the notion of temporality and change 'built-in'. Using Heidegger's notion of 'being-in-the-world' as a starting point means an approach that engages with psychology as something always bound up in temporal as well as social and bodily contexts.

(5) What is at stake here is an attempt at rethinking the role of science and expertise in the area of mental health. We seek an understanding of science as something that emerges from human concerns and interests. It is not a detached 'view from nowhere'. It cannot claim any authority other than that which it establishes for itself in regard to any particular problem. For example, simply because someone is a scientist does not give that person an automatic authority to make judgements as to whether experimentation with gentically modified foods should be supported or not. Such decisions have to be made democratically (see, for example, Chapters 9 and 10). The development of mental health services has to do with how we, as a society, wish to care for one another in times of distress. Our argument is that this is primarily a question of values and priorities and cannot be answered simply by a turn to 'evidenced-based' medicine. Postpsychiatry looks forward to a time when we become more comfortable with dealing honestly with different viewpoints and different ways of framing our problems, more comfortable with ambivalence. We will have moved beyond the idea that science has answers to our problems or even has the right questions. A more mature science will start with debate about meanings and values and then move to research and analysis. In Chapter 9, we will describe how community development and participatory action research can be used to address these issues with Black and minority ethnic communities. This is one emerging approach to investigating user and community needs that takes these issues seriously. It is time, we believe, that approaches like this will become the mainstream.

Losing Peter

You stormed out into the blizzard on your way to work. The door slammed in the gale, gagging me, unstuttered words stilled in my mouth. You died. I would never be able to say.

That night it began. Lying still and alone in the dark for the first time, I ached for you. I wanted you to hold and touch me. I mouthed those lost words to your dead ears. In the dark stillness I could not yet face your absence. You made me alive. Your fingers brought my body to life. I had never missed you or wanted you as much, and the more I missed you the more I hated you for not being there. And as I hated you I cried, and felt your closeness, not just felt it. I knew you were there. But I was alone. Your absence meant nothing to me until I wanted you to hold me and to love me. Solitariness. Your footsteps were still perceptible in the snow on the path outside. Do you know that piece by Debussy, Des Pas Sur La Neige? *My ponderous footsteps trudging through the white landscape of our past, wearily going over and over the same ground. What might have been said, what could have been said, what should have been said. In that frozen menacing waste I was lost.*

Do you remember the night on Cader Iris? We were mad, they said. You said the next morning we would wake up madmen or poets. After you fell asleep, I got up. Anything was possible at that moment. In the blink of an eye I counted every single star in the deep sky, before it fell upon me, and took me, made me forget everything. It sucked me into its great dark maw and I wondered and was lost. In that nothingness, I was alone, as alone as I am now, until you called me. You said you were cold. Hey! Come back here! It's freezing. I'm freezing without you. You ordered me. Hearing your voice brought me back. When we awoke, the madman was dead; the poet limped home. You were the voice I would be the ear. Forever.

Did you ever, when you were a child, play with a tooth that was loose, a small white dolorous peg wobbling from side to side? A presentiment of its own emptiness, imagining the chasm that would open up on its fall. But I never could, I could never bring myself to face what it would be like not to have the tooth there. I would try to guess what that new space in my body would feel like. I would run my tongue around the imagined negative image of its presence. But when it fell it finally relinquished its struggle to be a part of me; it freed up that space in me that was no longer part of me. How strange that feeling was! That a part of me is no longer there. Exploring the blank socket with my tongue I discovered that new emptiness with horror and curiosity. It made me think for the first time, what is it like to die? I remember thinking at the time, I could only have been 6, that at some point in the future I will no longer be, my body like my tooth, will no longer occupy this space that I am now in. But I knew without knowing that I could not know my own death. I can only know the death of another. And that is you. Now!

Gradually, I stopped crying. My chest heaved paroxysmally, sporadically; deep involuntary retches of raw feeling, dying away in the dark. At last I became still. In the dark, I tried to picture your face, but its familiarity was so great that you would materialize for one moment, only instantly to dissolve and morph into someone else, someone strange and different, but vaguely familiar. I kept still; stiller! To my right, the gaping void where once you lay. I turned to where you would have been, staring into the dark where your form had lain in rest next to me for 24 years. You were really there, weren't you? You were just lying still, not breathing, pretending to be dead like you did after the first time we made love. I tried to hit you and tickle you, pinch you and make you alive to respond to me. I tried to hold you and to have you hold me. There was nothing. First my fist hit the cold flat sheets. Then my hand clawed the cold air where you were. But as I turned away from you, and the sheets rustled over me, I heard you sigh. In that long blank night I froze, all my senses alert; I stopped breathing to listen more acutely. Outside the wind stirred the trees; the branches' dry crackle mocked my senses. My breath gasped out; I drew another and clung on to it with greater desperation. Again, your sigh! And this time more, for in the stillness there were waves breaking lazily on a shingle shore, the gentle rise and fall of your breast, your gentle, soothing breathing. I startled up, confused and mad with fear, snatching at the light switch to see the smooth untroubled counterpane flat and empty. You were not there.

That night I slept fitfully, with troubled dreams unremembered in the morning. I needed comfort. I wandered about aimlessly, went to the hairdressers; had a massage; I spoke to the undertaker. I needed desperately to talk with you about how Billy and Juliette were struggling. I fell asleep that night only to be woken by the soft snow lashing the windows. Barely perceptible above the muted storm I heard you breathe and sensed the rise and fall of the bedclothes, and now felt your warmth as I turned to where you once lay. And as I turned towards you, I found myself falling towards you, falling into your arms, rolling down the shallow depression in the mattress to where your body lay. I opened my arms to embrace you, and felt your warmth, and heard the catch in your breath as you felt mine. Your safe rhythm, falling and rising, marking out the seconds of our life together, calmed me, soothed me. I fell asleep.

It was only later, much later, months later in fact, that you changed. Things were not right when Billy saw the psychiatrist. I knew he wouldn't take the medication. He has very strong views about things like that; he always has. I knew he had started to smoke dope again. He'd smoked it on and off at college, but you had always put your foot down; you insisted that he stop it. I tried to turn a blind eye and ignore it, pretend that it wasn't going on, but they told me in the hospital that it would only make things worse. Make things worse? God! What did they think they were doing?

I turned to you again that night for comfort. I felt your warmth, your sweet breath on my face, but then you started. You're being stupid, you said. I froze, as I had done countless times when you were alive. This will not do. It's simply not good enough, you snarled. It's your fault his life's in the mess it is; yes, and you hammered in that fault as a nail into wood. I tried to defend myself. I told you that I was doing my best, that it was bloody difficult trying to be a mother and a father to two young people, especially with one struggling. But you wouldn't have it. Oh no, you wouldn't have it, because you hadn't changed. Besides, your hair's a mess, you said. But I needed to touch you, to feel in turn your touch and warmth, to take comfort from you. Instead you offered me your mark, your own special seal of disapproval. I have always found it so difficult to describe. I cannot mimic it. It has its own rhythm and cadence, uniquely yours. Tut, huh! Your hairs a mess, you said. That's how it goes, Tut, huh!

It was impossible for me to resist. You drew me on, inexorably. My reactions were shaped and honed as perfectly as the imagined negative image of the lost tooth, but created and hewn over 24 years. I'm not stupid. It's just bloody difficult. Stop going on at me like that! What've you done about it? All I wanted was your presence. Give me your presence instead. It was so wonderful when you were close, better even than when you were alive. You were never to know how much comfort I drew from feeling you there next to me. But as soon as you uttered a word, it vanished. Just as it was when you were alive.

You bastard!

In the morning, Juliette asked me what was the matter. I was worried that Billy wouldn't be allowed home for Christmas, I said, but she knew that there was more. She pushed me. I couldn't tell her. It's bad enough having a brother who's mad. God knows what she'd do if she knew that her mum was losing it. She told me that Billy had asked her to get him some dope yesterday when she visited. It helps him cope with the medication they're giving him, she smiled; he's a rebel isn't he? I sighed. He gets awful cramps on the drugs. They're painful. Dope eases it for him. What do you think, Mum? I couldn't reply. All I could hear was your mark. Your Tut, Huh!' Juliette sensed it. Dad wouldn't have been very impressed with this, would he? 'No I'm not', you replied.

I was channel hopping, unable to settle or concentrate that evening. Juliette had a piano lesson. I should have made an effort to put up the Christmas decorations but couldn't be bothered. Or so I thought at first, but then decided it was an act of rebellion. You always insisted on putting them up on the first day of Advent. I couldn't stand a house full of clutter for 5 weeks. This was the first time I could have it my way. You interrupted my reverie in the half light of the dying fire.

I know they do it.

I heard your voice so clearly, with such force and clarity I jerked awake. In the shadows by the window, I sensed your presence. You always stood there looking out into the garden when you pontificated and were laying down the law. Again, I wanted your love and comfort. I wanted you to hold me. Instead

I got your seal of disapproval. I said I know they do it. Can't you leave me alone, Peter? I need to rest; I'm tired. But you would not relent. They never did it when I was alive. It's your fault. The nail penetrated even deeper. I bit my lip. I waited. Tut, huh! Now you were mocking me, making me feel a fool. You have let things slip. You have been too soft on them. Maybe, I edged towards you; in the shadows I sensed you turning, towards me or away from me; I couldn't be sure. Outside the lights of Juliette's bike flickered behind the remains of the hydrangeas. And Billy, have you seen what has become of him? He respected me. I gave him discipline and self-respect, but... He was wary of you, frightened even. Stupid. You! Tut, Huh! His life now is in ruins with your indulgence. I knew this would happen, from the first minute... From the first minute of what, Peter? You shrank away. I heard the key turning in the back door. Your shadow withered. The light went on in the kitchen. Listen to me now you, you... bastard. You know that I'm the mother and the father now. You, you've just fucked off 11 months ago. You're not a part of this family anymore so how dare you criticise me. How dare you say what you said to me. Juliette came in. Are you okay mummy? Outside the wind stirred the hydrangeas. She hugged me. You vanished.

5   Mind, language, and meaning

Introduction

In the last chapter, we examined in detail the different meanings of phenomenology, dealing particularly with the limitations of the type of phenomenology
that has dominated psychiatry. We traced the origins of Jaspersian and
Husserlian phenomenology to the philosophy of Descartes, and drew attention
to the problems that arise from epistemological dualism, the Cartesian separation of the inner world of mind from the outer world. We noted that this is a
key feature of representational theories of mind that attempt to relate (inner)
experience to the outer world. Throughout the 20th century we can see a self-
consciousness and preoccupation with language permeating many areas of
thought, in psychology, philosophy, anthropology and literature. In psychology and philosophy, language came to have a central role in understanding
how it was possible for mental representations of the external world to be built
up, or 'processed', to use the jargon of the time. Some aspects of linguistic
theory became highly influential in shaping how we think about these inner
mental processes, and their breakdown in psychosis. The particular group of
theories we are referring to here may be loosely described as cognitivism. In
clinical terms, cognitivism, in the guise of cognitive therapy, is associated with
the work of Beck, and denotes a particular psychological therapy used
originally in depression, and increasingly in psychosis. In this chapter, we
shall consider the relationship between cognitivism and linguistic theory, or
more specifically psycholinguistic, and how, over the last 20 years or so, this
has influenced theories of schizophrenia[1], and resulted in new psychological
therapies in psychosis.

The problems we raised in Chapter 3 concerning phenomenology apply with
equal force to cognitivism. Indeed, in our view, Jaspersian phenomenology and
cognitivism, through their common heritage in Cartesianism, share a similar
set of assumptions and are closely linked. Language plays an important part in
forging this link. We shall argue that although cognitive theories of psychosis
can generate empirically testable hypotheses, they are in fact extremely

---

[1]Although we use the expression here, this does not mean to say that we accept the concept
uncritically. Here, a critique of the concept of schizophrenia is implicit in what we have to say
about cognitivism.

limited in terms of day-to-day clinical work. Furthermore, they also raise serious ethical questions when in the guise of cognitive therapy. Like phenomenology, cognitivism fails to recognize the extent to which human experience is contextualized and embodied. In this chapter, we shall briefly examine the link between Husserlian phenomenology and language, and then step back to examine the origins of cognitivism and psycholinguistics in the 20th century with reference to the work of Noam Chomsky and George Miller. This then leads us to consider recent cognitive theories of psychosis, particularly those of Chris Frith, Ralph Hoffman, Richard Bentall, and Derek Bolton and Jonathan Hill. To a greater or lesser extent, language lies at the heart of these theories, so we examine the implications of Ludwig Wittgenstein's later philosophy of language for these cognitive models of psychosis. The questions at issue here concern our understanding of mind, the nature of language and what it is possible or not possible to say about our inner mental worlds. Most important of all here is how we understand the relationship between mind and society, or the issue of epistemological dualism. Finally, we consider briefly the therapeutic implications of cognitivism. This is important because it brings us back to the issue of power and ethics.

Phenomenology, Language and Schizophrenia was the title of a symposium held 15 years ago in the psychiatric University Hospital in Heidelberg. The proceedings were published as a book with the same name, edited by Spitzer *et al.* (1992). This is steeped in the Heidelberg tradition, one that encompasses the work of Emil Kraepelin, Karl Jaspers, Kurt Schneider and Wilhelm Mayer-Gross. Two of its editors (Spitzer and Mundt) work in Heidelberg, and the text contains sections on phenomenology, language and cognition, and delusions. In their introduction, Spitzer *et al.* (1992) draw our attention to the inter-relatedness of mind, language and phenomenology, particularly in the study of schizophrenia:

> It must be emphasised at the outset that when we discuss schizophrenia we discuss the mind and its functions, and hence, that we are engaged in a psychological and also a philosophical enterprise. For the philosopher, phenomenology becomes important when we want to study these mental functions and their disturbances in detail. The psychologist will add that most of the thought processes mentioned are mediated (to say the least) by language, and therefore, that it is necessary to study language and its disorders in schizophrenia. (Spitzer *et al.* 1992: 4)

The authors point out that cognitive science has had an immense influence on our understanding of 'normal language processes', and that consequently most of the chapters on language and psychosis in the book are influenced by cognitivism. Our view is that the situation is more complex; cognitive theory and linguistic theory share a common heritage, a common set of influences and assumptions. As far as phenomenology is concerned, the authors firmly locate themselves in the Jaspersian and Husserlian traditions we considered in Chapter 3. For psychiatrists, phenomenology means '...*psychopathology in the Jaspersian tradition*', whereas for philosophers it means '...*philosophy in the Husserlian tradition.*' (Spitzer *et al.* 1992: 6). From a philosophical point of view, they point out that phenomenology is concerned with the specific problem of how it is possible to describe mental life, and it is here that we can see the importance of language beginning to emerge. In their view, language processes exist on interactional and social levels involving 'complex meaning structures' (stories), the sentence level (simple meaning structures) and at the phrase, word and sound levels. In other words, their view of the linguistic world is a broadly conventional one that sees language as an individual phenomenon, shorn of its communicative (social, historical and cultural) contexts. Such a view disregards the way in which an appreciation of contexts can render utterance meaningful. In order to understand more clearly the implications of this view of language and mind, we must explore the shared origins of cognitivism and psycholinguistics.

Language, philosophy and mind: the origins of cognitivism

Throughout the 20th century, linguistic science was divided as to whether we should account for language primarily in terms of its underlying biological substrate, or as a social phenomenon, a feature of the shared group functions of human life. There are good reasons to formulate questions about language in this way, in part because they also reflect a major preoccupation of 20th century philosophy. There have been three main lines of investigation in the relationship between philosophy and language. The first, exemplified by the work of the logical positivists including Wittgenstein's early work, deals primarily with the relationship between meaning and truth. The second, dominated by the ideas of Chomsky, concerns the relationship between mind and language. The third, identified with the work of Austin, Grice and Wittgenstein's later work, is primarily concerned with the relationship between language and meaning. Here, we shall explore in some detail the latter two approaches. Chomsky's work draws together linguistics, cognitivism and biology. We shall consider how language, through cognitivism, has come to play a central role in theories of psychosis, and seeks to move beyond 'descriptive' phenomenologies, to explanation.

Psycholinguistics and the origins of cognitivism

Chomsky's ideas revolutionized the way we think about language, and placed linguistics firmly in the domain of cognitive science. His idea that syntactic structures map directly onto the mind and brain opened up the field of psycholinguistics. His work begins with his celebrated critique of behaviourist explanations of language. In 1957, B.F. Skinner published *Verbal Behaviour*, in which he proposed a model of language acquisition from within a behavioural, 'learning theory' framework. Chomsky (1959) argued that behaviourism was incapable of accounting for the richly creative and diverse nature of human utterance. Learning theory might successfully explain how networks of associations of words are built up, but it was incapable of explaining the creative use of human language, the fact that from a limited number of words and rules, an infinite diversity of sentences is possible. He also argued that although the terminology of behaviourism sounds precise ('stimulus', 'response', 'reinforcement'), it becomes so vague when applied to language that empirical studies become meaningless. Chomsky's earlier work was influenced by the Bloomfieldian tradition which regarded linguistics as a self-contained, autonomous field. But with the publication of *Aspects of the Theory of Syntax, Cartesian Linguistics*[2] and *Language and Mind*, he opened up the frontier between linguistics and cognitive science, insisting that generative grammar played a central role in understanding the structure and organization of the human mind. In this view, the scientific study of language can make an important contribution to our understanding of cognitive processes.

American linguistics in the early 20th century had been dominated by the work of Leonard Bloomfield, the founder of American structural linguistics. Bloomfield adopted an empirical approach to the study of language and abandoned any interest in theoretical questions. Chomsky challenged this, proposing that the purpose of linguistics was to produce a general theory of human language. He argued that for speakers in all languages to be able to generate an infinite variety of sentences, all languages must share some common underlying principles that govern their structure and organization. He argued that certain features of language were universal, in the sense that they could be identified independently of their occurrence in any particular language, and on the basis of their definition in a general theory. Although languages such as Japanese, Urdu or Welsh may differ in terms of their syntax, lexicons, and so on, these are superficial formal differences. Chomsky argued that beneath these surface differences, all languages shared a common, under-lying deep structure, a universal grammar. This is illustrated in Fig. 5.1.

Universal grammar specifies a set of general rules for all languages that account for the relationship between deep and surface structure. Amongst other things, deep structure accounts for the relationship between active and passive sentences, by specifying a set of operations whereby the surface struc-ture of active and passive sentences can be derived from a common underly-ing deep structure. It is because active and passive versions of the same sentence (for example, John kicked the ball—The ball was kicked by John)

---

[2]Like Husserl, Chomsky paid respect to his Cartesian heritage in the title of one of his seminal works on linguistics.

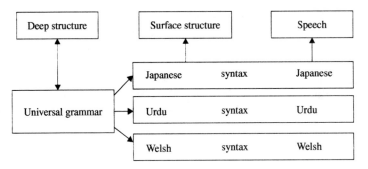

Fig. 5.1 Universal grammar.

share this same deep structure that they convey the same meaning. It should be apparent already that they are concerned with meaning only in the narrowest of senses, insofar as it could be modelled through deep (internal) universal linguistic or psychological processes, and, in this respect, the theory of phrase structure grammar played a critical role in forging the link between language and cognition. Chomsky and Miller were trying to understand the mental processes involved in sentence generation, and how memory capacity, storage and retrieval were related to syntactic structures. They (Chomsky & Miller 1963*a,b*) showed that context-free phrase grammars had similar properties to pushdown storage devices in automata theory. This model of information storage and retrieval, which is also a precursor of the concept of working memory, operates on the basis of 'last in first out'. When applied to model human memory, it accounts for the fact that we find it easiest to recall those items of information that we have stored in memory most recently. The capacity of short-term (or working) memory is limited, to use Miller's famous dictum, to seven plus or minus two items[3], a constraint that has implications for sentence generation, and in particular the structure of complex sentences. Chomsky and Miller used this early version of information processing theory to produce a rule-governed model of sentence generation. It is at this point that Chomsky's model of the formal properties of language becomes inextricably tied to the mental mechanisms that he considered essential for sentence generation. He used transformational grammar to explain the relationship between active and passive sentences, arguing that active sentences are transformationally simpler, because they require fewer rules or formal operations to generate them. By inference, he concluded that such sentences were also simpler in terms of the psychological processing involved, a view supported by empirical studies that showed that active sentences were indeed easier to remember than passives. However, as Lyons (1991) suggests, this could also be explained on the basis that active sentence structures feel more 'natural' than passive

---

[3]Miller argued this was why the optimum number of digits in a phone number was seven.

structures. Here, we would point out that Lyons' use of the word 'natural' refers to what feels right when speakers *use* language in the day-to-day task of communicating with others. In other words, social convention and cultural factors may influence the extent to which native language speakers find a sentence grammatically acceptable.

Cognitivism and psycholinguistics assume that mental processes underlie human intentional behaviour. Early cognitivists such as Miller and Chomsky believed that inner mental states and processes accounted for human thought, language and action. This raises a very real practical difficulty, since unlike phenomena in the physical world such as brain (*res extensa*), inner mental states or mind (*res cogitans*) is unobservable. How can mind be studied experimentally in order to test theory? They overcame this difficulty through positivism[4]. This makes the assumption that the mental processes involved in language must be the same for all humans; in other words, they must be universal. In other words, the differences described by linguists and anthropologists in people from different cultures or historical epochs are of little significance or interest. However, a fundamental problem with positivism remains. Because we cannot observe mental processes directly, we are forced to use metaphor, and invent expressions to conceptualize what might be going on in the mind.

We can see this in the endless use of metaphor to convey our feelings to others—'I was full of happiness' 'I felt empty inside'. We can also see this in the use of expressions such as 'information processing' in our attempts to express what we think is going on in the mind. It is also true of attempts to model the cognitive processes at work in generating sentences with varying levels of clausal complexity[5]. Chomsky would argue that the differences in processing these sentences are universal, common to all languages, because all human minds, irrespective of language and culture, use the same set of general principles to generate grammars to produce such sentences. This in turn opens up the possibility of generating a model of how the mind works, which will account specifically for the difficulties in processing left-branching sentences. This model in turn gives rise to a set of rules, or a set of operations that determine how information is handled in order to generate them. The cognitive metaphors of 'rules' and 'operations' also convey ontological assumptions, the most important of which is the very idea that mental processes can be explained by analogy with rule following. The positivistic underpinnings of cognitivism assume that, like natural systems, mental mechanisms must follow

---

[4]Positivism is associated with the work of the French sociologist Auguste Comte, who in the mid-19th century proposed that human thought evolved through a series of stages, the religious, metaphysical and scientific. Positivism stressed the unity of natural and human sciences, with the implication that human beings are suitable subjects for the formal methods of scientific inquiry.
[5]Chomsky and Miller demonstrated this in sentences with left and right branching clausal structure.

the laws of causality found in the natural sciences. Rules in cognitivism take many forms, and Chomsky's transformational grammar is but one example. We shall return to this point later when we consider the work of Bolton and Hill.

The next stage in the evolution of cognitivism was the computational model, which took the rule-following metaphor a stage further. This likened the brain to a computer (hardware) with cognitive processes as rule-governed software, and out of this came the various artificial intelligence (AI) models of mind. This led to belief in the possibility that all aspects of human behaviour and experience would become comprehensible through hypotheses about information processing mechanisms. Historically, Chomsky's work played a seminal role in the subsequent evolution of cognitive models of mind. Implicit in cognitivism is the idea that mental processes build up inner representations of the world outside. These representations may take a number of forms, such as schemas or maps, but they are built up through processing information governed by complex rules and formulae.

Chomsky's work also has implications for theories of language acquisition. If, as he argued, transformational grammar is a universal, then why should all languages have such similar structures? Empirically there are two explanations for this. First, all languages are used to refer to the properties of objects in the physical world, and these properties remain constant. We all refer to the physical world by describing it, making statements about it, asking questions of it, and so on. We shall see later that Wittgenstein offers some important insights here. Secondly, all languages must share the same structure because all languages are ultimately determined by the physical properties of matter (the biochemical and neurophysiological processes of our brain and speech apparatus). This reductionist view accounts for the innate 'language faculty' possessed by all human beings, and the universal structural features of deep grammar. In this respect, Chomsky may be described as a rationalist. He argued that it was only possible for children rapidly to acquire the highly restrictive principles of universal grammar if they were born with knowledge of these rules. In other words, language must be innate and dependent on mental structures. This is why we are able to acquire the rules of language. By implication, then, our enmeshment in the social and cultural world of language plays little or no part in language acquisition. Human relationships and nurturing, the social processes and interactions between children and parents, children and teachers, or children and peers, all the appurtenances of culture that frame our lives, are, in this nascent cognitivism, unimportant in language acquisition. Language 'grows' in the mind like a seed in a plant pot. In an interview with Brian Magee, Chomsky expresses it thus:

> We begin our interchange with the world with our minds in a certain genetically determined state, and through interaction with an environment, with experience, this state changes until it reaches a fairly steady mature state, in which we possess what we call knowledge. The structure of the mind, in this mature state (and indeed in intermediate states as well), incorporates a complex

> system of mental representations and principles of computation on these mental representations. This sequence of changes from the genetically determined initial state to the final steady state seems to me in many respects analogous to the growth of our organs. (Chomsky, in Magee 1978: 176)

In other words, our biological endowment is such that we are programmed to develop language. Language is innate, a biological system to be studied and understood in the same way that we might investigate the physical properties of any aspect of bodily function. This is not to say that environmental factors play no part in language development. Chomsky held that interaction with the environment is important at certain key periods, but language grows within the individual organism:

> ...it seems to me not only wrong to think of language being taught, but also, at the very least, misleading to think of it as being learned, at least if 'learning' is understood in any conventional manner. (Chomsky, in Magee 1978: 176)

Language, cognitivism, and schizophrenia

Examining the relationship between psycholinguistics and cognitivism is important for our purposes because the two have become influential in attempts to explain psychosis, most notably schizophrenia. Clinicians have long been intrigued by the utterance of people diagnosed as suffering from schizophrenia. For many years, the idea that there was a specific disturbance in thinking processes, so-called thought disorder, was immensely influential. Loosening of association, for example, was one of Bleuler's primary symptoms of schizophrenia. But, of late, 'thought disorder' has figured less prominently in research into psychosis, partly because it is notoriously unreliable and difficult to measure (Thomas 1995), and the fact that it is seen in 'normal' subjects (Chaika 1974). Instead, researchers have turned to linguistics and cognitive science in the hope that this is less subjective. This fruitful area has yielded many testable theories about the nature of schizophrenia. An excellent example of this is the work of Chris Frith, whose book, *The Cognitive Neuropsychology of Schizophrenia* (Frith 1992) is an ambitious project that sets out a cognitive model for the (descriptive) phenomenology of schizophrenia, and relates this to what is known about the neuropsychology of the condition. The role and structure of language is at the centre of his ideas.

Frith's theory tries to account for both positive and negative symptoms of schizophrenia. He proposes that we can think of the condition as a disorder of self-awareness, with related problems in the ability to represent other people's intentions and dispositions, or Theory of Mind (ToM). Neurologists have understood the importance of self-awareness for many years. In the 19th century, Helmholtz demonstrated the importance of self-monitoring in the neurophysiology of motor acts and perception. To initiate and complete a simple motor act, we must first form an intention or a plan of action (e.g. to pick up a cup) and then monitor what is going on accurately to coordinate the activity of many muscle groups. This occurs automatically and unconsciously in the cerebellum by internal proprioception from stretch receptors in muscles and tendons, which inform the brain of the exact position of the arm in relation to the plan of action. Frith argues that it is parsimonious to suppose that the brain developed such mechanisms solely for the control of motor activity. Take, for example, human action. There are two ways in which we may act in the environment, stimulus driven and intentional. In the first, action occurs in response to environmental stimuli. For example, I drive my car to work thinking about the problems that will face me when I get to my office. When I arrive, I may have little recall of the journey. My behaviour was determined largely by my responses to environmental stimuli and cues. I stop when the traffic lights turn to red, start again when they are on green, go straight ahead when I reach the New Beehive Pub, and so on. My familiarity with the route means that it is not necessary for me to make conscious decisions about my actions. I only have to respond to particular environmental events or cues. This is stimulus-driven behaviour. Now contrast this with my actions if I have to drive to a strange town. I have already obtained a map before hand, showing exactly where it is that I am supposed to be going. The map indicates my starting and ending points. As I drive, I carefully follow the road ahead looking for the junctions and road signs indicated by the map. My actions are carefully planned, and I make conscious decisions with the intention of ensuring that I follow the route on the map. I constantly monitor where I am on the road in relation to the plan represented by the map. This is intentional behaviour. Frith argues that it is the existence of the monitoring system which distinguishes between these two types of behaviour (stimulus driven and intentional), and the intact functioning of this system enables me to know that my actions are self-initiated and thus intentional. He proposes that such mechanisms must also exist for cognitive faculties such as thought, and that a break down in these mechanisms may explain how positive and negative symptoms arise. The first stage in this involves the formation of an intention to act, for example to communicate with someone. If this fails to happen, then I do not communicate, and I show evidence of the negative symptom poverty of speech. If I am responding to an environmental event, such as a request to pass someone a pen, my actions can be seen in response to an environmental stimulus. If my ability to monitor whether my behaviour occurs in response to environmental stimuli or whether it is self-initiated, breaks down then, according to Frith, my sense of intentionality is lost. Under these circumstances, I may incorrectly attribute my actions to external events, in other words, I have passivity experiences and believe my actions are being controlled by someone or something else.

Self-monitoring our intentions to act is a prerequisite for ToM, our ability to understand the intention, dispositions and actions of others. Frith proposes that we may understand positive symptoms such as verbal auditory hallucinations and delusions as a failure of ToM and self-monitoring. For example, let us assume that James is worried because he thinks his friend John believes that he is gay. Such a state of affairs may be represented in James' mind by the following statement:

5.1 (John thinks that [James is gay])

This sentence consists of two parts, a statement (*James is gay*) and a prefix (*John thinks that*), which indicates that the statement is an attribution made by James to another person. This sentence indicates that James is operating a ToM. The point here is that the sentence in parentheses is represented in James' mind, as part of his intention to talk with John. Now let us assume that there exists a cognitive mechanism that monitors our thinking processes. A failure of this could result in the first part of the sentence (*John thinks that*) becoming detached from the second (*James is gay*), in which case one of two things may occur. James might experience the second part of the sentence as a thought inserted into his head by John. Alternatively, he may hear a voice speaking out the words 'James is gay', possibly attributed by him to John. Either way the failure of a monitoring system means that a part of my conscious experience becomes detached from his sense of intentionality. This results in it being experienced as alien and not belonging to him.

Ralph Hoffman (1986) has proposed a similar model to account for verbal hallucinations. To communicate effectively, we must have a clear plan of what we intend to say, and we must monitor this plan to ensure that we are keeping to it. There are many ways of saying the same thing, and thus many plans that could be followed to achieve the same communicative goal. Planning and monitoring involve the selection of the optimal route, and rejection of less appropriate ways of saying something. If we fail to monitor our discourse plan, we may flit from unrelated topic to unrelated topic, leaving our conversational partner confused. Communication disorder arises as a result of a failure in planning and monitoring discourse. The rejected plans are normally discarded, but, in Hoffman's model, these discarded fragments of discourse are not inhibited, and are thus experienced as voices. These fragments of discarded discourse are then experienced as non-intended and therefore 'alien'. The 'parasitic' fragments are experienced as verbal hallucinations.

Cognitive theories of schizophrenia are becoming ever more sophisticated, with attempts to integrate cognitive theories and biochemical ones. For example, Cohen and Servan-Schreiber (1993) have adapted the concept of parallel distributed processing (PDP) systems from AI theory to develop a model of information processing, in terms of dopaminergic systems. Later, we shall return to the models developed by Bolton and Hill, and Bentall, but there are questions of a philosophical nature that are outstanding from our examination of cognitivism. This concerns the influence of Descartes, and again, as in Chapter 3, the main aspect of his philosophy that we are interested in here is epistemological dualism. True to the tradition of Descartes, cognitivism maintains that we make sense of the external world through internal *representations* of the world outside. It is this aspect of cognitivism that gives rise to what we refer to as the 'interiorized' view of language and the mind, and which we shall now examine critically.

Philosophical critique: Wittgenstein and the question of mind

In his early work, *Tractatus Logico-Philosophicus* (Wittgenstein 1961), written after he studied logic with Russell in Cambridge, Wittgenstein explored the relationship between language, the world and thought. In the *Tractatus*, he proposed that language represents the world by depicting it in much the same way that a picture may depict a real life scene. Thought is expressed through propositions. He argued from first principles that any utterance about the world could be reduced to names of objects in the world, with the propositional or structural relationship between the words in the sentence corresponding directly to the physical relationship between the objects that the words represented in the world. In other words, Wittgenstein proposed that there is a one to one relationship between the propositional structure of sentences that we use to describe the world, and the aspect of the world that is being described. Thus the propositional structure of thought mirrors the state of affairs in the outside world. For this reason, his earlier theory of language is sometimes referred to as the 'picture' theory of meaning. It is clear, though, that this view imposes restrictions on what we consider language to be, the implication being that language can only be meaningful if it relates to factual states of affairs in the world. This means that a great deal of human communication, such as the use of language to convey emotional states, or to talk about ethics and values, is impossible to fit into this view of language.

His later theory, although very different, and although it reaches a completely different set of conclusions about the nature of language and its place in our lives, nevertheless follows on from the *Tractatus*[6]. (Perhaps it is this that makes Wittgenstein such a deeply fascinating philosopher.) Instead of describing a set of abstract principles that specify the relationship between language, world and mind, he comes to regard language as a human and social phenomenon. If the metaphor of language developed in the *Tractatus* is that of a picture, then that developed in *Philosophical Investigations* (Wittgenstein 1967) is of language as a tool, in which the meaning of an utterance is to be found in the great variety of uses to which it may be put. This is a fundamentally different view of language. The *Tractatus* specifies a representational model of

---

[6]The seventh and final section of the *Tractatus* consists of the famous aphorism 'Whereof we cannot speak, thereof we must be silent'. In a sense, this opens the way for *Philosophical Investigations*, which deals with those things that the language he describes in *Tractatus* finds it impossible to speak of—values, feelings, belief, ethics, and so on.

language that sits comfortably alongside cognitive models of mind. *Philosophical Investigations*, on the other hand, opens up a view of language in which its social use is seen to be of paramount importance. He arrives at this position in the following way. First, language is only possible if we accept that speakers share sets of rules[7] that govern the *use* of language. But here, Wittgenstein is not so much interested in rules in terms of their formal or structural properties, but their place in human life and activity. In this sense, he argues that we may think of language 'rules' in terms of games, and he introduces the expression language games to account for the great many uses to which the tool of language may be put.

> But how many kinds of sentence are there? Say assertion, question and command?—There are *countless* kinds: countless different kinds of use of what we call 'symbols', 'words', 'sentences'. And this multiplicity is not something fixed, given once and for all; but new types of language, new language-games, as we may say, come into existence, and others become obsolete and get forgotten . . .

> Here the term 'language-game' is meant to bring into prominence the fact that the *speaking* of language is part of an activity, or a form of life . . . It is interesting to compare the multiplicity of the tools in language and of the ways they are used, the multiplicity of kinds of word and sentence, with what logicians have said about the structure of language. (Including the author of the *Tractatus Logico-Philosophicus*.) (Wittgenstein 1967: para. 23; emphasis in the original)

Games are rule governed, but rules are flexible. They are not universally fixed for all time. They may change with time, and in different places in the world and, although some games may resemble each other, there is no common characteristic to all games other than a general family resemblance.

Here, Wittgenstein is moving us away from the idea of psychological universalism and the representational view of language. Next, he deals with the problems of interiority, Descartes' epistemological dualism. In *Philosophical Investigations*, Wittgenstein went to considerable lengths to move away from the idea that the primary function of language is to enable us to talk about our

---

[7]Of course, we saw earlier that rules played an important part in Chomsky's theories. For Chomsky, rules in language were prescriptive. Their purpose was to specify the syntactic (structural) transformations necessary to relate deep and surface grammar. In Wittgenstein's philosophy, rules do not prescribe. They are there for guidance. If language is a human activity, then rules must be flexible; in language games, they may even be made up as we go along:

> 'Doesn't the analogy between language and games throw light here? We can easily imagine people amusing themselves in a field by playing with a ball so as to start various existing games, but playing many without finishing them and in between throwing the ball aimlessly into the air, chasing one another with the ball and bombarding one another for a joke and so on. And now someone says: the whole time they are playing a ball-game and following definite rules at every throw.

And is there not also the case where we play and—make up the rules as we go along? And there is even one where we alter them—as we go along'. (Wittgenstein 1967: para. 83)

inner mental lives. His argument here concerns the difficulties that arise if we assume that we can use language to talk about our inner worlds *in the same way that we use it to talk about the external world*. By pointing this out, he lays open the assumptions that lie beneath the interiorized view of human experience. Let us take sadness. In Western cultures, we accept as 'given' the existence of internal states such as sadness, but there is a serious difficulty with this. How am I to know, or for that matter infer, that others have the same experience that I have when I am sad? And if I am able to know, or infer, that others are sad, how am I to know that it is exactly the same experience as mine? We assume that our private, inner worlds are much better known than the public, the mental better than the physical. Wittgenstein says that there can be no such thing as inner knowledge. He points out that since Descartes, this inner knowledge has been privileged, not only as the basis of empirical knowledge about the world, but also as the foundation for our understanding of language. We assume, for example, that word meanings must stand in a fixed relationship to inner experience, such as sadness, but there is absolutely no way that we can be certain that this is the case[8]. He describes the problematic nature of this assumption in the following way, using pain as an example:

> If I say of myself that it is only from my own case that I know what the word 'pain' means—must I not say the same of other people too? And how can I generalise the *one* case so irresponsibly?

> Now someone tells me that *he* knows what pain is only from his own case!— Suppose everyone had a box with something in it: we call it a 'beetle'. No one can look into anyone else's box, and everyone says he knows what a beetle is only by looking at *his* beetle. —Here it would be quite possible for everyone to have something different in his box. One might even imagine such a thing constantly changing. —But suppose the word 'beetle' had a use in these people's language? —If so it would not be used as the name of a thing. The thing in the box has no place in the language game at all; not even as a *something*: for the box might even be empty. —No, one can 'divide through' by the thing in the box; it cancels out, whatever it is.

> That is to say: if we construe the grammar of the expression of sensation on the model of 'object and designation' the object drops out of consideration as irrelevant. (Wittgenstein 1967: para. 293)

Thus the representational model of language breaks down when it comes to attempts to convey anything about our inner worlds. The importance we attach to our inner experience is problematic, because to declare that we are sad does not depend on verifiable factual evidence. This places my own knowledge of my own sadness in an epistemologically privileged position. Yet, on the the other

---

[8]It is worth recalling here from Chapter 3 that it this is the same certainty that so concerned Descartes.

hand, denying that I am sad makes no sense, as does denying that anyone else can experience sadness. Wittgenstein argues that the problem arises through the inappropriate use of language games that are applied to the reporting of inner states, as though they were the same as states of affairs in the external world. Because I can examine the external world, and name the objects on my desk to another person—'That is a pen', 'That is a book', 'That is a computer'—I assume that I can participate in the same language game to report my inner state to another person—'That is sadness'. Wittgenstein points out that this is a profound error, because the two are very different types of operations, or language games. If we self-report inner states, we are not simply engaging in the language game of listing the things and experiences we find within ourselves, as I would if I were to describe to you what I see on my desk before me. If we are to avoid making serious errors in the way in which we use and participate in language games, we must have a sense of the appropriateness of an utterance within a particular context. This means that the social contexts in which people say things, as well as the actions that typically accompany a particular utterance, are important in understanding an utterance. For this reason, uncoupling language and speech from the social contexts in which it takes place can be seriously misleading.

Wittgenstein's brilliant insight about what we might reasonably expect from language in talking about our experiences is of immense importance in psychiatry. When we come to apply positivism to human subjects, tragic human stories, experiences and emotions, we are immediately confronted with this dilemma. Take, for example, the use of rating scales to measure mood. A great deal of work has been devoted to the construction of scales such as the Hamilton scale, the Beck Depression Inventory or the Montgomery–Åsberg scale, all of which attempt to quantify feelings of sadness. Although much of this work was undertaken for research purposes, it has also influenced our daily clinical practice. Most of us at some time have asked our patients to say how low or high they feel on a scale from +10 to +10. Wittgenstein's point about the use of language in this context is that psychological or social facts are not 'things' that can be talked about in the same way as facts in the physical world. Consider the two sentences:

5.2 Water is in the jug.

5.3 Sadness is in my heart.

These sentences are very similar. They are both declarative. Their syntactic structure is identical. But there is a profound difference between them. We can see the jug and the water it contains. We can describe the water, whether it is clear or dirty. We can measure its volume, and analyse precisely its chemical constitution. We simply *cannot* do the same with sadness. To describe sadness, we must rely on metaphor and pretend that our hearts are vessels like jugs that can contain sadness. Nobody really believes that sadness is a physical thing contained within our hearts, so it is not possible to measure sadness in the same way we can measure water in a jug. The problem arises because we assume that because it is possible for us to talk about our emotional worlds, our beliefs, values and experiences as if they were physical entities, this means that they must indeed be physical entities.

There is another vital consequence of Wittgenstein's insight. It means that it is not possible for us to talk about our knowledge of the mind in the traditional Cartesian way, with the assumption that the world consists of two very different phenomena—the external world of matter in space and time, of the natural world, of mountains, oceans, animals and forests, of other human beings and the inner worlds of thoughts and feelings. Wittgenstein's work implies that these two worlds, rent asunder since the Enlightenment, are intimately bound together, and that there can be no consideration of what we have to say about our inner, mental lives, *without* considering the outside world, especially the social, historical and cultural contexts, to which the thoughts, percepts and feelings which constitute our inner lives are indissolubly tied. A direct consequence of this insight is that we are above all else embodied social and cultural beings, each of us with a unique history and story to speak of through language. Consider this with reference to our earlier sentence 'John thinks that James is gay', which we used to demonstrate how a failure in monitoring could result in the emergence of either a delusional belief or a verbal auditory hallucination. Cognitive theory says nothing of why James might be concerned that John believes he is gay in the first place. To understand this, we need a shift from the epistemological (knowledge of the world) framework of cognitivism to an ontological (understanding our existence in the world) framework. And to achieve this, we need an approach that considers the nature of James' relationship with John, its development, their respective life histories and life circumstances. This is exactly why, in our view, the Cartesian framework that has been so influential in Western thought, particularly in phenomenology and cognitivism, is so restricted.

Button and colleagues (1995) have developed Wittgenstein's later philosophy of language into a powerful critique of cognitivism and Chomskyan linguistics. They point out that although language occupies an important position in the debate about the relationship between brain and mind, they raise the important role of language in meaning. They counter Chomsky's view of language as a mental operation by reformulating the question of meaning in the following way; is the meaning of a language-user's utterance located inside the head of the speaker, or in the speaker's social environment? They argue that most philosophical and empirical investigations disregard the fact that language is a social institution. As we have seen, cognitivism assumes that the understanding of language between humans is dependent on internal psychological processes and inner representations of social reality. Ultimately the implication here is that language is determined physically by the laws of nature. It also implies that the human capacity for language is innate, and hard-wired into the central nervous system. The problem here lies with the Chomskyan (and cognitivist) claim that the existence of neuropsychological structures instantiate a knowledge of language, and the related assumption that language acquisition is dependent on the possession of an innate set of rules. Button *et al.* contest this, arguing that whilst it is undeniable that language has a biological basis, the language we actually speak is not innate, neither is it something that has developed out of an individual psychology:

> It is *within the collective lives* of human beings that language has been developed, and it is as a phenomenon *of life and activity rather than that of neurophysiology* that Wittgenstein and Ryle invite us consider language. (Button *et al.* 1995: 6; emphasis in the original)

The implication here is that language cannot be regarded simply as a property of an isolated human mind, cut off and isolated from human activity. Because Chomsky argued strongly that language cannot be 'learnt' in the behaviourist sense, he ruled out the possibility that we might ask questions about the importance of social processes in language acquisition. This is the fundamental difference between Chomsky's view, and that of the 'discursive psychologies'[9].

It is important to bear in mind that we are contrasting two very different views of language here: whether we consider language to be little more than a vehicle for internal thought—the 'software' or programs which run on the hardware of the brain, or whether we regard language as being to do with our participation in the social world:

> Those of more or less mentalistic persuasion will perhaps admit that language is a social matter, but such acknowledgement will be at best perfunctory, and the role of language as a part of social life will be treated as a secondary, derivative feature which can be treated as incidental to the understanding of language. (Button *et al.* 1995: 220)

Button *et al.* argue that cognitivism relegates the role of language to that of providing a commentary upon intentionality and human action, with the implication that the external world would somehow carry on even if there were no such thing as language. This we have seen in the monitoring function ascribed to language by Frith, which sees language as nothing more than an expediency for monitoring or predicting human behaviour. Button *et al.* draw an analogy with a game such as tennis. It is impossible to disengage the history and development of the game, including the human actions out of which it developed, from the specialist words and expressions that are used in association with it. We did not invent the game of tennis, and at the same time fabricate a new vocabulary, which conjured the words 'deuce' 'love' and 'set' out of thin air to describe the rules of the game. The game, its rules, the human activity of

---

[9]In addition to Wittgenstein, the ideas of the Russian Marxist psychologist Lev Vygotsky (1978) have influenced discursive psychology. Vygotsky's studies of the acquisition of language in children provide empirical support for the Wittgensteinian view of language as a social tool, and run counter to the Chomskyan view that language is innate.

playing tennis, the historical and cultural contexts in which all this took place shaped the vocabulary associated with the game. In the same way, human language is intertwined with and inseparable from culture, human action and history. Chomsky transformed language into psychology, with the result that the study of language structure became the study of mental phenomena, but as Button *et al.* point out:

> The effect of this position is, however, the *dissociation* of speaking a language from the *other* activities in which people engage, as if the *system* of language could be described and understood in complete abstraction from the patterns of life in which the speakers of the language otherwise engage. (Button *et al.* 1995: 217; emphasis in the original)

The implication of Wittgenstein's later philosophy view is that we cannot think of language simply in terms of a set of rules, or mental operations, locked away inside the head of a speaker. Language is primarily a tool in our social and cultural processes, and as such it is indissolubly tied to meaning in human life.

Meaning and the limits of cognitivism

Recent developments in philosophy and cognitive science have attempted to find ways around the limitations of representational models of mind, and their failure to grasp the importance of meaning and contexts in understanding human life. In their book, *Mind, Meaning and Mental Disorder*, Derek Bolton and Jonathan Hill (1996) argue that meaning *can* be encompassed by a modified cognitive framework. They acknowledge the importance of Cartesianism in cognitive science and, like us, they are dissatisfied with the way that Cartesianism privileges mental states as private. They claim, however, that cognitivism can overcome this by subjecting mental states to scientific enquiry, something that becomes possible if we blur the Cartesian distinction between *res extensa* and *res cogitans* and regard thought and matter as one and the same thing:

> ... a defining attribute of the Cartesian mind was *thinking*, which is closely linked to representation, meaning, and intentionality, and these are none other than the characteristics of mental states which are essential for the purposes of cognitive explanations of behaviour... what was essential to the Cartesian mind is essential also to mind as posited by cognitive-behavioural explanations. This means that the latter will not be satisfied with any definition of mental states that makes them 'material' *as opposed to* 'thoughtful' ... if mind is going to be identified with the material brain, then the material brain will have to be—like Cartesian mind—a 'thinking substance'. (Bolton & Hill 1996: 74–75)

In other words, meaning is encoded in the brain. This implies that brain activity cannot simply be grasped in terms of conventional causality, and for this reason they propose the existence of intentional causality, a property of physical systems including organic molecules such as DNA and haemoglobin, as well as human thought and reason. The transitions between the physical and the realm of thought are said to be 'seamless' (Bolton & Hill 1996: 260). This makes it possible to talk in terms of a 'predictive' science of psychology, albeit one which pays attention to human meanings. While they reject the idea that human reality can be explained by reference to 'physical laws', they nevertheless assert that cognitive psychology establishes 'natural laws' and 'norms of function' in the mind. They write, unproblematically, about people who develop psychotic episodes as possibly exhibiting a 'design fault' (Bolton & Hill 1996: 284). If psychology can describe what the 'normal design' of a human being actually consists of, and can describe 'norms of function', then it can predict what will happen under particular conditions, given that the system is functioning 'normally'. They are quite clear that once such norms are established, psychology becomes a true causal science. They maintain:

> ...the idea that the causal status of cognitive explanations derives from their place within a well-entrenched systematic empirical theory about relations between stimuli, cognitive states, and behaviour. There is something correct about this suggestion, but it is not yet complete. It omits special features of descriptions of functional systems, namely, that they essentially invoke *norms* of function, and that this accounts for their necessity. (Bolton & Hill 1996: 200).

Asserting that there are 'norms of function', which can be established, leads Bolton and Hill to elaborate an account of human beings as 'rational agents'. Unless human beings act in a rational and consistent way, the predictive power of psychology starts to evaporate. Because of this, they propose that there are 'laws of reason', according to which particular behaviours can be judged to be rational or otherwise. In doing so, they take us back to the problem of universalism that we encountered in relation to Chomsky. Thus:

> If a person believes such-and-such, then she *must*, in appropriate circumstances, act in a way that accords with that belief. This 'must', however, has nothing to do with scientific theory or natural law. If the consequent of the hypothetical fails, no scientific theory has been refuted, still less has there been a miracle! Rather, the inference would be that, for one reason or another, the person has apparently acted irrationally. The nomological character of the prediction pertains to the 'laws' of reason, not to laws of an empirical science. (Bolton & Hill 1996: 201).

The problem with this theory is that there simply are no universally accepted 'laws of reason'. There are only human judgements about what it is to be rational or irrational. Anthropologists have long debated the supposed universal nature of rationality. Hobart (1985) describes how Balinese epistemology is highly sophisticated and subtle. In Balinese culture, language is recognized as polysemic, 'double-edged', and always influenced by the interests and intentions of both speakers and listeners. Truth is always relative to context. Hobart writes:

> Balinese ideas of what is manifestly so or not so cannot be grafted onto our model of propositions being true or false. Scepticism over human abilities sets the Balinese sharply apart from Hellenic, and later, traditions of the omnipotence of reason. (Hobart 1985: 113).

If this is the case, and complex and different rationalities exist in different cultures, it is very difficult to see the value of talking about 'laws of reason' at all. Any proposed set of 'norms', 'rules' or 'laws' of thought will always be the product of a particular perspective. This is the central difficulty with the approach of Bolton and Hill. While they claim to endorse a 'post-empiricist' epistemology, they appear to locate this epistemology solely in the *subjects* of psychological research, and not in the *researchers* themselves. What a researcher puts forward as 'normal functioning' may well be uncontentious and generally agreed in the world of biology, but *disagreement* about the nature of normality is the *usual state of affairs* in the world of psychology and psychiatry. Bolton and Hill admit that generalizations in the area of human psychology are 'vague' and 'non-specific' (p. 207). Nevertheless they argue that such generalizations do exist and can be used scientifically. For example, they refer to Seligman's work on 'learned helplessness'. This developed out of an animal model (dogs in cages), but the concept has been widely adapted as a model for depression in humans. Bolton and Hill argue that:

> ...the cognitive-affective state of helplessness (which) results from persistent or traumatic (perceived) lack of control over major aversive events, such as pain, or deprivation, and ensues in behavioural inertia .. (Bolton & Hill 1996: 206)

...is an example of a generalization over a cognitive-affective state. This 'learned helplessness' which results from negative life events is understood by many to lead to a state of intense hopelessness and, through this, is held to account for many features of the syndrome of depression. Presumably this would be an example of what Bolton and Hill mean by 'intentional causality'. In a similar vein, one could develop 'causal' theories about the origins of depression from the work of Brown and Harris. The Sri Lankan anthropologist, Gannanath Obeyesekere, quotes the following passage from their work:

> The immediate response to loss of an important source of positive value is likely to be a sense of hopelessness, accompanied by a gamut of feelings, ranging from distress, depression, and shame to anger. Feelings of hopelessness will not always be restricted to the provoking incident—large or small. It may lead to thoughts about the hopelessness of one's life in general. It is such *generalization* of hopelessness that we believe forms the central core of depressive disorder. (Brown & Harris 1978: 134)

However, Obeyesekere makes the following observation:

> This statement sounds strange to me, a Buddhist, for if it was placed in the context of Sri Lanka, I would say that we are not dealing with a depressive but a good Buddhist. The Buddhist would take one further step in generalization: it is not simply the hopelessness of one's own lot; that hopelessness lies in the nature of the world, and salvation lies in understanding and overcoming that hopelessness. (Obeyesekere 1985: 134)

In other words, hopelessness is not something that has a fixed meaning. How it relates to sorrow and loss is determined by cultural context. Thus the relationship between life events, states of helplessness and hopelessness and the syndrome of depression cannot be stated in terms of an acultural, decontextualized law. States of depression can be interpreted in terms of life events, but such interpretations emerge in the context of a particular culture which places certain values on affective states and differentiates such states in particular ways. Janis Jenkins and Marvin Karno make a similar point regarding 'expressed emotion'. This is, currently, one of the most researched constructs in psychosocial research and is cited by Bolton and Hill. High 'expressed emotion' in the families of patients with schizophrenia is understood to be causally related to relapse in such patients after they leave hospital. However, Jenkins and Karno demonstrate that there are substantial cultural influences on the way in which family context, symptoms and relapse are related. Because most researchers in this area of research are committed to psychology as a causal science, they have assumed the universality of the 'expressed emotion' construct and failed to see the cross-cultural difficulties:

> Quite striking from a cross-cultural psychiatric point of view is the neglect on the part of expressed emotion researchers in calling for a systematic examination of the relationship between culture and expressed emotion. Since the anthropological and cross-cultural psychiatric literature of the past several decades has documented substantial cultural differences in conceptions of psychosis, display of emotion, behavioral rules and norms, and family structure and identification, it is reasonable to expect that features such as these are of key relevance to the explication of expressed emotion. In our view, it is these features that go to the very heart of what the construct of expressed emotion embraces. (Jenkins & Karno 1992: 19)

One can only speak confidently about 'norms of function' and 'rational action' in the human world, after one has bracketed out contextual phenomena such as culture, language, gender, social and political circumstances. However, as we saw in Chapter 4 in hermeneutic philosophy these phenomena actually *constitute* the meaningful reality of human beings. When one enters debates about cultural norms, beliefs and practices, and how these relate to metaphysical and ontological assumptions, one has *de facto* moved away from any sort of causal framework. This is a realm of interpretation and hermeneutics.

In his book *Madness Explained*, Richard Bentall sees cognitive explanations of psychosis as a means of overcoming the shortcomings of Jaspersian phenomenology that we described in the previous chapter, but he remains intent on explaining the experiences of psychosis in terms of faulty 'schema' or reality testing. He attacks psychiatry as being unscientific, and implies that cognitive science, unlike psychiatric diagnosis, is value free, and universal. He uses the composite noun 'mind–brain' to side-step the issue of ontological dualism, and thus lapses into an uneasy dualism that leads nowhere in terms of understanding experience. For example, in Chapter 13 of his book, he presents a cognitive model of paranoia in which he describes the 'attributional style' of paranoid patients, and the results of functional magnetic resonance studies in these patients, as if somehow the two are related, and together they will reveal more about the meaning of their experiences. This in part is because he fails to engage with the problems of epistemological dualism. Such an approach is no more likely to reveal the meaning of these experiences than knowledge of the circuits inside a television is likely to help us to understand how the characters in a television soap opera feel. We might know the current in this transistor and the impedance of that capacitor, but this does not help in understanding the plot of *Coronation Street*. We understand others through the human processes of telling stories.

Ethics and cognitivism

So far our arguments have largely concerned the philosophical limitations and drawbacks of cognitivism, but there is something vital missing from our exegesis. Cognitivism has come to represent more than yet another set of abstract theories used to model psychosis. It has deeply influenced a new form of therapy that has gained wide currency in mental health practice over the last 20 years. So, to end this chapter, we want to examine the implications of our analysis for this new therapy. This is important because it raises the twin issues of power and ethics. Psychologists and psychiatrists have adapted Beck's cognitive behaviour therapy for use with people who hear voices or have unusual beliefs. Good examples of this are to be found in the work of Richard Bentall (2003) and Chadwick & Birchwood (1994). Their work is indebted to that of Beck[10], and draws on cognitive and information processing models of psychosis, such as those by Frith and Hoffman we described earlier. Chadwick and Birchwood argue that changing the subject's beliefs about voices may reduce the distress associated with them:

> The cognitive treatment approach to hallucinations involves the *elucidation and challenging of the core beliefs that individuals have about their voices.*

---

[10]Beck wrote the foreword to Richard Bentall's book.

> The weakening or loss of these beliefs is predicted to ease distress and facilitate a wider range of more adaptive coping strategies. (Chadwick & Birchwood 1994: 195; emphasis added)

The origins of their way of working with people who hear voices is deeply influenced by Beck:

> ...the belief that a voice comes from a powerful and vengeful spirit may make the person terrified of the voice and comply with its commands to harm others; however, if the same voice were construed as self-generated, the behaviour and affect might be quite different. This cognitive formulation of voices was inspired by Beck's cognitive model of depression (eg. Beck *et al.* 1979)...(Chadwick & Birchwood 1994: 190–191)

They propose that the distress associated with voices may be reduced by changing the subject's beliefs about the voices. First, they produce empirical evidence from interviews with voice hearers, which suggests that beliefs about voices' identities (whether they are malevolent or benevolent) determine how people respond to the voices. Their subjects engaged with positive voices; they resisted malevolent ones. This observation establishes a rationale for the intervention:

> The cognitive treatment approach to hallucinations involves the *elucidation and challenging of the core beliefs that individuals have about their voices.* The weakening or loss of these beliefs is predicted to ease distress and facilitate a wider range of more adaptive coping strategies. (Chadwick & Birchwood 1994: 195; emphasis added)

Therapy consists of three stages. In the opening phase, the therapist engages the voice hearer, and establishes rapport. Education is an important component, and a tone of what is described as 'collaborative empiricism' (Beck *et al.* 1979) is established. The second stage involves disputing the subject's beliefs about voices, using two techniques drawn from cognitive therapy, hypothetical contradiction and verbal challenge. The former 'measures' the voice hearer's willingness to accept evidence that challenges their beliefs, by considering their responses to hypothetical contradictory evidence. A verbal challenge is then used to challenge the subject's beliefs directly:

> The next stage in therapy is to question the beliefs directly. This involves first *pointing out examples of inconsistency and irrationality, and then, offering an alternative explanation of events:* namely that the voices might be self-generated and that the beliefs are an attempt to make sense of them. (Chadwick & Birchwood 1994: 196; emphasis added)

Finally, the therapist tries to test the subject's beliefs about voices by setting up situations in which the subject can discover that, for example, control can be exerted over the voices.

There are several ways in which our critique is relevant to this work. First, is the importance attached in getting the subject to agree that voices are self-generated. The assumption here is that voices arise through faulty internal mental mechanisms. As we have seen, cognitive science has expended much effort in establishing the nature of these internal faults, and as far as therapy is concerned, the subject has to be persuaded that the voices are located internally, even though in many cases the subject's *reality* is that they are located externally. Subjects then have to be convinced by the therapist that their beliefs about voices are erroneous, and that if the correct beliefs can be established, then distress will be reduced. Thus the therapist has an important role, that of an arbiter, or judge, as to what might be rational or irrational beliefs for subjects to hold about voices.

Now there are serious difficulties here. The insistence that voices are internally generated directs attention away from the possibility that voices may be related in some way to events that have occurred in the voice hearer's social reality. In Chapter 6, we shall see very clearly that voices certainly can be aligned in meaningful ways with characters and events from people's personal and social lives. This is important because there is evidence to link hearing voices and other first rank symptoms of schizophrenia to trauma, such as sexual abuse (see, for example, Ensink 1993). It also disregards the possibility that voices may have metaphorical significance for subjects, and that understanding this by relating the identity and content of voices to past experience may be a vital part of coping (Romme *et al.* 1992; Davies *et al.* 1999). Gillian Proctor (2002) argues that the use of cognitive–behavioural therapy obscures the power relationships that exist between patient and therapist. She points out that the authority of the cognitive therapist is founded on an appeal to rationalism and science, based on the questionable assumption that the therapist is objectively placed to decide what is best for the patient. This view downplays the power dynamics that exist between the two. Cognitivism holds patients to a moral imperative; their view of the world, their understanding of themselves is at fault. They must rectify their faulty thinking processes, their errant reasoning.

To work in this way raises serious ethical issues, particularly if cognitive therapy is used in a way that really fails to contextualize voices[11], and thus precludes the possibility of understanding voices in terms of experience, usually painful. This is likely to arise if the therapist strives to convince subjects that their beliefs about voices are wrong. Someone who has been abused in childhood may well report hearing the voice of the devil telling them they are evil. Such a voice may share pragmatic features of the abuser (Leudar *et al.* 1997) which suggests that the identity of the voice (devil) is aligned with the abuser. From the voice hearer's position as an abused person, it is quite true to say that the voice represents the devil. Most people would agree that abuse is evil. If we

---

[11]We express this conditionally because many psychologists are fully aware of this difficulty, and use cognitive therapy in flexible ways that explore meaning and contexts.

attempt to persuade the subject that they are not really hearing the devil, and the voice comes from within, we are denying that aspect of the subject's reality that signifies the abuse. Is not such an act abusive? Cognitivism's preoccupation with internal thinking processes, their rationality or 'rightness' means that it is in danger of being blind to the social world in which we co-exist. There is no possibility for understanding voices or, for that matter, any aspect of human experience, within shared human contexts. To be fair, many psychologists are aware of this shortcoming. A subject in a study by Haddock *et al.* (1993) found it extremely difficult to accept that his voices were internally generated. The authors noted that his voices were largely understandable in terms of the depressing social and material circumstances in which he was living at the time. This highlights the futility of trying to make psychological interventions without acknowledging the subject's social reality.

In Chapter 3, we pointed out that in psychiatry the content of experiences such as voices and unusual beliefs is widely held to be meaningless. In contrast, cognitive psychology holds that such experiences are not necessarily meaningless, but the meanings attributed to them by those who experience them are simply wrong. In our view, both these positions are unethical. It is just as wrong to say that someone is mistaken to believe in what they think is true about themselves, as it is to say that there is no meaning in what they say[12]. In Chapter 6, we shall explore the issue of ethics and technology in greater detail.

---

[12]Or, to put it another way, that a delusion is an 'empty speech act' (Berrios 1991).

Beetles

final. I missed the

that I did, the question that I asked him, you know, a question

the question him

that's all that I did, and the question that I put to him was a simple

and all that it was, this simple enough question, the question that was simple enough was as follows

as following

the following is an utterance that takes the form of a question, that's all it was a question, you know a simple enough question, a sentence of a certain and particular type of syntactic structure,

a specific and particular type of order of clauses and structure of a clausal manner for the organization of utterance

that differs from other sentences of slightly similar but specifically different syntactic structures,

and which is marked by a simple convention orthographically, that is to say in a manner of speaking in terms of the mark

that is placed at the end of the sentence so as to indicate orthographically that it, the sentence, is a question,

but the question I gave to him,

or rather should I say the question that I put to him in the form of a specific and particular order of clauses, was a question that was along the following sort of lines

how do you know that the beetle in your box is the same as the beetle that is in my box?

he looked at me,

he looked at me and I didn't understand why, but the

question was the question

that I put to him and which I have already just mentioned to you a simple enough question a moment ago, the question that I put to him

this question although simple enough is a

matter of doubt and certainty

it is a perfectly simple question

I have a box you have a box we both have boxes

a box, a container a rectangular box-like object that has boxness usually,

with a lid for the keeping of objects in

not the lid, the box in its boxness is for keeping objects in, you know a box, a box can be of many shapes and sizes

do you know do you understand do you know what I mean

so

you have a box and I have a box, and the question is, the question that I put to him is

a perfectly simple enough question how do I know that the beetle that is in your box, the oblong container usually fitted with a lid is the same as the beetle in my box, the oblong container usually fitted with a lid?

I don't know

he answered, that is to say in reply he confessed

ignorance to the knowledge of the answer to my question

but how can you not know I said, how can you confess to

ignorance of the knowledge of the answer to the question that I put to you

that's not important he said

that's not important?

then he said, following on from that which he had just said about that not being important

look! I haven't got much time, and

he looked at the watch on the wrist that I could hear ticking like a wrist watch on a wrist, or was it

LOOK

I said you haven't got a lot of time, you have just said that you haven't got a lot of time

that's right, he said I haven't got a lot of time

then he turned to the student and said note the thought disorder particularly poverty of content of speech, the empty repetitiousness and philosophizing and then I said is this your poverty of content of speech or thought or both or maybe one or the other, if

my verbal utterance is characterized by a marked degree of prolixity, this circumlocutiousness or if you prefer to call it circumstantiality has a purpose

the purpose for which my verbal utterance is marked by a considerable degree of verbosity is for the following reason

the reason, that follows, is quite precisely, specifically but uncertainly related to the simple enough question that I placed before him and of which he confessed, complete ignorance of the knowledge of the answer to

the question of course being whether, I could know that his beetle in his box is the identical self same beetle in my box this is

this is

this is

really

really important for me this is,

a matter of DOUBT AND CERTAINTY because the words are the pictures that deceive and,

all that I am left with and all,

that you are left with and all that,

everyone is left with is that each and every single one of us
has a box and not one single alone one of us knows whether the beetles in our
  boxes are the exactly self same identical beetles that are in the one single
  alone one's other boxes and I don't
I don't
I don't
I DON'T WANT TO BE ALONE
in a box a lonely, single and alone small beetle in a box that no one knows is
  the same as their small lonely little beetle in their box because,
my words and your words and everyone's words are forming
and the words that are formed in my mouth and
in your mouth and in
all our mouths and, the words in my mouth
become grey shapes and shadow phantoms of truth in your mind's mouth
and in all our mouths these shifty shifting words change
shape and become grey wraith shapes and shadows on the borders of many
worlds, many single alone word worlds,
my word world, your
word world, all our word
worlds.
and words
as they leave my mouth have cheated me these grey phantom shadow word
  worlds retreat from my cheated mouth and disavow our beetles, this
AWFUL WONDERFUL
beetle thing that the shadow words retreat from is in a box, was there for an
  instant of tick tock wristwatch time it was in a box, my box was it in your
  box.
I know he said
I said I think therefore I am a person
and I know he said I am thought
disordered, so does
this mean I am not a person?
anyway how did Tim Henman get on I missed the

6 Ethics before technology

Is 'treatment' the best way to think about mental health work?

Introduction

In previous chapters, we raised questions about the appropriateness of the concept of 'diagnosis' when it comes to psychiatric assessment and understanding. We argued in favour of a different way of framing and interpreting the experiences of people in states of distress. We argued that when we use the adjective 'mental', we are indicating some aspect of the meaningful world in which we live. This world has an obvious biological dimension (if I pass too much alcohol through my brain I stop making any sense!) but when we talk about 'mental health' or 'mental illness', we are automatically moving beyond the biological world of cells and circulation, hormones and nerve pathways. We are in the realm of thoughts and feelings, beliefs and behaviours, reasons and relationships.

Our argument has been that while some aspects of this 'mental' world can be illuminated through scientific experimentation and discourse, in a very important way, the world of meaning resists analysis through the methods of positivist science whether this is biological, psychological or social. We believe that this conclusion resonates with the insights of Wittgenstein and Heidegger (arguably the two most important philosophers of the 20th century). However, this conclusion runs against the modernist urge to frame all our problems as technical, all our suffering as medical, ultimately something open to cure through some expert intervention or another. Postpsychiatry is about thinking beyond this modernist preoccupation with technical framing and expert interventions.

In this chapter, we continue the argument and raise questions about the concept of 'treatment'. We challenge the idea that successful mental health work is always best understood as 'treatment'. Instead, we make the case that, whether we like it or not, most good mental health work is actually based on meaningful relationships between helpers and clients, professionals and patients. In other words, this work involves in some central way a human encounter focused on issues such as hope, trust, dignity, encouragement, making sense, empowerment, empathy and care. We shall argue that whatever model it works to, successful mental health work always involves a positive engagement with these matters. On the other hand, if they are marginalized and neglected, no treatment will be experienced as helpful. Of course, modernist psychiatry acknowledges the importance of these aspects of care but sees them as somewhat marginal to its essential task: the development of treatment technologies designed to eliminate disease entities, the latter being identified through the discourse of psychopathology.

These questions are of great importance at the moment as we live through the era of 'evidence-based' medicine. In essence, this is the belief that medical practice consists of a number of different discrete interventions that can be compared with one another as to efficacy, cost and safety. Good 'evidence-based' practice involves using the interventions that are judged best by 'consensus' panels of experts. We have seen that psychiatry understands its endeavours as being essentially medical in nature. It has embraced the notion of 'evidence-based practice' and sought to examine the effectiveness of various interventions [drug treatments, therapy and electro-convulsive therapy (ECT) in the main] in the same way that oncologists examine the difference between their interventions for cancer.

The arguments here link very clearly to the matters raised earlier in the book, matters relating to the framing of mental health problems. If one begins by framing mental health problems as discrete disease entities, one moves to push the ethical and contextual issues that we are trying to foreground to the sidelines. Once these problems show up as 'depression', 'panic disorder', 'schizophrenia', etc., medical thinking has come to the fore. The next logical move is to ask 'what treatment would be best?'

Our main argument in this chapter is that, whatever their supporters may claim, current interventions are not, in reality, simply based on detached objective science. Current psychiatric technologies are themselves deeply laden with assumptions, priorities, meanings and values, and a great deal of their success is determined by the relationships in which they play a role. *In reality, current psychiatric interventions are based on the manipulation of meanings, hopes and expectations.* If this is accepted, then it supports our case to foreground discussion of these issues, to see them as primary. We shall focus on drug treatments, but our assertions about the importance of meanings and relationships apply equally well to the field of psychotherapy. In his book *Persuasion and Healing*, first published in 1961, the psychotherapist Jerome Frank surveyed the world of psychotherapy. He came to the conclusion that all forms of therapy, even those with very different theoretical frameworks, work on the basis of a common set of essential elements. These are: a helping relationship with a thoughtful and concerned listener, a clearly defined space in which healing can take place and the use of some 'ritual' or other which serves to strengthen the relationship between therapist and client (Frank 1961).

Frank's conclusions have been supported by a body of more empirical research in which comparisons of different types of psychotherapy have been made (e.g. Luborsky *et al.* 1975). In a meta-analysis of 375 studies of different sorts of psychotherapy, Smith & Glass (1977) found that therapy was generally very effective; the typical patient who received therapy was, on average, 75% better off compared with untreated individuals. However, echoing Frank, they concluded that:

> Despite volumes devoted to the theoretical differences among different schools of psychotherapy, the results of research demonstrate negligible differences in the effects produced by different therapy types. (Smith & Glass 1977: 760)

Therapy works. But it does so through the generation of hope, through establishing relationships and by working on meanings. Our argument is that these are best understood as hermeneutic and ethical phenomena and as such cannot be conceptualized adequately through a depersonalized, technical language. We shall now make the case that the discourse of modern psychopharmacology is a sort of social movement premised on such 'ethical' matters as power, profit, priorities, values, relationships and what has become known as 'spin'! We believe that an examination of the available evidence points to the fact that drugs such as antidepressants work largely to the extent that we (as professionals, patients and as a society) believe they do, and want to believe.

To a considerable extent, the benefits of these drugs depend on two factors. First the creation of a *social milieu* where different states of mind are understood to result from the workings of our neurotransmitters. This understanding extends way beyond the consulting room. It is bound up with other cultural ideas about who we are and the nature of suffering and healing. Secondly, it depends on a *therapeutic milieu* in which doctors present drug treatments to their patients with confidence and leave the benefits of other forms of help out of the picture. Of course these are flip sides of the same coin. We shall see that the drug industry has worked with (and 'on') the medical profession *and the public* to generate a set of background cultural assumptions and orientations through which we as individuals experience and understand our different states of distress.

At the end of this chapter, we look at one of the most important moments in the history of mental health care. This was the advent of 'ideas about humane treatment' at the end of the 18th century. Our point is that a major advance in the care of mad and distressed people was made, not through the development of some new medical breakthrough but by a different way of ordering the relationships between carers and those cared for. We believe that the impulse that gave rise to moral treatment is similar to the impulse behind postpsychiatry. Both involve an explicit move to assert the primary importance of ethics in the field of mental health.

Psychiatric drugs work: but largely on account of meanings, expectations, and relationships

The context in which doctors prescribe and patients consume

Psychiatry presents its use of drugs as scientific, rational and technical; very much 'evidence-based'. The 1990s saw a number of major developments in psychopharmacology. Most important was the introduction of the selective serotonin reuptake inhibitor (SSRI) class of antidepressants and the 'atypical' antipsychotic drugs. The decade saw these 'new' and more expensive drugs replace older and therefore cheaper drugs that had been used for the previous 20 years. These 'new' drugs were presented to psychiatrists and other doctors, governments and patients as 'wonder drugs'. Their advent represented major 'breakthroughs' in the treatment of depression and schizophrenia. They were 'revolutionary' agents that would change patients' lives forever. Brought to the market after years of costly pharmacological research, they would be expensive but 'worth it'. Most psychiatrists were happy to see drugs on the market that they could present to patients and families as 'new'. They also liked the idea that these agents were perhaps more effective and safer than older drugs. Their advent also boosted the status of psychiatry within medicine. Articles and advertisements in medical journals presented the new drugs as specific treatments for discrete diseases. Maybe psychiatry could make diagnoses in the same way as other branches of medicine after all? Maybe their theories were scientific and had brought real innovation? It seemed like there were winners all around. Psychiatry could jettison the vague theories of the past (such as psychoanalysis) and embrace the 'new psychopharmacology'. Its treatments were now essentially technology based.

Four years into the new century, things do not look so clear cut. There is mounting evidence that this representation of psychopharmacological 'innovation' is far from the truth. The side effects of these new drugs are now recognized to be very severe and there is no evidence that their efficacy is superior to older drugs (Moncrieff 2003). A growing number of doctors and patient organizations are asking: does the hype surrounding these 'new' drugs represent simply the triumph of marketing over research, mythology over science, profit over medicine? In fact, the last 5 years have witnessed a growing disillusionment within medicine more generally about the pharmaceutical industry and the way it relates to the profession (Abbasi & Smith 2003). Doctors prescribe drugs according to what information is available to them in books, medical journals or directly from representatives of drug companies. Increasingly, the nature of this information is being questioned. More and more medical journalists, doctors and researchers are pulling back the rocks to reveal the murky reality of drug company research, publication and sponsorship. Hardly a week goes past without one scandal or another breaking in the news pages of medical journals. A former editor of the *New England Journal of Medicine*, Marcia Angell writes:

> This is an industry that in some ways is like the Wizard of Oz—still full of bluster but now being exposed as something far different from its image. Instead of being an engine of innovation, it is a vast marketing machine. (Angell 2004: 20).

On one level, this is hardly surprising. The pharmaceutical industry realized about 20 years ago that it could make more money through investing in marketing instead of researching new drugs. It is now one of the biggest industries on the planet. It is certainly one of the most profitable. In the context of a series of articles about drugs for HIV/AIDS in Africa, Julian Borger wrote in the *Guardian* newspaper in 2001 about the power and influence of the Pharmaceutical Research and Manufacturers Association (PhRMA):

> There was a time not long ago when the corporate giants that PhRMA represents were merely the size of nations. Now, after a frenzied two-year period of pharmaceutical mega-mergers, they are behemoths which outweigh entire continents. The combined worth of the world's top five drug companies is twice the combined GNP of all sub-Saharan Africa and their influence on the rules of world trade is many times stronger because they can bring their wealth to bear directly on the levers of western power. (Borger 2001: website)

Selling drugs to the postmodern self

There is a lot at stake when doctors prescribe. This hugely powerful industry depends almost entirely on the sort of decisions doctors make. In turn, these decisions depend on what ideas are in the head of the doctor as well as what the patient expects. So-called 'blockbuster' drugs have become increasingly important to the industry and psychiatry one of its biggest growth areas. A number of commentators have pointed to the importance of 'market expansion' for the drug companies. In their book, *Making us Crazy*, Kutchins and Kirk write of how pharmaceutical companies were directly involved in the development of the DSM, the diagnostic manual for psychiatry in the USA. Every edition of the DSM has seen more disease entities described, more areas of life brought within the embrace of psychopathology. It has clearly been in the interests of the pharmaceutical companies to support the development and the uptake of the DSM.

Rather than witnessing cut-throat competition between different companies selling similar products, we see a deal of cooperation in order to expand the overall consumption of the particular class of drug. Antidepressants provide a good example of this. Fluoxetine (Prozac) was the first SSRI on the market. Through the 1990s, sales of the drug rose continuously in spite of a series of other SSRI drugs appearing on the scene. In the UK alone, prescriptions of antidepressants rose by 173% in the years between 1991 and 2001 (Department of Health 2002). From the point of view of the companies involved, more was to be gained by working (together) to expand the overall numbers taking these drugs instead of aggressively competing with one another. This lack of genuine competition also meant that the manufacturers of different antidepressants did not exert a great deal of effort pointing out the faults of the other drugs. Although the pharmaceutical industry has directly supported the Republican Party in the USA (advocates of 'free market capitalism'), in practice it is debatable whether the public has really benefited from a genuinely free market when it comes to pharmaceuticals (Borger 2001, website).

The public understanding of states of sadness and distress has been a clear target for the industry. Expansion of markets has involved working on the different ways in which members of the public (potential consumers) register and think about their emotions, their relationships, their priorities, in short: them*selves*. The New York-based psychiatrist Bradley Lewis talks about an 'epidemic of Prozac signification'. In other words, the selling of Prozac is not just about a product and information about its use. It is about changing 'significations', changing meanings, changing our background cultural assumptions about states of pain and suffering and what we can do about them. Lewis writes:

> a major effect of Prozac is to support a psychopharmacologic, or biopsychiatric, discourse of human pain and suffering which has deeply conservative political ramifications. Biopsychiatry as a way of talking and organizing human pain minimizes the psychological aspects of depression—personal longings, desires, and unfulfilled dreams—and it thoroughly erases social aspects of depression—injustice, oppression, lack of opportunity, lack of social resources, and systematic denigration. (Lewis 2003: 56)

This discourse is a public, shared orientation, not simply a *medical* ideology foisted on a resisting public. In some ways, the reduction of our emotional states to chemicals in our brains fits easily with the consumerist logic of postmodern society. We encountered the article 'From vastation to Prozac nation', by Alice Bullard (2002) earlier in the book. Bullard argues that culturally there has been a shift from 'deep' notions of the self and its psychological complexity in the modern period to more superficial concepts of the self as something that is open to change through consumption. Just as we can change our identity through the purchase of new designer clothing and change our lifestyles through some other purchases, so too the biological narrative of the self opens up a world where rapid changes in mood, personality and outlook can be induced by consuming chemicals. The message of the drug companies fell on fertile soil. With the more psychological self of the modernist period, change was slow and difficult. Depression and anxiety were deeply meaningful. Their origins were in the conflicts and complexities of our earliest relationships. Now they show up culturally as aberrations; biological malfunctions like diabetes.

In the consumerist culture of postmodernity, the self that we are offered is able to choose its moods and switch off its past. The pharmaceutical industry has capitalized on this cultural shift and promoted it. The following are some of the practical ways in which this powerful industry has driven a particular idiom of distress.

Promotion through the media

During the 1990s, psychopharmacology went public. Millions of people throughout the world started to think about their periods of low mood in terms of neurotransmitters in their brains. Serotonin levels became the stuff of dinner party conversations. The era of Prozac (fluoxetine) had arrived. Although there has never been any evidence that fluoxetine has more efficacy that older anti-depressant drugs such as amitriptyline or imipramine, massive media attention greeted the arrival of this drug. A number of books, penned by journalists, simply assumed that this drug made people happy, contented and confident. They assumed that its beneficial effects were due to its pharmacological action and not due to other factors such as a placebo effect. We will look at a Swedish study below that showed no significant difference in efficacy between active drug and placebo, in 50% of the antidepressant drug trials submitted to the Swedish regulatory authorities (Melander et al. 2003). Media hype can rapidly establish something as 'given', an assumed 'reality', very quickly.

One of the most influential books aimed at public consumption, mainly in the USA, was Peter Kramer's *Listening to Prozac* (1993). This played a major role in the early 1990s in convincing the public that changing one's serotonin levels had powerful effects on mood and personality. Kramer simply assumed that the effects of fluoxetine were pharmacological and raised a somewhat spurious debate about whether (what he called) 'cosmetic psychopharmacology' was ethical. As Elliot Valenstein notes, the effect of this sort of writing was simply to promote the drug:

> ... most readers who are exposed to all the descriptions of people who have had their lives turned around by Prozac—people claimed to have been made happy, productive, and successful for the first time in their lives—are likely to request the pill and leave Peter Kramer to worry about the ethical questions. (Vallenstein 1998: 103)

Unlike most other new drugs, the public were made aware of fluoxetine, not by their doctors or pharmacists, but by news magazines. On the March 26, 1990, the cover of the magazine *Newsweek* pictured an enlarged Prozac pill with the heading: 'A Breakthrough Drug for Depression'. The same magazine devoted a further cover to the drug on the February 7, 1994. The heading this time ran: 'Shy? Forgetful? Anxious? Fearful? Obsessed? How Science Will Let You Change Your Personality With a Pill'. Science had nothing to do with this. There was no breakthrough. In reality, the new SSRI drugs were no more successful in treating depression than the older drugs that had been around for the previous 20 years. If there was a benefit, it was in side effect profile not in efficacy. In spite of this reality, media hype convinced the public that the answers to many of life's difficulties lay in altering serotonin levels. In their book *The Serotonin Solution: The Potent Brain Chemical That Can Help You Stop Bingeing, Lose Weight, and Feel Great*, Judith Wurtman and Susan Suffes state confidently that:

> Serotonin was one of the key neurotransmitters that seemed to malfunction in people who are stressed, anxious, depressed, tense, irritable, confused, angry, or mentally fatigued. (Wurtman & Suffes 1996: 18)

While psychopharmacologists and the drug industry cannot be blamed for all of this, no major campaign was launched to correct the inaccurate portrayal of scientific knowledge in the field. Instead, the 'serotonin solution' was promoted as a simplistic explanation for states of sadness, and the public grew to believe that there were chemical answers to life's problems. In fact, many doctors were happy to tell patients that their painful moods were due to a 'chemical imbalance' even though there was no real scientific basis for this claim.

Direct-to-consumer advertising

The drug industry has long campaigned for direct-to-consumer advertising (DTCA) of their products. In 1997, this was made legal in the USA. The industry's spending on ads went from US\$266million in 1994 to nearly US\$2.5billion in 2000, according to the Kaiser Family Foundation (Boseley 2001: 17). They are now campaigning for direct advertising to patients in Europe. They argue that the patient should have more information about what treatments are available. Consumer organizations who usually spend a great deal of energy campaigning *for* more information are not convinced. In Britain, the respected Consumer Association is leading resistance. They distrust 'information' that comes from companies whose central focus is profit. This suspicion would appear justified given experience in the USA and New Zealand, the only two countries to allow DTCA. In an editorial on this issue in 2002, the *Lancet* wrote:

> DTCA is also often inaccurate. The FDA regulates such advertising in the USA. From 1997 to 2001, the FDA issued 94 notices of violations, mostly because benefits of the drug were hyped up and risks minimised. (*Lancet* 2002a: 1709)

Funding of patient and relatives' organizations

The ban on DTCA has not stopped the industry working on patients and their families in other ways. Very many organizations representing patients and family members receive direct funding from the industry. The European-wide organization GAMIAN Europe (Global Alliance of Mental Illness Advocacy) was actually founded by Bristol-Myers Squibb (Herxheimer 2003: 1209). In the USA, the organization NAMI (National Alliance for the Mentally Ill) is closely associated with the pharmaceutical industry. In a 2003 review article on this issue, Andrew Herxheimer, who is an emeritus professor of the Cochrane Centre, wrote that:

> ... between 1996 and 1999 [NAMI] received almost $12m from 18 drug companies, led by Eli Lilly. The organisation promotes the nationwide expansion of PACT (Program of Assertive Community Treatment), which includes home deliveries of psychiatric drugs backed by court order. (Herxheimer 2003: 1209)

Through these pathways, the pharmaceutical industry works to shape what sort of discussions take priority in such patient groups. As a result, organizations that represent patients and families can end up doing advertising and promotion work for the industry without the latter having to engage in direct adverts to consumers. In turn, stimulating demand amongst patients and their carers for certain drugs can have an effect on doctors and their prescribing.

The drug industry and psychiatry

Establishing a public demand for 'brain chemicals' is one half of the equation, convincing doctors to go this route is the other. However, this is not simply about getting psychiatrists to prescribe. They have always been happy to do so. This is also about narrowing the vision of psychiatry, ruling out other approaches so that the huge cost of the newer drugs is not spent elsewhere. This has meant massive investment in the promotion of reductionism and in particular biopsychiatry (see Introduction). There are essentially three pathways through which the drug companies exert influence on the theory and practice of psychiatry:

(1) Direct funding and control of the research process relating to psychiatric drugs.
(2) Influence on the regulation process.
(3) Direct links between the drug industry and psychiatry.

Direct funding and control of the research process relating to psychiatric drugs

Drug trials

Because drug trials are expensive, very few are now carried out in any sort of independent fashion. While in the 1960s, large clinical trials were funded through state money in the USA and the UK, at present 70% of research into drug treatments is funded by the industry (Bodenheimer 2000). The actual research is carried out by a mixture of academic institutions and private research organizations; in the USA, most drug trials are now performed by commercial organizations called Contract Research Organizations (Angell 2004). These bodies are in competition with each other and so there is a direct incentive to perform trials in a way that favours their customers: the drug companies. Thomas Bodenheimer, writing in the *New England Journal of Medicine*, concluded that:

> trials conducted in the commercial sector are heavily tipped towards industry interests. (Bodenheimer 2000)

Industry-funded researchers usually design trials in a way that will maximize the benefits of the new product. This was famously the case in the early trials of the atypical antipsychotic drugs (Whitaker 2002). One study design technique used to maximize the seeming benefit of the drug was to put patients through a 'washout' period prior to the actual study period. This meant that the 'placebo' group in these studies consisted of patients who had been abruptly withdrawn from previous treatment and given no active replacement drug. (Sometimes extrapyramidal side effects of antipsychotic agents become more severe when the active drug is withdrawn.) These patients were effectively in a withdrawal state, unlikely to do very well. Furthermore, in an effort to show a benefit in terms of side effect profile, researchers compared their drugs with an older antipsychotic, haloperidol, *known* to induce extrapyramidal symptoms in a significant number of those taking it.

In a 2003 study, Lexchin *et al.* looked at the outcomes and quality of industry-sponsored research. They concluded that:

> Research sponsored by the drug industry was more likely to produce results favouring the product made by the company sponsoring the research than studies funded by other sources.

Furthermore:

> All the evidence reported in our meta-analysis... suggests that there is some kind of systematic bias to the outcome of published research funded by the pharmaceutical industry. (Lexchin *et al.* 2003: 1169)

Drug company sponsorship was associated with a greater reported benefit of the particular drug in studies of clozapine (Wahlbeck *et al.* 2000) and antidepressants (Freemantle *et al.* 2000).

Publication of results

An extension of this control of study design is control of publication: the way in which the results of drug research find their way into the scientific literature. Evidence-based medicine is very much dependent on experts carrying out meta-analyses of all the individual studies of a particular treatment. If a company only publishes those trials that are favourable to its products or if it publishes the results of positive outcome trials more than once, then the outcomes of such meta-analyses are systematically distorted. In addition, results of drug trials can be analysed in different ways, e.g. according to an 'intention to treat' framework as opposed to a 'per protocol' one, the latter being usually more favourable to the drug involved.

Hans Melander and his colleagues from Sweden studied the bias produced by these processes in relation to studies of SSRI antidepressants. They examined the research on these drugs placed before the Swedish drug regulatory authority, between 1983 and 1999. Companies are required to submit all the information available to them about their product, including studies with a negative outcome, when they are seeking approval. As a result, it can be assumed that the information submitted was *not* subject to selection bias. Melander's group compared this data set with the results made available to the medical community (through publication in the scientific literature) and thus accessible to experts carrying out meta-analyses. Of 42 submitted studies, 21 found the test drug significantly more effective than placebo. An equal number, 21, did not show significant results; in these, the drug had no greater effect that did the placebo. However, 19 of the positive studies were reported in the form of stand-alone publications while only six of the negative studies were published in this form. Four studies were not published at all. All of these were negative from the companies' point of view. The authors found:

> . . . evidence of duplicate publication, selective publication, and selective reporting.

They conclude:

> Without access to all studies (positive as well as negative, published as well as unpublished) and without access to alternative analyses (intention to treat as well as per protocol), any attempt to recommend a specific drug is likely to be based on biased evidence. The probable choice of a specific selective serotonin reuptake inhibitor based on pooled analysis of publicly available data is not likely to be supported by an analysis considering the total body of evidence. (Melander *et al.* 2003: 1173)

Influence on the regulation process

USA

In the USA, the regulation of prescription drugs is in the hands of the Federal Drug Administration (FDA). Since 1992, under the terms of the Prescription Drug User Fee Act (PDUFA), the FDA receives a substantial portion of its funding directly from the industry. In addition, FDA policy is (to some extent at least) subject to political influence. We noted above that the pharmaceutical industry has been a large corporate sponsor of the Republican Party. In 2002, Dr Paul Stolley, a former senior consultant with the agency, claimed that the FDA had become a:

> servant of the industry, where dissenting voices are intimidated and ostracised and where scientific debate is repressed. (quoted in Moynihan 2002: 593)

Dr Stolley was involved in the post-marketing surveillance of the controversial drug alosetron (used in irritable bowel syndrome). In a *British Medical Journal* editorial relating to this drug and the concerns raised by a number of doctors about its safety profile, Professor Michel Lièvre wrote that:

> With massive direct industry funding of the FDA through the Prescription Drug User Fee Act, some doubt can be expressed about the ability of the agency to resist pressure from industrials.

Furthermore, he noted a shift in the FDA from being:

> traditional and paternalistic to holding a more republican view of public health. The agency would now rather provide the best information for patients and doctors to make their own decisions than to make the decisions in their name.

The problem with this is that:

> Most patients obviously lack the background and training necessary to assess correctly the balance between risk and benefit, and they may be misled by self help groups that have financial ties with the pharmaceutical industry. (Lièvre 2002: 555–556)

In relation to this controversy about the licensing of alosetron, the *British Medical Journal* front page carried a photo of the FDA building over the heading: 'Who owns the FDA, the drug industry or the people?'

Specific concerns about the approval of antidepressants are raised by Irving Kirch and Thomas Moore in a paper that we shall examine in more depth later. They question the licensing of the SSRI drug Celexa (citalopram) when only two out of five efficacy studies submitted to the FDA showed a significant antidepressant effect. These authors quote an FDA official essentially arguing the company's case when justifying the approval.

Europe

Concerns about close links between the drug industry and European regulatory bodies has also been raised. In a review article exploring these links in 2002, Professor John Abraham wrote that:

> As the regulatory agencies in the European Union are now largely funded by industry, and because companies look for fast approval rates as a key criterion when choosing where to submit the application for approval of a new drug, regulatory agencies are, in effect, competing with each other for 'regulatory business' by attempting to approve drugs at an ever faster pace. (Abraham 2002: 1166)

Two French commentators on his paper agreed:

> Drug regulation has gradually moved away from its public health mission. National medicines agencies and the European agency are now serving first and foremost the pharmaceutical companies, who provide their main funds. (Bardelay & Kopp 2002: 1167)

Direct links between the drug industry and psychiatry

An editorial in the *Lancet* in 2002 was titled: 'Just how tainted has medicine become?' (*Lancet* 2002*b*). Their reply: 'Heavily, and damagingly so, is the answer' (p. 1167). An entire edition of the *British Medical Journal* in 2003 was titled: 'Time to untangle doctors from drug companies'[1]. One of the articles in this edition identified 16 ways that doctors are entangled with the industry (Moynihan 2003: 1190). We list these in Table 6.1.

Moynihan quotes Arnold Relman, a professor at Harvard and a former editor of the *New England Journal of Medicine* as saying:

> The medical profession is being bought by the pharmaceutical industry, not only in terms of the practice of medicine, but also in terms of teaching and research. (Quoted in Moynihan 2003: 1190)

These are voices from the heart of medicine, sounding the alarm. Increasingly, doctors are moving to disengage. We believe that psychiatry has been particularly targeted by the industry. The successful marketing of 'new'

Table 6.1 Drug Industry links with Medical Profession

- Face to face visits from drug company representatives
- Acceptance of direct gifts of equipment, travel or accommodation
- Acceptance of indirect gifts, through sponsorship of software or travel
- Attendance at sponsored dinners and social or recreational events
- Attendance at sponsored educational events, continuing medical education, workshops, or seminars
- Attendance at sponsored scientific conferences
- Ownership of stock or equity holdings
- Conducting sponsored research
- Company funding for medical schools, academic chairs or lecture halls
- Membership of sponsored professional societies and associations
- Advising a sponsored disease foundation or patient's group
- Involvement with or use of sponsored clinical guidelines
- Undertaking paid consultancy work for companies
- Membership of company advisory boards of 'thought leaders' or 'speakers' bureaux'
- Authoring 'ghostwritten' scientific articles
- Medical journals' reliance on drug company advertising, company purchased reprints and sponsored supplements

---

[1]This was the May 31st 2003 edition. The cover contained a cartoon by Malcolm Willett showing a group of pigs (some in white coats with stethoscopes) eating and drinking at a large table. At the end of the table a lizard-like creature is writing a cheque!

antidepressants, 'new' antipsychotic drugs and, more recently, 'mood stabilizers' has meant huge profits for the companies involved. This has been accompanied by a massive effort to steer psychiatry in a biological direction.

There are a number of ways in which the industry has a direct effect on psychiatry.

Funding of academic work

We have seen above how most drug trials are directly funded by the industry. We have noted reports of 'systematic bias' in these studies. However, it is in the industry's interests not just to fund drug trials but also to encourage the biological reductionism we noted in the Introduction more widely. If doctors are trained to encounter mental health problems as largely the result of disturbed brain biology, it is a short step for them to see the solutions in terms of chemicals of one sort or another. We have pointed out above that a great deal of pharmaceutical promotion activity is aimed at market expansion. Thus it is in the interests of the industry to fund research on non-drug aspects of psychiatry (such as genetic research and the development of diagnostic tools) that encourage this biological perspective.

Joanna Moncrieff writes that:

> ... marketing strategies now include attempts to shape psychiatric thought through the academic arena. This is done by a strategy that is conceived long before a product is officially marketed and may involve the promotion of disease concepts and their frequency. A recent guide to pharmaceutical marketing suggests the need to 'create dissatisfaction in the market', 'establish a need', and 'create a desire'. (Moncrieff 2003: 5)

It is estimated that 60% of all biomedical research and development in the USA is now privately funded and two-thirds of academic institutions have shares in outside sponsors (Beckelman *et al.* 2003). The industry directly funds university posts, sponsors academic lectures and provides grants for the infrastructure of academic departments. As most doctors in training receive their academic inputs from these departments, it is hardly surprising that most psychiatrists understand nearly all mental illness as being essentially a biological problem. As a result, few patients leave a psychiatric consultation without a prescription. An academic department of psychiatry not dedicated primarily to biological research is now a rarity!

Development and sponsorship of 'opinion leaders'

Academic departments of psychiatry are also the main source of 'opinion leaders' in the field. These individuals write review articles, chapters and summaries. These often act as unofficial guidelines for the profession. Busy clinicians look to these works for a sense of 'what the profession thinks' about particular problems and so they are highly influential. In an article titled 'Are you being duped?' published in 2001, Trevor Jackson reviewed the May 2001 edition of the industry journal *Pharmaceutical Marketing*. This contained a 24 page supplementary guide headed 'effective medical education'. This gave interesting insights about what it called 'the tricks of the trade'. As well as describing medical education as 'a potent weapon to be used by the marketer in supporting promotional activities', apparently the guide had a lot to say about the cultivation of opinion leaders. It warns its readers not to waste their time dealing with just any old academic but instead to concentrate on 'the editorial boards of key publications for ultimate target audiences', on doctors who sit on scientific committees, members of important professional societies and those who are representatives of national and international guideline committees. Jackson quotes the guide:

> Marketers are advised to ask opinion leaders for their advice. 'The advisory process is one of the most powerful means of getting close to people and of influencing them. Not only does it help shape medical education overall, it can help in the process of evaluating how individuals can best be used, motivate them to want to work with you—and with subliminal selling of key messages ongoing all the while'. (Jackson 2001: 1312)

We believe this last quote betrays exactly what is going on when drug companies work 'closely' with the profession. We believe that through its influence on the academic world of psychiatry, the industry has effectively brought about a sort of 'normal science' of psychiatry that is favourable to its ends. This is based on certain assumptions, supported by selective overviews of the literature. We believe that this influence has contributed substantially to the dominance of biological reductionism within academic psychiatry.

Clinical practice guidelines play an important role in shaping 'normal practice' in any branch of medicine. In a 2002 paper published in the *Journal of the American Medical Association*, Choudhry *et al.* surveyed 192 authors of 44 guidelines endorsed by North American and European medical societies between 1991 and 1999. They found that 87% of authors who responded had some sort of interaction with the pharmaceutical industry. A majority had received financial support to perform research and 38% had served as employees or consultants for a drug company. In spite of this, specific declarations concerning drug company involvement were made in only two cases.

Relationship with professional organizations

In a very hard-hitting article published in the journal *The American Prospect* in 2002, the prominent American psychiatrist E. Fuller Torrey described his attendance at the 7th World Congress of Biological Psychiatry. He wrote:

> Until about a decade ago, pharmaceutical companies passed out pens or notepads with their companies' logos at such events, and most speakers presented data and opinions based on their true scientific beliefs.
>
> That all changed when Big Pharma took over. At the congress, I counted 15 major displays on the way to the lunch area, including an artificial garden

(Janssen-Cilag), a brook running over stones (Lundbeck), and a 40-foot rotating tower (Novartis). Almost all offered free food and drink, T-shirts, or other inducements designed to get psychiatrists to pause so that an army of smiling sales representatives could give their sales pitch. (Fuller-Torrey 2002; viewed on website).

The title of Fuller-Torrey's article is 'The going rate on shrinks: Big Pharma and the buying of psychiatry'. This title is very similar to Joanna Moncrieff's Maudsley Discussion Paper 'Is psychiatry for sale? An examination of the influence of the pharmaceutical industry on academic and practical psychiatry'. These are both prominent psychiatrists. Both are sounding alarm bells. In her book on the drug industry, Marcia Angell makes the point that there is so much commercial involvement in medical meetings at present that:

> Instead of sober professionalism, the atmosphere of these meetings is now trade-show hucksterism. (Angell 2004: 145)

Angell points out that membership fees for the APA (American Psychiatric Association) are falling because of massive industry sponsorship of their 'scientific' meetings. The big illusion (or *lie* depending which way you look at it) is that this sponsorship is about promoting 'education'. As we have seen above, this activity is actually about market expansion. By funding scientific meetings, the industry is effectively able to set the clinical and research priorities of the profession. This is not education but manipulation. Angell quotes Stephen Goldfinger, chairman of the APA's Committee on Commercial Support:

> The pharmaceutical companies are an amoral bunch. They're not a benevolent association. So they are highly unlikely to donate large amounts of money without strings attached. Once one is dancing with the devil, you don't always get to call the steps of the dance. (Goldfinger; quoted in Angell 2004: 147)

The benefits of antidepressants

Antidepressants work; to some extent at least. It would appear from the research literature that a majority of patients who take them feel a bit better after a couple of weeks. However, evidence is accumulating that little if any of the improvement seen is due to specific chemical effects. In placebo-controlled trials, the placebos are usually nearly as effective as the active drug. In some trials, they have been more effective. In the Swedish study of Melander and colleagues, quoted above, only 50% of the drug trials examined showed a significant difference between active drug and placebo. In the other 50%, placebos had the same effects as the active drug. In 2002, the American psychologist Irving Kirsch and colleagues used the Freedom of Information Act to gain access to all the efficacy data submitted to the FDA for approval of the six most widely prescribed antidepressants (Kirsch *et al.* 2002). These drugs were approved between 1987 and 1999. The drug companies are required by law to submit *all* their data to the FDA when seeking approval, not just the results of trials that they judge to be favourable to their product. In all, data on 47 randomized placebo-controlled trials were studied. In all trials, the Hamilton Depression Scale (HAM-D) was used to assess clinical change and so it was possible to make direct comparisons of outcomes. The Hamilton scale is a physician-rated scale and one of the most widely used rating scales in psychiatry. Longer (21-item) and shorter (17-item) versions of the scale were used. Kirsch *et al.* found that 82% of the drug response was duplicated by the placebo response. In other words, it would seem that only 18% of the drug response in these antidepressant trials was due to pharmacological effects of the medication. This is substantially less that what is generally claimed by the drug companies. However, it is in keeping with a previous analysis of the FDA data by Khan *et al.* (2000) who estimated that 76% of the antidepressant response was duplicated by placebo. Furthermore, in the Kirsch *et al.* study, the difference between drug response and placebo while *statistically* significant was on average less than 2 points on the HAM-D and thus of questionable *clinical* significance:

> The range was from a 3-point drug/placebo difference for venlafaxine to a 1-point difference for fluoxetine, both of which were on the 21-item (64 point) version of the scale. As intimated in the FDA memoranda...the clinical significance of these differences is questionable. (Kirsch *et al.* 2002, viewed on website)

The authors also make the point that these studies were carried out using inert placebos. It is possible that some, if not all, of the small difference between active drug and placebo was due to breaking of the blind in these trials. In other words, some patients given the active drug might well have been able to guess correctly that they were getting the active compound from the side effects experienced. Active compounds usually produce more side effects than placebos. In a study in the 1980s, Rabkin and colleagues (1986) showed that the ability of doctors and patients to guess correctly whether active drug or placebo was being used exceeded chance. Knowing that one is taking the active drug leads to an *enhanced placebo effect* in such conditions and so will work to exaggerate the positive effects observed with the active drug.

Furthermore, one of the most common side effects of psychotropic drugs is sedation. For patients who have problems relaxing or going to sleep, taking a chemical that causes sedation might well be experienced as a positive. Combined with an enhanced placebo effect, the sedative power of most antidepressants might also explain some of the 'left over' differences between active drugs and placebos. If this is the case, true pharmacological antidepressant effects brought about by these chemicals might be very small and clinically irrelevant.

It would seem that, in reality, antidepressants work largely because both patient and doctor want them to work. However, this wish for efficacy would probably not be sufficient on its own. The other key ingredient is a shared set of assumptions and expectations about the nature of our mood states and their responsiveness to chemical manipulation. Traditional healers from different societies effect cures in many ways. However, one important method is the manipulation of shared cultural beliefs about the spirit world, the nature of illness and bodily forces. Healers everywhere draw on background cultural beliefs when they offer explanations and interventions. When the modern psychiatrist or general practitioner talks to her patients about their sadness being due to a 'chemical imbalance' or a 'lack of serotonin', she is drawing on background ideas that have been promoted at many different levels by the pharmaceutical industry over the past 20 years. The point is that not only do doctor and patient *want* the ingested chemicals to work, they also *expect* them to effect change.

A different way of understanding the biological effects of antidepressants

This is not to say that the changes brought about by antidepressants are purely *psychological*. As we have stated before, we are embodied creatures. Our states of sadness, distress and despair always have a biological dimension. It is not hard to imagine how a severe lowering of mood, motivation and activity can itself bring about pronounced effects on our biological systems and that these changes in turn make it difficult for patients to move on. In our experience, patients who are depressed feel genuinely 'stuck', lost and overwhelmed. There is clearly a biological dimension to this. Sleep and appetite are often reduced and activity lessened. In severe states of depression, the individual can come to find all activity difficult and many people simply want to retire to bed. Some people can become virtually mute, finding the effort involved in conversation excruciating.

Overcoming depression often involves a struggle with one's own biology. Traditional psychiatry works with different theories about how this happens. As we have seen above, the 'serotonin story' is the latest. From this angle, antidepressants work because they raise serotonin levels in the brain. There is very little evidence that this actually happens (Valenstein 1998). Furthermore, antidepressants that do not affect serotonin levels or receptors are marketed alongside the SSRI drugs. The biology of overcoming depression is obviously more complicated.

If the studies by Kirsh, Melander, Khan and colleagues discussed above are taken seriously, then placebo preparations would appear to be effective in helping people overcome states of depression. Could it be that a substantial proportion of the *biological* effects of these drugs are, in fact, brought about by the response of the person's body to the simple fact of taking a pill? We believe that the answer is yes. There is evidence from other branches of medicine that placebos work *biologically* as well as psychologically. In his book on the subject, Daniel Moerman (2002) quotes a major trial comparing the efficacy of the drugs lansoprazole (Prevacid) and ranitidine (Zantac) in the treatment of peptic ulcers. This was published by Lanza *et al.* in 1994. Three hundred people entered the trial. They were all diagnosed as having ulcers by endoscopy. The study was a radomized control trial with a placebo arm. They found that after 2 weeks about 30% of people in the two drug groups had healed ulcers. After 4 weeks, two-thirds of the people taking ranitidine had healed ulcers, while this was the case with 88% of the people taking lansoprazole. The trial demonstrated that these are highly effective drugs. However, in the group of 44 patients given placebo, a third had healed ulcers at 2 weeks and this had occurred in nearly 50% at 4 weeks. There can be no dispute: this was biological healing of ulcers; confirmed by endoscopy. It must have combined a coordinated response from various systems in the patients' bodies: endocrine, neurological, haematological, immunological, etc. It would appear that simply taking a pill in the right circumstances, with the right motivation, can have a powerful effect on our bodies.

Our proposal is that a substantial proportion of the healing effect of antidepressant drugs is also biological: bringing about physical changes in the body of the person taking them. However, the healing involved happens through pathways other than the ones put forward by most psychopharmacologists. It does not start with drug effects on neurotransmitter levels but with the instillation of hope, the mustering of courage and generation of motivation. Any nerotransmitter changes observed are most likely to be secondary to this process.

So far in this chapter, we have looked at how psychiatric treatments work mainly through non-specific pathways. These pathways involve meanings, values and relationships. Although current interventions are promoted as being treatment technologies, in reality the specific effects of these technologies are of limited importance. Psychiatry, and medicine more widely, does not generally like to admit this. Professional prestige is predicated on having knowledge that other people do not have. Corporate profits are dependent on the illusion that drugs work through highly specific pathways that take huge companies to research them properly. We want to challenge these illusions and the power that goes with them. Postpsychiatry seeks a discourse of mental health that is more honest about healing and more modest about the importance of professionals. In the next section, we look at a previous mental health movement that worked with similar ideals. We believe that the philosophy of care developed by English Quakers at the end of the 18th century also worked to challenge the idea that mental illness was *primarily* a question of technology. It also worked to foreground the question of ethics.

A lesson from history

The madness of King George: madness and its treatment in the Age of Reason

At the end of the 18th century there was a great optimism amongst the physicians who cared for insane people in England. This was the Age of Reason and Enlightenment. These physicians saw themselves as engaged in a battle to overcome unreason. There was a consensus at the time that physical treatments such as bleeding, spinning, and dunking the patient in freezing cold water were effective cures and were widely prescribed.

Such 'mad-doctors' were given a great boost by the apparent cure of King George III by Francis Willis in 1789. The king had developed a variety of symptoms the year before: extreme agitation, talkativeness, hoarseness, colic, insomnia, anorexia, fever and copious sweating. But the most distressing problem was his periods of confusion. This caused great distress for the King himself, the Queen and of course for his Ministers who were worried that if his condition became chronic the King's son, the Prince of Wales, would seek to obtain the throne for himself. He was likely to make some major changes at court.

Willis was a clergyman and a 'mad-doctor'. He ran an asylum for 30 patients in Lincolnshire. Of all the doctors interviewed by the government ministers, Willis was the most optimistic and maintained that nine out of ten of his patients recovered. The regime he instituted for King George was very severe. He put emetics in his food and, as a result, the King was continually sick while not realizing the cause of this. Willis also made regular use of a 'straitwaistcoat'. The King was punished for any 'non-compliance' by being bound in this and virtually tied to his bed. King George eventually improved and recovered. Willis and his interventions were given the credit and the social position of 'mad-doctors' was given a great boost. Their harsh and brutal treatments were assumed to work.

In spite of this confidence on the part of their doctors, the patients concerned were more sceptical. They experienced these treatments as nothing short of cruelty and were doubtful of their benefits. With the benefit of hindsight, we concur with the patients and wonder at the arrogance of our medical predecessors. We now believe that George III was probably suffering from a form of porphyria that caused delirium. The interventions of Willis, if they did anything, probably only served to aggravate his condition. Macalpine and Hunter write that:

> a great deal of the trouble and violence that ensued was in direct response to the control and coercion to which he was subjected and against which he rebelled. (quoted in Glover 1984: 100)

We question the morality of these doctors who proudly proclaimed their knowledge of madness while overseeing institutions that were actually characterized by torture, deprivation, neglect and death.

Another side to enlightenment: the York Retreat

It took the establishment of the Retreat in York, in 1796, to challenge this contradiction. We believe that that there are many lessons still to be learnt from the
history of the Retreat. The incident that was the impulse behind its creation was
the death of a Quaker widow, Hannah Mills, in 1790. Hannah was from Leeds
and attended the Quaker meetings in that city. When she became unwell, her
friends brought her to the York Asylum and asked the Quakers in York to visit.
They attempted to do so but were not allowed to see her when they called. Some
months later, she died. The Quakers in York were outraged and one of their
members, William Tuke, a tea merchant, put forward the idea that they should
establish their own asylum in York. The Retreat opened its doors 4 years later,
initially to Quaker patients alone but later to the wider community. William's
grandson, Samuel, published his *Description of the Retreat* in 1813. A modern
edition of this work was published in 1964 with an introduction by Richard
Hunter and Ida Macalpine. A further edition with a foreword by Kathleen Jones
appeared in 1996 (Tuke 1996). An account on the history and philosophy of the
Retreat and its influence on psychiatry in the 19th century was written by Mary
Glover and published in 1984 (Glover 1984).

From the start, William Tuke was clear that the Retreat was to be based
on a different philosophy from that at work in the York Asylum and other
mad houses. Tuke was not opposed to doctors as such but was sceptical of their
various treatments for mental illness. While it was accepted that a doctor
should be recruited to the staff, they chose for the job a man who had not been
trained in the field of insanity. In fact, Dr Thomas Fowler was chosen for the
job precisely *because* of his inexperience and because he was also a modest
man with an open mind. When he began work at the Retreat, not surprisingly
he read what he could about the various medical technologies available at the
time. Initially he used these on patients so that:

> Bleeding, blisters, seatons, evacuants, and many other prescriptions, which
> have been highly recommended by writers on insanity, received an ample
> trial. (Tuke 1996: 111).

Dr Fowler kept careful notes on the condition of his patients before and after
these treatments. Eventually he concluded that most were simply ineffectual.
Furthermore, their administration often involved a great deal of distress for
patients and staff alike. Soon Dr Fowler gave instructions that no patient should
be compelled to undergo such interventions if they objected. Eventually, he abandoned their use altogether. The one treatment that he thought was helpful was the
provision of warm baths, particularly for patients with 'melancholia'. Letting go
of the traditional treatments created a relaxed and therapeutic environment and
patients did very well. The focus was on nursing *care*, not medical treatments.
The head female nurse was Katherine Allen. Mary Glover writes:

> It was said that William Tuke was much impressed by this success. One
> might guess that the most creative thing Dr. Fowler did during his short

> time at The Retreat was his courageous abandonment of traditional treatment.
> Once these recurrent crises of treatment were abolished for good, Katherine
> Allen and her nursing staff could get on with their business of calm, good-
> tempered routine, and Fowler gave them consistent support. (Glover
> 1984: 54).

The regime at the Retreat was explicitly based on kindness and non-restraint.
George Jepson, the first Superintendent, was opposed to the use of fear in
relation to mental patients. He is described as treating patients with kindness,
gentleness and respect. Quaker values were the guiding principles not medical
doctrine.

Samuel Tuke's *Description of The Retreat* was published in 1814. A very
positive review of the book appeared in *The Edinburgh Review*, written by
Reverend Sydney Smith who visited the institution in the same year and was
struck by its tranquillity. Smith's article attracted a stream of visitors, some of
whom travelled from abroad. Many 'mad-doctors' visited the Retreat and were
also impressed.

The reforms introduced 200 years ago by the Tukes in England coincided
with developments elsewhere. In 1793, Philippe Pinel was appointed by
the revolutionary government in France to oversee the insane of Paris who
were housed in the twin institutions of the Salpêtrière (for women) and the
Bicêtre (for men). When he took over, Pinel found his patients kept in very
poor conditions and generally treated like animals. Chains, fetters, hunger and
disease were the norm. Pinel was inspired by the ideals of the revolution
and set out to change things. Like the Tukes, Pinel became very sceptical about
the value of medical interventions. Such treatments were:

> 'rarely useful and frequently injurious', methods that had arisen from 'preju-
> dices, hypotheses, pedantry, ignorance, and the authority of celebrated names'.
> (quoted in Whitaker 2002: 21)

Pinel set out to talk to and listen to his patients. He focused on the 'management of the mind' and coined the term *'traitement morale'*. As in York, by treating his patients with some degree of respect and avoiding physical 'treatments',
Pinel was able to establish a more positive and nurturing environment.

The ideas of Pinel and the York Quakers travelled to North America and
were taken up enthusiastically there. By 1817, the Quakers in Philadelphia had
opened an asylum modelled on the project in York. Others followed. A major
change had occurred in the social perception of insanity. A real opportunity
to overcome exclusion had arisen. However, as the 19th century progressed,
in Britain, Europe and America the medical profession again asserted its
authority and gradually the focus shifted back to interventions centred not on
ethics but on technology. Huge asylums were built across the Western world.
While some of these were built because of altruistic motives, they soon
became almost as terrible as the mad houses of a previous era. Our contention
is that if the focus had remained firmly on the importance of relationships,

respect, comfort and dignity as pioneered in the York Retreat, this could not have happened. In other words, if the care of mad people had remained a *moral* issue, the disasters of the asylum era may well have been avoided. With the ethics of care to the fore, attention is focused on the behaviour of the *care-givers* and the sort of environments constructed by them. With a medical logic in ascendance, these move to the background and only the disturbed behaviour of the *patient* is visible. Analysing this behaviour and its response to different treatments become the priority. In the 19th century, the focus returned to debates about the biological causes of insanity, and again medical technology came to the fore.

Our sympathetic account of the Retreat and 'moral treatment' contrasts with that of Foucault. In *Madness and Civilisation*, Foucault argued that the moral therapy developed by Pinel in France and the Tukes in England was not really a movement towards liberation at all but an 'instrument of moral uniformity and of social denunciation'. The essence of Foucault's work is an invitation to question the project of Enlightenment: the replacement of religious revelation with human reason as the path towards truth and progress. In *Madness and Civilization*, moral therapy is seen very much as an Enlightenment phenomenon. He argues that Pinel and the Tukes were centrally focused on engaging with and expanding the reason of the patient.

We believe that while there is some truth in this, Foucault is overly negative in his writing about the Tukes. In our opinion, their efforts were more complex than his account allows. Their work embodied Enlightenment ideals but was not a one-dimensional phenomenon. As we have seen above, religion, friendship and community were as important as reason in the quest for therapy.

Foucault did not get everything right. His work changed emphasis and direction at many junctures. While it is important that we 'listen' to his critique, it is equally important that we do not treat it as some sort of postmodern canon. We continue to believe that we have much to learn from the tea merchants of York.

Conclusion

We are essentially arguing that postpsychiatry involves a different way of understanding our priorities. It does not mean an abandonment of science, technology or even control, but it does mean a reversal of the traditional order of priorities. We believe that the first move in mental health work should be an exploration of how we, as a community, want to care for one another in states of madness, distress and alienation. This is primarily about what values we wish to attach to such states of mind. This is not a technical issue but an ethical one, and so one that should be open to democratic debate and discussion. In this debate, there will be different perspectives. These will be multiple and diverse. We use the word 'democratic' to indicate openness to difference and respect for alternative perspectives. There will not be one answer but many, some conflicting. Democracy is always messy. This is a move away from the univocal 'consensus' statements of modernist psychiatry which ignore differences and usually seek simply to silence alternatives.

Our argument is that the field of mental health treatment is best understood as being *primarily* about values, meanings and relationships and only *secondarily* about questions of treatment efficacy and outcomes.

Traditional psychiatry

Primary concern: understanding based on science
Treatment based on technology

Secondary concern: meanings, values and relationships

In Chapter 4, we worked out these arguments in relation to issues around the question of understanding; in this chapter, we turned to interventions and treatment. We examined the relationship between technology and ethics. We do not want to get rid of psychopharmacology and psychotherapy but we believe that decisions about the use of various techniques and interventions should be *secondary* to a more original discourse based on the 'ethical' encounter between helper/care-giver/professional and the user/client/patient.

Postpsychiatry

Primary concern: ethics and hermeneutics of madness, distress and alienation

Secondary concern: development and analysis of specific technologies

---

For the pioneers of moral treatment, progress was not about an increase of knowledge but rather about a different sort of encounter between patients and those who provided care. If anything, it was predicated on an increase in humility above all else. Our argument is that something similar is needed now.

7 Narrative and the ethics of representation

'I couldn't write about the people (in my plays) if I didn't care about them. I have to become them.'

(Edward Albee interviewed on *Channel 4 News*, 15 April 2004)

This chapter marks an important transition in this book. In it, we are moving away from academic critique to raise some important questions about the seemingly neutral, practical activity of writing in psychiatry and medicine. We also want to raise questions about the different ways in which we may be permitted to present evidence about the way we work. This means we move beyond the question of evidence-based medicine (i.e. effectiveness) to question the nature of evidence itself. To some extent, we have already dealt with the different types of evidence that are admissible in psychiatry, and although we won't dwell on this in detail, here we want to consider the nature of evidence in the light of recent debates about the nature of truth. At issue here are the implications of how our positions as doctors influence how and what we write about our work, our patients and, more rarely, ourselves. We want to question what the act of writing in such circumstances is really all about. This means we must consider the relationship between the *way* we write (or genre, to use the literary expression) and the worlds we are attempting to describe. In short, the key issues we want to explore at this point are those of truth and representation. The questions we explore here are related to matters we have explored earlier, but here we turn the critical gaze on ourselves as potential writers about our own *oeuvre*.

The problems of truth and representation are, in our view, closely related to the problems of modernity, and deal particularly with the problems of epistemology—the nature of knowledge. Here we want to develop our earlier arguments about the nature of knowledge in psychiatry in the light of our struggle throughout this book to convey something of how postpsychiatry relates to practice. This, as we shall see, has implications for the particular genres of writing we have adopted in our attempts to represent our ideas. To make our case, we have searched far and wide in other disciplines. We find a particularly rich seam of ideas in the expanding overlap between medicine and the humanities, especially literary and aesthetic theory, as well as anthropology. Our view is that medicine, and psychiatry in particular, has much to learn from these disciplines, since all three have had to grapple with the issues that preoccupy us in this chapter. Consequently, there is a great deal that medical, especially psychiatric, writing can gain from an encounter with the arts and humanities.

To begin with, we focus on the most traditional and widely established genre in medicine and psychiatry—the case history. This has a particularly important position in biomedical psychiatry. We examine the notion of case and case history critically through the work of Robert Barrett, who trained as both a psychiatrist and an anthropologist. We then scrutinize what has been called the narrative turn in medicine and psychiatry. This has been widely adopted by those disenchanted with the sterility of positivism in medicine, particularly the influence of positivism on evidence, medical practice and medical writing. Thinking about the practice of psychiatry as narrative raises the possibility of thinking about psychiatry as a discursive (and thus social) practice. Although we welcome the narrative turn in medicine, we are not convinced that its advocates have fully thought through the implications of their position. In particular, we believe that if we are to engage seriously with the ethical implications of narrative, we must be prepared to engage with the problem of truth and representation. What is narrative? Who authors it? What is it trying to say? How does it relate to the worlds that it speaks of? It is here that recent developments in anthropology, literary and aesthetic theory are helpful. Finally, we consider how this analysis influenced the choice we made about how we would try to write about postpsychiatry.

The case history

It is said that Hippocrates introduced the case history as a way of systematically describing the natural course of disease, so-called pathography. In the 19th century, the case history reached its apogee. Psychoanalysis and neuropsychiatry were founded upon case histories. Freud and Breuer's book *Studies on Hysteria* epitomizes this tradition. In it we see the origins of psychoanalysis unfolding in a series of detailed case histories, with descriptions of the technical procedures that were to constitute psychoanalysis. The focus in *Studies of Hysteria* is primarily on the scientific analysis of the mind. It is less a patient's, or even a doctor's story than a great adventure story, a heroic account of the exploration of uncharted territory, the story of the discovery '...of a succession of obstacles that have to be overcome' (Strachey 1955: 35) in exploring the unconscious. Out of this psychoanalysis evolved the method of free association, which depended on the patient's spontaneous outpourings which psychoanalysis transmuted through the mechanisms of transference and interpretation. The technology of psychoanalysis became the end, not the human story on which this operated. Indeed, in his letters to Fliess, Freud expressed concern that his case studies were not sufficiently scientific (see Roberts 2000: 432).

Today, the case history is little more than a form of natural history, for there is, as Oliver Sacks observes, little or nothing of the human being to be found in it. The subject, her/his unique life story, the personal battle to cope with, survive and recover from illness, plays little or no part in the modern case history. We might as well be talking about laboratory animals. As Sacks puts it:

> To restore the human subject at the centre—the suffering, afflicted, fighting, human subject—we must deepen a case history to a narrative or tale: only then do we have a 'who' as well as a 'what', a real person, a patient, in relation to a disease—in relation to the physical. (Sacks 1985: x)

The ubiquitousness of impersonal scientific and technological medicine over the last 50 years has been at the expense of a richly descriptive and humanistic tradition of medical story telling that was an important feature of 19th century medicine. Stories become meaningful for us through our ability to identify with the dilemmas and experiences represented in the lives of the characters portrayed. This act of identification with other human beings, in suffering, in illness, is of fundamental importance to the ethical aspects of narrative in medicine. Sacks' own richly descriptive case histories exemplify this. He points out that his neurological patients assume prominent archetypal roles—heroes, victims warriors and martyrs, but they become something more. There is a fabulous quality to their worlds that *compels* him to write in terms of 'tales and fables as well as cases'. He invites us to stand in awe[1] and wonder at the lives he describes. This is an important aspect of Sacks' book. He invites us into an ethical space in relating to illness, one that should also be a feature or our clinical encounters with our patients. We are drawn to illness not with fear, nor with the objectifying gaze of science, but with the sense of wonder that might be evoked by the Shaman.

The case history, narrative, and the medical model

It is quite obvious that our attention has been drawn from the tradition of case history and case, to narrative, but then the case history is a form of narrative. Robert Barrett's (1996) participant observer study of the 'schizophrenia team' at 'Ridgehaven', an Australian state hospital, yields powerful insights into the role of case history in biomedical psychiatry. Talking and writing about patients, constructing a story about illness is exactly what a case history is. But a 'case' is much more than an illness. It is also a way of constructing a person[2]:

> When a person is rendered into a case format, a particular temporal framework is invoked. The person is shaped into a 'case history'. He or she becomes an

---

[1]His use of the word *awe* is important for us. The meaning of the word originally implied terror and dread (*Shorter Oxford Dictionary*), but also carries strong spiritual connotations, as standing in awe of a Divine Being, or solemn and reverential wonder.

[2]Or perhaps, in the light of Bakhtin's work with which we end this chapter, a character, not a person.

evolving narrative that begins with genetic endowment and proceeds through each stage of the person's life—gestation, neonatal period, childhood, adolescence, adulthood—culminating in the onset of the psychiatric illness. (Barrett 1996: 13)

Psychiatrists use indeterminate knowledge in their 'construction' of case[3], and Barrett's description of this process is powerful. A 'case' has a deep interior core (in psychodynamic terms) and a temporal dimension extending back in time. Case space and time are the secret domain of psychiatry, which also patrols the boundary between body and mind, personality and illness. There is also a tension between objectivity and subjectivity, relating to the distinction between psychiatry as technology (medical model) and psychiatry as moral enterprise. On one occasion, a 'case' may be treated as an object without consciousness or intentionality. At other times, it may be seen as a person endowed with subjectivity and intentionality. Disciplinary institutions such as asylums constitute their subjects through narrative processes such as the interview, the examination, the entry in clinical notes, and the personal biography of the subject. Barrett demonstrates how these narrative processes are the means through which the institution exercises its power.

Written case notes play a particularly important role in these processes. Ricouer (1979; quoted in Barrett 1996: 108) points out that the meaning of a text lies in its possible future interpretations. Case histories are written so as to influence future readers' interpretations, which in turn determine the questions that clinicians put to patients. Thus arises a circle of writing and speaking in psychiatric narratives. The interpretation of written knowledge determines what was said, and the interpretation of what was said shapes what is written. Patients usually have no access to what is written about them, yet the clinician in interviewing the patient will have access to what was previously written, and will question the patient in the light of this. Barrett points out that patients adapt to this, and learn what is relevant in the circle of writing and speaking. In other words, this circle influences how patients articulate their accounts of their lives and their experiences. In addition, individual entries are aligned with past entries, so that what was already in the record is reinforced, through the cycle, by subsequent entries. In other words, the cycle results in patients reiterating a narrative that has already been established in the notes. Although superficially they appear to be active participants in generating a written account of themselves, the real power in defining the case lies in what is written in case notes by the clinician.

---

[3]Here he uses Jamous & Pelloile's (1970) distinction between technical knowledge, the type of knowledge that can be set down rationally and set out by prescriptive rules to be handed on to others, and indeterminate knowledge, which is much more a feature of the professional's biography and personality. Indeterminate knowledge cannot be codified and passed on in the same way as technical knowledge, and is very much a feature of medical knowledge. Medical knowledge, being by and large indeterminate and thus located in the characteristics of doctors, allows the profession to exert a monopoly over its field, and thus control and limit external appraisal.

Barrett compares an interview between a psychiatrist and a newly admitted patient, with the case records made by the psychiatrist of the interview. He shows that the complexity and great variety of meanings of the patient's narrative is truncated in written record in the notes[4]. This is achieved through a number of mechanisms, such as the use of closed questions to truncate the patient's account when it fails to fit in with the psychopathological framework of the clinician. Ambiguities are cut out, so that the patient's account fits the clinician's framework '...a stripping away of the lifeworld contexts of patient problems.' (Mishler 1984; quoted in Barrett 1996: 130). Patients make sense of their experiences through a variety of frameworks, including spiritual ones, not in the psychopathologically weighted categories of *Appearance*, *Behaviour*, *Conversation*, *Perception*, *Affect*, *Cognition* and *Insight*. This process reveals again the preoccupation of psychiatry with depth, and the distinction between inner and outer, and the nature of the relationship between these two. These headings, according to Barrett, fill out the 'depth dimensions' of the case, with the implication that what is situated deep inside operates causally to determine what appears on the surface. Barrett's work is valuable because it shows how narrative functions as a tool which psychiatry uses to shape the subjectivity of those diagnosed as suffering from schizophrenia. Narrative functions not to liberate, but to control, define and constrain. It demonstrates how narrative in psychiatry is 'constructed and transacted' to serve the interests of professionals.

Narrative, medicine, and psychiatry

Although the case history has played an important historical role in the evolution of our understanding of disease and illness, as well as providing evidence for the effectiveness of different types of treatment, evidence-based medicine (EBM) now dominates clinical practice. This reflects a fundamental shift in the profession's values over the last 50 years or so. The organizing principle of EBM is hierarchical (see, for example, Yusuf *et al.* 1998) in which meta-analyses and randomized controlled trials are seen as more 'robust' because they are believed to represent more faithfully some underlying objective 'truth' about illness and its treatment. In epistemological terms, this is, of course, a product of modernism in medicine. EBM is founded in a belief that there is such a thing as a single objective truth about the treatment of a particular disease. It relied upon the techniques of positivism, such as the development of statistical theory and mathematical methods grounded in this. Through its positivist roots, it also maintains a distinction between expertise and expert, knowledge and knower, a distinction that mirrors the Cartesian split between the subjective and objective we described in detail in Chapter 4. EBM in psychiatry has

---

[4]It is well worth comparing this observation with Mary O'Hagan's story which we referred to in Chapter 2.

created a space in which clinical practice is dominated by the elucidation of 'facts' by an expert about another human being.

EBM also represents an attempt at standardization, or, if we may put it this way, the imposition of the grey sheen of uniformity on doctors and patients. It strives to overcome the *differences* and *disagreements* that occur naturally between doctors, and between doctors and patients, in the course of the complex negotiations that constitute day-to-day clinical work. A good example of this is the notoriously poor reliability of psychiatric diagnosis. The process is now governed by criteria drawn up by international consensus. However, Sackett (a founding father of EBM) *et al.* (1991) argue that we should show more interest in disagreements between clinicians rather than trying to make them disappear as if by magic. Disagreements reflect our different views of the world, our different perspectives. They originate in the subjectivity of individual clinicians, and in clinical settings they say a great deal about the profound uncertainties and ambiguities that lie at the heart of all human encounters. Thus we would argue that disagreements between professionals about treatment, or how best to handle a clinical problem, primarily relate to problems of interpretation. In other words, they are disputes about the meaning and significance of human encounters, about what stands out and makes sense for us. We can see now where this is leading us. What takes place in clinical encounters between doctors and patients may be seen as a form of narrative. A patient tells a story; a doctor listens and makes an interpretation. In this case, the interpretation may be a medical history or a diagnosis but, as Greenhalgh (1999) points out, this is narrative because the act of interpretation and the creation of meaning is a fundamental feature of narrative. We know this from studies in literary criticism, and we shall see later that there is much to be gained from examining clinical work from this perspective.

A great deal has been written of late about the distinction between EBM and narrative-based medicine (NBM), but there is one thing worth highlighting[5]. EBM moves us from the general to the particular. The statistical and mathematical processes involved in randomized controlled trials and meta-analyses, for example, consist of stripping away the particular and rendering the individual without identity and human uniqueness. This has to be so to make it possible to reduce the complex human experience of illness to the bare essentials, so that these crude signifiers may be pooled and operated on mathematically. What matters in such an approach is not the individual, but the idealized outcomes of hundreds and thousands of individuals. Out of this, we develop generalized notions of effectiveness, widely suited to the greatest number. NBM operates in the opposite direction. It begins with the particular, indeed it may never leave it. Its primary concern is the uniqueness of each human being, the details of life history and circumstances,

---

[5]What follows is one way of describing the difference between nomothetic and ideographic approaches to research in medicine.

and reactions of joy, despair, hope and tragedy that arise in human responses to illness.

In practice, the boundaries between EBM and NBM are fluid and not sharply defined. But there is a growing awareness of the limitations of EBM, and a realization that we must pay more attention to the values attached to different treatments from patients' perspectives (Faulkner and Thomas 2002). What point is there in knowing which is the most effective drug for the treatment of an illness if we are blind to the subjective effects of medication, issues such as side effects, and subjective effects on well-being, that influence whether patients are likely to take the drug? There is a strong case for the integration of the two approaches (Reis *et al.* 2002).

From our perspective, the real value of narrative in medicine and psychiatry is its potential to contextualize practice. We agree with Greenhalgh & Hurwitz (1999) who point out that all illness can be considered in terms of narratives that are located within the wider narratives of people's lives. They argue that the use of narrative in clinical settings results in a more holistic approach to the person's problems, and a means of dealing with the existential significance of illness.

However, there are also serious difficulties here, not the least of which concerns what we mean by narrative. So far, we have used the word loosely, but we have to be more specific if we are to argue the case for the way we use narrative in this book. Brown *et al.* (1996) point out that in general, clinicians' understandings of what narrative is tend to be much broader than definitions of narrative formulated by academic socio-linguists. Here, we want to make a not too rigid distinction between what we regard as the largely practical activity of NBM (i.e. understanding day-to-day clinical practice in terms of the processes of story telling, in negotiating understandings and meanings of illness), and medicine as narrative (i.e. largely conceptual explorations of medicine as a narrative form in its own right, which includes the overlap between medicine and other forms of literary narrative, and especially the ethical implications of understanding medicine as narrative). The former is hands on, engaged with the world of patients, illness and practitioners. The latter is reflexive and critical. It involves clinicians and non-clinicians, especially those with a background in literature and the humanities. It is particularly interested in the way doctors' accounts of illness stand in relation to other accounts. We will see that it can make useful contributions to critical perspectives on the former.

Narrative-based medicine

General practitioners (GPs) have been at the forefront of NBM in recent years. In part, this may be understood as an attempt to re-assert the unique role of the GP within our culture as a healer rather than a doctor, a tradition that is threatened by the domination of technologies such as EBM. Some psychiatrists, too, especially those working in psychotherapy, child and family psychiatry and primary care, have written about the value of narrative in their clinical work.

Launer (1999) points out that in practice, adopting a narrative approach means setting aside the view that there is a single 'truth' which has to be either the doctor's or the patient's. It is no longer possible to maintain the view that the talk that takes place between doctor and patient is a means of revealing previously hidden truths about the patient's life. He suggests that narrative serves the purpose of exploring and developing 'better' stories.

For Holmes (2000), narrative is a central feature of clinical practice in psychiatry and psychotherapy, and is a particularly important aspect of history taking, formulation and engagement. When we take a history, we construct a story from a sequence of seemingly unrelated events. We encourage our patients to become the authors of their own stories, and in doing so we start from a position of puzzlement similar to that we experience when we begin reading a novel. In this clinical sense, narrative:

> ...leads the listener deeper and deeper into the causal chain of events—both intentional and non-intentional—which underlie the presenting problem. (Holmes 2000: 94)[6]

Glenn Roberts (2000) makes some valuable points in his paper on the use of narrative in rehabilitation psychiatry. He describes a journal club in which two editorials from the journal *Evidence Based Medicine* were presented alongside Trisha Greenhalgh's short story about a GP reluctantly called out to attend an elderly dying woman, *The Conker Tree*. The story provides no evidence for the effectiveness of different ways of managing terminally ill patients, but generated a reflective discussion in which those present spoke in personal terms about the things that mattered to them. In other words, the story focused participants' attention on values, especially the importance of being more in touch with people's lives. He also points out that the use of narrative in psychiatry results in plural, not single, truth. The patient's story and medical interpretation of this in the form of the case history co-exist independently.

Again, we find ourselves in partial agreement with this. The difficulty is that not all narrative does convey plural truth. Barrett's work demonstrates very clearly how narrative in mainstream biomedical psychiatry closes down truth and meaning, presenting a single view. The critical point for us in this chapter is to explore this issue, and in particular understand how narrative can either open up or close down meaning. At the end of this chapter, we will argue that the ideas of Mikhail Bakhtin can assist us in this task.

Medicine as narrative: towards a new ethic

In its simplest form, a narrative is a story, and is found in novels, short stories, adverts, photography, film and television. Jones (1997) draws our attention to

---

[6]We would take issue with the implication here that narrative is best approached through the notions of causality and 'chains of events'.

the growing interest in medicine and narrative, which in her view covers a wide area, from the work of doctors as writers and poets, the application of insights from literary criticism to our understanding of medical ethics, and the features of different genres of medical writing. Of particular importance in our view is the recent convergence of narrative and ethics. Jones comments that this is because medical knowledge and practice are, as we have seen, essentially narrative in nature. McLellan (1997) describes three types of literary narratives in medicine. First is the extended case history that we have already encountered in the work of Freud and Sacks. Next is what she describes as a hybrid form, a mixture of imagination and experience in which fact and fiction are combined. A good example of this is the story 'The case of George Dedlow', by the American neurologist Weir Mitchell (1915) in which he describes the psychological trauma of having all one's limbs amputated, and the altered sense of self that ensues. Another example is the work of Richard Selzer, whose writing also takes us into the grey area between the factually based case history and fiction[7]. Finally, McLellan refers to fiction written by writers who have had medical training. Examples here include Chekhov, Somerset Maugham, A.J. Cronin and Sir Arthur Conan Doyle. She makes the interesting and important point that narrative is the most important link between being a physician and a writer. She describes the commonality as follows:

> Both are engaged in an often complex process of identification with and detachment from their subjects—close enough for compassion, both distanced enough for critique. And both are involved in making meaning of experience, in ways they may not even fully understand. Formulating a diagnosis, like constructing a text, can be a complicated task, involving experience, intuition, and interpretation. (McLellan 1997: 566)

She suggests that the fundamental tasks of clinical medicine, history taking, making a diagnosis and presenting a history have much in common with the processes of story telling found in novels and short stories.

This is fine to a point. But we believe that there are shortcomings with the position of those such as McLellan, Greenhalgh and Holmes, who draw analogies between the practice of medicine and narrative. In particular, recent work in anthropology and philosophy raises difficult issues for those who see their work in terms of story telling, or who, like ourselves, aspire to tell stories about their work. In our view, these issues concern whose perspective matters or, more accurately perhaps, whose interpretation really counts. This is pre-eminently an ethical matter because it involves the use (or abuse) of power. This matter is fundamental to our view of narrative in clinical or research situations, or in academic texts such as this. Any attempt to use narrative without taking these points into account is deficient.

---

[7]Selzer's work is arguably better described as case stories rather than case histories.

Critical perspectives on narrative in medicine

> The Enlightenment is dead, Marxism is dead, the working class movement is
> dead and the author does not feel very well either. (Smith 1992)

Thinking about the practice of medicine and psychiatry through the eyes of
narrative is seductive. Whilst we would not argue with the proposition that -
narrative in medicine is a powerful antidote to positivism, all narrative
approaches should carry a government health warning. They have their own
risks and pitfalls, and it is vital that we now examine these in some detail.

Truth, representation, and the Other

Barrett's empirical work has strong affinities with recent critical conceptual
critiques of narrative in medicine. The critique of Brown *et al.* (1996) highlights the epistemological assumptions of much of the work that has been
written on narrative in psychiatry. It deals with what we would call the power-
shaping activities of narrative, especially the editorial role of therapists and
psychiatrists, and the related matter of the culturally available discourses that
are available for clients to understand their problems[8]. In addition, they point
out that there are many different ways of understanding how narrative operates in therapy, some of which have more in common with foundationalist
cognitivism than with what we would regard as a hermeneutic approach. An
example of this is Wigren's (1994; quoted in Brown *et al.* 1996) work on the
narrative processing of trauma, which identifies the role of narrative in therapy as the location of 'incomplete' narratives in the individual's mind that
require 'processing'.

Brown *et al.* invoke the concept of genre as a means of understanding how
psychiatric languages operate. Genre is a literary concept used to describe the
language styles that are understood by members of a professional or academic
community. They are highly structured, with particular constraints imposed
on who may contribute, how, for what purpose and in terms of the form the
communication may assume. Members of professional communities use these
constraints for private purposes (Bhatia 1993; quoted in Brown *et al.* 1996).
In other words, within professional narratives, genres serve the purpose of
maintaining professional power and control. Thus, as Barrett has shown, the
narrative and textual processes of psychiatry, history taking and writing, case
presentation and the use of case histories are important parts of these processes
of control and exclusion.

Thus far, our concern with narrative has overlooked the role of the author.
Postmodernism has resulted in an acute self-consciousness about the position

---

[8]This particular aspect of narrative we have already considered in some detail in Chapter 3 in
which we considered the work of Foucault, the power of psychiatry to *create* subjectivities, and
the idea of technologies of self. For this reason, we will not go into this here.

of the author. When we describe patients, or write about them in the processes of clinical narrative, we do so believing in our own neutrality. It is as though the patient, the 'Other' about whom we write, is described from a disembodied view suspended outside time and space, what Haraway (1988) has described as 'the God trick'. The supposedly 'neutral' features of academic and clinical writing in psychiatry, which is stylistically detached and objective, purports to tell the truth, but it hides the identity of a narrator who is telling a story about someone else. In psychiatry, that someone else will be drawn from a marginalized and excluded group—mental health service users, women, members of our Black and minority ethnic communities, and so on. Brown *et al.* point out that the genre of scientific psychiatry restricted to clinical settings of out-patient and in-patient is an important element in the process of 'othering'. As a result, we fail to see the person as a contextualized being whose life is meaningful in worlds outside the clinical setting[9]. The assumption here is that:

> ... knowledge is not neutrally describing the 'patient' but that it is created by and interacts with other kinds of social business which is being conducted in the clinical or research context. Indeed, there is some suggestion that the very categories of 'patient' and 'clinician' are afforded and sustained by this social interaction. (Brown *et al.* 1996: 1574)

Brown *et al.*'s critique is helpful, but it only takes us so far. In our view, there are more fundamental problems with narrative. Let us assume for the moment that we are fully aware of the power that narrative has, in clinical settings, to shape, define and control the experience of others as Barrett so vividly illustrates. We would like to believe that this is not how the narrative of postpsychiatry functions. We would like to see it as an emancipatory narrative, one that creates an ethical space in which people can safely explore their own understandings of their experiences, that foregrounds patients' narratives. Let us assume for the sake of argument that it manages to achieve all this (we are certainly not making these claims), and that we want to write about it, to describe it. We would thus write our own account of our work with patients. We might do this in a number of ways. For example, we might write about

---

[9]It is worth briefly considering the nature of narrative in academic psychiatry to make this point more clear. Some years ago, one of the current writers (P.T.) was co-author of a scientific paper describing the pedigree of a Welsh hill-farming family in which those family members who suffered from Darier's disease (a rare, genetically transmitted skin condition) were also afflicted with affective disorder (Craddock *et al.* 1994). The purpose of the paper was to point to a new genetic locus for affective disorder. To do so, the authors had to conform strictly to the house style of the journal, *The British Journal of Psychiatry*. The genre of academic psychiatric discourse, with its insistence upon brevity and a particular style of writing, for example the use of impersonal agentless passive sentence structures, imposes major limitations on what can and cannot be said. Thus only the sketchiest outlines of the lives of the family members was possible, and it was impossible to say anything at all about the socio-historical context in which individual members of the family, as Welsh hill-farmers, lived their lives at the time the study was written. This served to emphasize the importance of biological factors in depression at the expense of social and cultural factors that made the mental health problems of family members understandable.

a series of cases we were involved with. Let us for the moment set aside the obvious practical difficulties that this would entail; how we would identify suitable 'cases', their representativeness of our work as a whole, the basis on which we would select them, the problems of consent and confidentiality, and so on. Let us say that we were able to overcome each and every one of these problems, and presented in this book a series of stories—a collection of clinical narratives that represented postpsychiatry. Is this really what we would have? How true a representation of postpsychiatry would these narratives be? How would we know that they genuinely reflected what happens in our clinical work? The answer to these questions is that we have no way of knowing the answers because the questions concern the problem of writing, representation and interpretation. This problem has figured prominently in recent debates in film studies, art and anthropology. Although the medium of expression is different, the problem of representation and narrative is a crucial aspect of modern aesthetic and literary theory. Here it concerns the position of the subject of study, whether in writing, in painting, photography, or for that matter in film, and particularly the power relationships that exist between representee (the subject who is represented), the representer (artist, photographer, writer) and audience. Our position is that the problem of writing about our work is a complex ethical one that can best be understood through recent work in aesthetic theory and anthropology.

Representation and complexity in art and anthropology

The ethics of representation are complex as can be seen in the response of the Black gay writer and critic Kobena Mercer to the White photographer and artist Robert Mapplethorpe's portrayal of Black male nudes[10]. Initially, Mercer's response to Mapplethorpe's work was an angry rejection of the artist's objectification of his subjects. However, in his later readings of this work, he (Mercer 1992) argued that to interpret Mapplethorpe's work simply in terms of the objectification of Black men by White men overlooked a degree of mutuality and complicity between subjects and photographer. As long as he (Mercer) maintained his position of power and authority as a Black critic, he was only able to see the subjects of Mapplethorpe's photographs as disempowered Black male objects. In other words, the processes of representation and our relationships as portrayers, subjects or objects of portrayal, and interpreters of portrayals are ambiguous and uncertain. They also shift depending upon the position we adopt in relation to what is seen.

A similar issue arises in different readings of Australian film-maker Dennis O'Rourke's controversial film *The Good Woman of Bangkok*. O'Rourke is well

[10]See, for example, http://www.mapplethorpe.org/malenudes8.html accessed August 4, 2004.

known in Australia for his critical documentaries about the baleful consequences of Western neo-colonialism in the Asia-Pacific region. In *The Good Woman*, he tells the story of his involvement with Aoi, a Thai prostitute working in Bangkok, after the break up of his own marriage. The film sets out how he became one of her clients, but then charts the development of their relationship through the process of making a documentary. In fact, 'Aoi' is not her real name (it means 'sweet') but is the one she chooses to use in the film. He documents aspects of her life, including her family, her work, her feelings about her clients, and so on. Towards the end of the film, she declines his offer to buy her a rice farm so that she may give up her life as a prostitute. Feminist critics have attacked the film as an example of patriarchal exploitation of women, but in doing so they fail to see the film as an attack on Western neo-colonialism, as exemplified by sex tourism. In aligning themselves with Aoi, their position is similar to Mercer's initial response to the representation of Black men in Mapplethorpe's photographs (Berry 1994).

There is uncertainty about the status of O'Rourke's film; is it documentary fiction, or fictional documentary? Berry puts it this way:

> It crystallises all the ambivalences in the film that the various positive and negative responses (to it) block; the ambivalence of being both artist and part of one's art; both documentarian and part of what one documents; both female and Western; both male and oppressive. In each case, failing to take on board both aspects of the ambivalence defends the legitimacy of a certain power. What may be more difficult to see is that these powers are defended at a price; that something is lost in this defense. (Berry 1994: 32)

This analysis is helpful. It draws our attention to a number of ways of interpreting O'Rourke's film, particularly the controversial manner of his portrayal of Aoi. Some of these interpretations are situated within contemporary debates about Australian identity in relation to colonialism and post-colonialism. These debates resonate with our own dilemma over our right (or otherwise) to represent psychiatric patients as others, and also how these representations may be interpreted. The point we want to draw out of these examples is the impossibility of addressing these issues without considering our own positions and identities as writers.

For our purposes, this analysis relates to how, through narrative, we might represent psychiatric patients in our work. For us to do so as psychiatrists means that we would constitute the patient as other, through the difference of madness and irrationality; historically excluded, devalued and oppressed. Barrett's work shows how psychiatric narrative in the form of the case history seizes the patient's subjectivity, twisting and moulding it for its own purposes. Berry's analysis helps us to see that the enmeshment of our own histories and subjectivities as white male doctors and psychiatrists, with the power and authority associated with this, makes it impossible for us to write about madness from a neutral position. This holds if we write a case history from a traditional biomedical position, or from the perspective of postpsychiatry. That in itself is not a problem; we can open ourselves up to criticism and become aware of our assumptions. The real problem arises if we believe or pretend that an awareness of our own assumptions entitles us to represent the other. As psychiatrists or postpsychiatrists, we write from an epistemologically privileged position of enlightened rationality. In presenting 'case studies' of our work, those about whom we write become objects to be known about by others.

Schwartz (2003) sees the problem of representation in terms of the objectification of the subject through the act of portrayal[11]. She points out that that there is a parallel here between this appropriation and the misuse and violation of personal narratives that can occur in qualitative research and NBM. Stories of suffering may be transposed, transformed and decontextualized to serve the researcher's purposes. Furthermore, the use of anonymity in the presentation of personal stories is a double-edged weapon:

> In research as in art it is the anonymity of the subject that erases the control the subject has over her own image. The moment a subject becomes the object of interpretation she loses control. Her identity is veiled either behind interpretation or research protocols which eliminate what is specifically hers in favour of attempted universalisation and generalisation. (Schwartz 2003: 63)

The point here is that representation is not a neutral act. It is not value-free. We shape the image (or account) we produce with our own desires, expectations and prejudices. Many qualitative researchers are now aware of this problem, and the difficulties posed by taking extracts from depth interviews with a research subject and using them out of context to convey meanings that were not in the original. Again we emphasize that in our view this is an ethical issue. What we

---

[11]Feminist critiques of representations of women in art point out that their involvement is restricted to the role of artist's model, the object of male gaze. Kelly (1987) points out that the character of female models is, through the male gaze, emptied in the interests of male desire. This is a powerful point. We have only to consider Gainsborough's *Mr. and Mrs. Anderson*, which portrays a man and his possessions (land, dog, gun, and woman). The model in Titian's *Venus of Urbino* is portrayed as a voiceless, characterless figure, an idealized male view of the female body. Her physical attributes have been taken over and controlled by the artist. According to Fisher (1987), this is a doubly violent act:

> 'Representation is double appropriation: firstly, the possession of the object by the image maker himself; and secondly by the spectator, who through theft and possession of the image perpetrates a further act of violence.' (Fisher: 322–323; quoted in Schwartz 2003: 64)

The argument of feminist artists, therefore, is to give the female model a voice, as a participant in art as a discursive practice. Consequently, the work of artists such as Hannah Wilke is concerned to present self as model, thus giving control over how self is represented in art. In doing so she of course challenges male ideals of body display and beauty. Her exhibition Intra-Venus chronicles the ravages of chemotherapy on her body as she undergoes treatment for the cancer that killed her (available at http://www.feldmangallery.com/pages/exhsolo/exhwil94.html accessed February 28, 2005). She photographs herself semi-nude, in poses that mimic Old Master portraits, but in ways that disclose the effects of treatment on her breasts, tongue, and hair.

think we present in the guise of truth and objectivity may be a travesty of this. Indeed, it is arguably more 'truthful' to be translucent about one's desires, expectations and prejudices so that they are absolutely clear. Indeed, this was one of Dennis O'Rourke's intentions in *The Good Woman of Bangkok*. Schwartz proposes a collaborative way forward, citing as an example the work of artist Christine Borland. Her work, *From Life* (http://www.gene-sis.net/ artists_borland.html), attempts to recreate (with the help of a forensic sculptor) the face of a skull used originally for educational purposes. The point here is an attempt to reconstruct the subject's unique identity from the anonymous and generalized. An important feature of her experience in this work was how much interpretive freedom there was in re-creating a face. On the basis of this comparison with recent development in aesthetic theory, Schwartz proposes collaboration between researcher and research subject[12]. But we disagree with the interpretation of Borland's work as collaborative. It was never possible for Borland to ask the person whose skull she used how they felt about their involvement in her work. If it had been possible, Borland's work would not have been possible in the first place. Her work is an act of re-creation, not one of collaboration, but it is no less valuable for this. Indeed, our argument is that in terms of case history NBM, we remain unconvinced that true collaboration is possible[13].

There is an interesting parallel here with an exhibition held at the New York State Museum in 2004 organized by one of the curators at the museum, with Darby Penney, a mental health official, and Peter Stastny, a psychiatrist. In 1994, when part of the old Willard Psychiatric Centre in New York was being demolished, a collection of nearly 500 suitcases was discovered in the attic of one of the buildings. Many of them were empty, but many contained personal items and possessions of former inmates, the majority of whom had since died. Stastny and Penney went through these items, old clothes, photographs, diaries and letters, in an attempt to piece together some of the personal stories signified by these possessions, by juxtaposing personal items against extracts taken from their psychiatric case notes[14]. One view of this work is that like Christine

---

[12]We would broadly agree with Schwartz as far as research is concerned. Indeed, the research methodology of action research has exactly such a collaborative intention at its heart.

[13]Neither are we convinced that the joint construction of narratives by patient and doctor, as Brody (1994, *vide infra*) suggests, shifts power. One of us (P.T.) has attempted this in the past in a published scientific paper (Davies *et al.* 1999) describing our work with Peg Davies, a voice hearer and a patient of P.T. Peg's narrative, in the form of her diary entries during the course of 2 week's intensive work on her voices, were an integral part of the work, and the narrative processes describing the work. In the process of writing the paper, Peg had full editorial control and used this to good effect, but the paper could not honestly be described as co-authored. This is because it was primarily written for the technical purpose of demonstrating a way of helping people who hear voices, and illustrating the value of a dialogical approach to understanding human experience. We might say, therefore, that Peg's role in writing was as the subject of the study, a role that is analogous to the patient who willingly consents to examination by medical students under the eye of the consultant.

[14]At the time of writing, this fascinating and moving project has not been written up. Further information is available at http://www.nysm.nysed.gov/press/2004/willard.html accessed on February 28, 2005.

Borland's work, it is not a collaborative act. The Willard patients gave no consent to the inclusion of their personal material and case histories in the exhibition, even though their identities are not fully revealed (only first names are used). However, another way of looking at the project is as an act of remembrance for lives wasted and lost in the old asylums. In this sense, we may see it as an act of reparation. The creative processes involved in respectfully imagining another's life, a life that in its time was seen as valueless and meaningless, are transformative, and call to mind the Edward Albee quote at the head of this chapter.

Over the last 20 years, anthropology has also had to confront the problem of representation as part of what has been called the crisis of ethnography. This has much in common with the way we see the problems of narrative in medicine. Some anthropologists have expressed concern about the authority of Western academics to write about non-Western people, given the historically and culturally contingent nature of cultural representations, and the history of colonialism. Of particular importance here are Edward Said's (1978) insights about the way that cultural representations of the Orient are textualized in Western literature. As part of the legacy of colonialism, Western culture confers on the Other its own identity, but does so from a position of power and authority, a perspective from which it can gaze without being seen. Writing and the creation of texts are central aspects of the work of anthropologists. Anthropology, like medicine, is part of a range of linguistic and historical practices that constitute culture, and both disciplines are open to postmodern questions about authority and authorship. Narratives in ethnography and medicine (such as case histories) both masquerade as fact, things that are heard in dialogue or written down as text. In anthropology, the traditional divisions between biological anthropology, archaeology, social anthropology and linguistics have largely disappeared, and there is no longer a sense of a coherent unified approach to the subject. The forces that have wrought these changes were described in a series of essays, based on seminars at the School of American Research in Santa Fe in 1984, published under the title *Writing Culture*. As a result of the crisis of representation, anthropology is now fragmented as a discipline, and draws on literary criticism, cultural history, semiotics, hermeneutic phenomenology and psychoanalysis (Clifford 1984).

Our infatuation with the author has blinded us to the extent to which texts are put together from many different accounts. We think of authorship in terms of a single voice speaking knowledgeably, truthfully, authentically. The power relationship between writer and subject may become a microcosm of the wider socio-historical power relationships embedded in colonialism; 'They are constituted . . . in specific historical relations of dominance and dialogue.' as Clifford has put it (Clifford 1988: 23). He points out that a classical anthropological account of Sioux culture was constructed from dozens of sources, including field notes, personal accounts of ritual and autobiographies. The question— who writes—is inescapable here, with the result that the ethnographer no longer has unchallenged authority to bring tradition, culture and custom into a written form. The same question may be asked of NBM. When we write a case history we draw on many sources—the patient, the family, employer, teacher, GP and colleagues in other disciplines. Yet the case history, as Barrett has shown, emerges as though through a prism from these tellings and retellings, in which these multi-hued sources are refracted back into the pure, monological white light of the authoritative medical case history. For us, the problem of narrative in medicine *is* that of the author. This does not mean that we must reject the idea of progress through a search for truth and science; it does mean, though, that we must build up our understandings of the world carefully over time, understandings sourced in many voices. Problematizing authorship means that we challenge the grounds on which one group or individual may represent or talk about another group or individual. This is particularly important when those who do the representing are powerful, privileged professionals, and those who are represented are members of socially excluded groups.

There is another aspect to this, for the way we understand truth, and the relationship between representations of the world (whether in anthropology, medicine, literature or art) and truth is closely related to the problem of knowledge and knowing. In the same collection of essays, Rabinow (1984) draws on the ideas of Rorty and Foucault who see the problems of representation as part of Western philosophy's preoccupation with epistemology. Since the Enlightenment, knowledge has been equated with internal representations of the world, and judgements as to the correct evaluation of those representations. Rorty puts it this way:

> To know is to represent accurately what is outside the mind; so to understand the possibility and nature of knowledge is to understand the way in which the mind is able to construct such representations. Philosophy's eternal concern is to be a general theory of representations, a theory which will divide culture up into those areas which represent reality well, those which represent it less well, and those which do not represent it at all (despite their pretence of doing so). (Rorty 1979: 3; quoted in Rabinow 1984: 235)

Rabinow argues that in the 19th century, philosophy was largely concerned with writing its own history, a history in which it saw itself as the arbiter of truth and reason. The 20th century saw a revolt, brought about (as we have seen) by the philosophies of Heidegger and Wittgenstein[15], who challenged the notion of knowledge as accurate representation, and in doing so shifted the ground from epistemology to hermeneutics, from knowing to interpretation. Rabinow's point is that even if we reject epistemology, as Rorty would have us do, this does not entail the rejection of concepts such as truth, reason and

---

[15]Rabinow also includes the work of the pragmatist Dewey along with Heidegger and Wittgenstein, but space precludes exploration of his work here.

judgement. We can, as Ian Hacking suggests, see truth as contingent upon prior historical and cultural events that set out the conditions we require to be fulfilled in order to decide whether a given proposition or fact is true in the first place. Hacking puts it this way:

> By reasoning I don't mean logic. I mean the very opposite, for logic is the preservation of truth, while a style of reasoning is what brings in the possibility of truth or falsehood. ... styles of reasoning create the possibility of truth and falsehood. Deduction and induction merely preserve it. (Hacking 1982: 56–57; in Rabinow 1984: 237)

Thus how we think about truth and falsity are social facts. Because the styles of reasoning we employ differ across our historical epochs[16], the conditions necessary for establishing the truth of a statement change with time. This way it is possible to avoid a relativistic free for all, or turning different ways of thinking about truth and falsity into subjectivity. However, there is a problem with Rorty, who, according to Rabinow, fails to account for the relationship between thought and social practice. This is where Foucault's ideas are helpful. Unlike Rorty, Foucault regards philosophical ideas as social practices. He sees the problem of representation as emblematic of a large number of related modernist concerns, especially those relating to order, truth and the subject.

The literary critic Terry Eagleton (1983) has argued that since the Enlightenment, science has restricted itself to the expression of transparent objective truth and facts. Rhetoric, fiction and subjectivity have all been excluded and consigned to the 'literary'. But literature and science are in any case transient categories. We are concerned here with a struggle, as Clifford (1984: 6) puts it, *against* the received definitions of art, literature, science and history, and to which we would add medicine and psychiatry. In literary criticism, the word 'fiction' does not imply falsehood or untruth. It refers to the contingency, partiality and incompleteness of any attempt at representation and interpretation, and it is this incompleteness that gives rise to the need for interpretation, and the uncertainty and lack of fixity inherent in interpretation. For this reason, we do not consider it possible to render a transparent and authoritative 'truth', or representation, of postpsychiatry by writing a series of case histories based on our clinical work. Instead, we have felt compelled to move to a variety of genres in our attempt to say something about postpsychiatry, the nature of which remains elusive.

The core project of representation, whether in literary fiction, art, cinema, ethnography or NBM, is the description of the other. The hermeneutic turn

---

[16]Ivan Leudar and one of the present writers (P.T.) made a similar point in *Voices of Reason, Voices of Insanity* (Leudar & Thomas 2000). Our socio-historical analysis of the meaning of Socrates' *Daemon* (in Chapter 1) involved analysing the implications of saying, as the French proto-psychiatrists Brierre de Boismont and Lelut did, that Socrates' experience was an hallucination. In other words, the meaning of saying that Socrates was hallucinating depended upon the historical and cultural context in which the statement was embedded.

means that there are times when it is necessary for us to divest ourselves of the protective garb, ritual and mysterious vestments of scientific (and philosophical) authority and objectivity, and write about our subjects as subjects. This means that like the anthropologists, we are engaged in a quest for different ways of writing. But at this point, we feel we are now in a position to answer the question we posed earlier. How can we know whether narratives open up or close down the possibilities for truth and meaning?

Narrative, ethics, and the problem of authorship

The critical question 'who writes?' that confronts ethnographers also confronts those of us interested in medicine and narrative. Bolton (2003) asks who speaks when we read? Whose voice is expressed within the writing when we write? Jones (1999) makes the point that narrative approaches to ethics in medicine make possible the formulation of the same questions. In our view, the ideas of Mikhail Bakhtin can help us in this task. According to Jones (1996), his work can also help us to be more sensitive to the position of the patient as Other. Although his influence in medicine has been restricted to medical ethics, our view is that his ideas have wider relevance, and may be applied to many aspects of narrative in medicine.

A recurring theme in much recent literature on medicine and narrative (see, for example, McLellan 1997; Jones 1999; Holmes 2000; Puustinen 2000; Kottow and Kottow 2002) is what has been called the multi-voicedness of literary fiction and the significance of this for narrative in medicine. Kottow & Kottow (2002) propose that literary fictional narratives provide a valuable way of counteracting the medical profession's '... rigidly unilateral description of itself' (p. 43). Puustinen (2000) uses Chekhov's short story *A Case History* to show how fictional accounts of illness open up the networks of relationships that give distress meaning. His analysis relies heavily on Bakhtin's work and, although it is beyond our remit to give anything like a full account of this, we will focus on those aspects that are specifically relevant to the problem of authorship[17].

Like many thinkers in the 20th century, Bakhtin, a literary and classical scholar, was preoccupied with the problems of language, and its organizational role in the 19th century novel. In *The Dialogical Imagination*, Bakhtin (1981) stresses the ineluctable cultural and historical nature of language. He refers to language not in a restricted, linguistic sense, but as an infinite variety of genres, stratified into not only dialects, but socio-ideological languages belonging to

---

[17]Bakhtin's work is immensely influential in literary theory and literary criticism, but it has also had very strong influences, along with the ideas of Lev Vygotsky, on what might broadly be described as discursive psychology. Wertsch (1991) is an excellent example of this. Excellent overviews of Bakhtin's work can be found in Holquist (1990), who translated many of Bakhtin's texts from the original Russian, and Dentith (1995).

professions, or to different cultural groups[18]. In other words, language (and language in the novel) reflects the infinite variety of human life. This great diversity of languages *is* our human condition. It is inescapable. It influences how as individuals we choose to use, interpret and experience language. Holquist (1981) likens this to two opposing forces, one centrifugal that separates out and stratifies all human differences as manifest through language, the other centripetal, attempting to impose an unnatural single unitary language on human reality. Centripetal forces find expression in languages that seek to articulate a single, absolute truth. They thus share much in common with the grand narratives of the Enlightenment (see Rorty earlier in this chapter) that posit a single, absolute truth. Bakhtin maintained that unitary (or what we would call universal) languages stand in contrast to the reality of heteroglossia (literally, 'different tonguedness' or voicedness) or the diverse nature of language as spoken and used in real life, in an infinite variety of cultural and historical contexts.

Bakhtin's ideas have implications for our understanding of consciousness, and particularly our awareness of difference. His view of language and consciousness originates in two people in dialogue with each other, in a particular place and at a particular time. He asks the question how do they organize themselves into an 'I' and an 'Other', and what role does language play in this? Thus Bakhtin's view is that language deals fundamentally with the issue of alterity. He points out that there is no such thing as a neutral language spoken in a detached impartial voice devoid of context. By virtue of the fact that we are embodied beings, we speak from a specific position in space and time[19]. Thus the act of perception is not a pure act, but one in which as human subjects we make of necessity constant judgements about what we see or hear. These judgements originate in our unique positions in culture and history. In his book *Problems of Dostoevsky's Poetics* (Bakhtin 1984), he uses Einstein's relativity theory as a metaphor for how all aspects of our being, our speech, perceptions and actions are bound to a specific position by virtue of our embodiment. He also contrasts Einstein's understanding of the Universe with Newton's.

---

[18]We are reminded here of Wittgenstein's notion of language games.

[19]Bakhtin uses the expression chronotope to explicate the infinite varieties of ways in which our position in space (culture) and time (history) contributes to the meaning of our utterances. But we use the expression embodiment deliberately here to convey something of the affinities that exist between Bakhtin and the hermeneutic phenomenologies of Heidegger and Merleau-Ponty. Both attend to the role of the body in specifying our unique location in space and time. The related issue of human finitude is as much an issue for Bakhtin as it is for Heidegger. In Bakhtin's view, the reality of our finitude contributes immeasurably to the uniqueness of the person. In my own consciousness, I am unaware of my birth and I will be unaware of my death. He argues that because the consciousness of the person has no fixed beginning or end, it is experienced from the inside as '...infinite, revealing itself only from within, that is, only for consciousness itself.' (Bakhtin 1984: 290; quoted in Holquist 1990: 165). Holquist points out that beginnings and endings belong to the objective world of others, so that from an external, objective position each person is unique, but this uniqueness is one of many.

Newton's view of the Universe was God's view, an absolute and certain truth predicted by Newton's mathematical model of the Universe. God authored by Newton. There could never be any doubt about events in the Universe because everything was seen and judged from the same viewpoint—that of God[20]. Time and space are seen as fixed and absolute referents for all that was, all that is, and all that ever shall be. In Bakhtin's metaphor, Einstein's rejection of the Newtonian Universe forces us to see time and space as relative, so we are all forced to make judgements about how we should choose our reference points in culture and history, in much the same way that astronomers now have to specify how our positions as observers alter the way we see events unfolding in the Universe. Holquist (1990) points out that both dialogism and relativity (albeit in different domains) can be seen as metaphors in human thought for dealing with the question of alterity. How do we understand our tendency to see people and events as different and distinct from ourselves, yet at the same time being bound together with us in time and space?

The concepts of sameness and difference are fundamental to how we understand identity[21]. Any concept of sameness must be posited in relation to a difference—a here requires a there, a then a now, a me a you. We have seen that the dialogical consciousness has no access to a pre-existing set of absolute referents, so we constantly have to make judgements about value in relation to the dialogical consciousness of the Other. This has important implications for our understanding of what it means to be a person, especially the distinction Bakhtin makes through his analysis of the novel[22], of the crucial distinction between character and person. This may be understood as a special case of the more fundamental distinction between 'I' and 'Other'. A character is a superficial, monological, fixed, unvarying and static category that may be assigned to describe generalized features of otherness. In contrast, a person is truly dialogical, an ever unfolding set of infinite possibilities, unfixed and dynamic, unpredictable and indeterminate.

---

[20]This has echoes of the magisterial male gaze, supposedly for all and but from nowhere, that Haraway refers to as the 'God trick'.

[21]It is worth referring back to O'Rourke's film here. For O'Rourke, any notion of sameness has to be posited in relation to a difference. He does this by looking at the relationship between film-maker and subject. O'Rourke's critics saw him as arrogant because they believed that he had forced his subject to participate in the film against her wishes. Aoi, as Berry points out, was complicit and accepted his stylized narrative of her experience. This problematizes the postmodern view of the author as all-powerful. A critical and reflexive self-awareness of our use of power is clearly important, but we must be careful that we do not deny the perceived subject's agency (again, see Mercer's point). There is a problem with reflexivity. We are privileged to be able to scrutinize our own positions, but this should not be an end in itself. The real world is one in which we are all bound in endless webs of power relationships.

[22]Bakhtin does this in his book *Problems of Dostoevsky's Poetics* (1984). In it, he describes how monological (or 'Newtonian') authors such as Goethe perceive the relationships between characters in their novels in terms of a unified development. On the other hand, he sees Dostoevsky as a dialogical author who portrays the relationships between his characters in terms of an endless series of struggles to reconcile their different positions and interests (chronotopes).

Thus dialogism has implications for our understanding of what is meant by the expression 'point of view', and again Einstein ventriloquates[23] through Bakhtin's words. Because there is no such thing as an absolute referent in time and space, there can be no such thing as an absolute point of view. Any point of view is by definition a point of view from somewhere. Any event is seen from a particular socio-historical position imbued with its own set of values, and must thus be understood in relation to an infinite variety of other possible positions, each bringing its own set of assumptions. Texts have their own (linguistic) means for separating different points of view, such as first, second and third person pronouns in grammar, or specific ways of delimiting the words of others through punctuations, or references so that we may quote from others. In fiction, these devices operate so as to ensure that the speech and actions of protagonists are marked off from each other. However, Bakhtin maintains that these devices are insufficient to account for the distinctiveness and indeterminacy of the person. The problem here is in part to do with the inadequacy of visual metaphor of 'point of view', or the aural metaphor of 'voice' to convey differences of relations between persons. For this reason, Bakhtin develops new metaphors such as polyphony and dialogism to convey the idea that what is seen or heard is a unique point in an infinite spectrum of possible positions.

So, what conclusions are we to draw from Bakhtin's ideas? Puustinen (2000) argues that multiple voices and perspectives make up narratives of illness, reflecting a great diversity of beliefs, values, convictions and fears. His arguments are made through an analysis of Chekhov's short story *A Case History*, but in our view Bakhtin's insights apply more widely to narrative in medicine, and should not be restricted to literary fiction. This means that we can think of doctor–patient communication in dialogical terms. Thus the danger with biomedical theory is that it can reduce the polyphony of doctor–patient communication to a monologue. Puustinen suggests that the incorporation of the patient's voice within a monological biomedical case history reduces the patient to a solely biological object. We would agree with this, but our examination of Bakhtin's ideas enables us to take this a stage further. Within the biomedical discourse of the case history, the patient functions as a character, not as a person. We have seen this already in Barrett's account of psychiatric narratives, and Sacks's plea to restore the human subject to the centre of medical narratives.

For us, the most important aspect of Bakhtin's work is his distinction between character and person. Medical narratives that see the person as the passive matrix in which disease takes place, fixed and static (or as 'voiceless objects', to use Bakhtin's expression), see patients as monological characters. The first danger in writing about postpsychiatry, the task of presenting 'evidence'

---

[23]We use Bakhtin's expression here to refer to how the words of one person may speak through those of another.

about the way it does or does not work, is that we fall into the trap of EBM, that we produce an account saturated with the pure white light of monological reason. One that is written from nowhere but everywhere, that stifles and suffocates difference. The second danger lies in writing case histories. That way we run the risk (as Barrett has shown) of not writing about our patients as persons, but as characters. This way does not stifle difference. Instead it controls it and misappropriates it. It presents difference as our own likeness (like God created man), as we would wish the subjects of our narratives to be. We present our subject matter not as living, different beings, full of contradictions for us, of complex, endless possibilities for *becoming*, but as one of Damien Hirst's dead animals fixed and preserved for eternity in formaldehyde, fascinating, grotesque, dead and commandeered, something that we gawp at in horror.

So, we have had to find a way of expressing postpsychiatry that acknowledges the dialogical nature of human experience; one that acknowledges that like our patients, we too are human beings with our own interests and concerns. This means that we must engage with the ambiguity, contradiction and uncertainty that are ineluctable aspects of human encounters and of otherness. In particular, it means that we must have a willingness to engage with the other's reality, to imagine those realities, to enter into those worlds without judgement or prejudice. We have left the questions 'Who speaks?' or 'What is postpsychiatry?' open for readers to interpret. We have tried to write about postpsychiatry in such a way that makes it possible to ask these questions in the first place, and not to disavow the endless possibilities of reply.

8   Meaning and recovery

The struggle against power is the struggle of memory against forgetting.

(Milan Kundera 1996)

In the last chapter, we considered the complexities of narrative. In this chapter, which is written in two sections, we try to consider the role of narrative in recovery. In the first part, we develop a theme that emerged in Chapter 6 concerning the cultural aspects of healing. Here we are particularly concerned with the role played by doctors, as healers, in the narrative processes that are thought to be important in recovery. In the second, we draw attention to the importance of narrative in survivors' experiences of recovery, especially the importance of having a voice and being heard. We juxtapose these two perspectives because we consider them to be related. They also disclose a deeper moral struggle, one that we had to engage with in a very personal sense in writing this chapter. Our position as clinicians is that we cannot remain neutral in the face of suffering, and our own complicity in suffering. We are writing here about a conflict that lies at the heart of our work as psychiatrists. It is only possible for us to understand the moral functions of recovery, which we describe towards the end of this chapter, if we are prepared to grapple with the contradictions and inconsistencies of what it means to be a psychiatrist. To put it glibly, we might say that another theme running through this chapter concerns the conflict between care and coercion that is a feature of much of our work. We want to explore this by first considering what it means to be a healer, but at the same time we must draw attention to the potential that healing has for harming those whom we think we are healing. We use the word 'healing' deliberately because, as the late Roy Porter points out (1997), its root relates both to 'holiness' and to 'wholeness'. People come to us with their lives in shards. As we shall see, the theme of 'wholeness' is intimately tied to the notion of recovery.

Many colleagues will find it hard to accept the perspective we adopt here. This is because it is very difficult to accept the idea that something you genuinely believe that you are doing for the benefit of others is not experienced that way. We draw attention to Gillon's (1985) point that the extent to which we have a duty to do good is contested. Our primary duty is to do no harm (*primum non nocere*).

In Chapter 6, we examined critically some of the assumptions that lie behind the use of drugs in medicine and psychiatry. We argued that to a large extent the benefit people gain from medication has less to do with science than it has to do with the placebo effect, less to do with nature than with human nature. The benefits of drugs such as antidepressants depend to a considerable extent on shared cultural understandings about the nature of suffering and healing, and particular features of the relationship between doctors and patients. We argued that antidepressants seem to be effective largely because doctors and patients generally want and expect them to work. Shared assumptions and understandings about mood and the readiness of mood to be manipulated pharmacologically are of great importance here. In other words, there are powerful non-pharmacological factors at play that influence outcome when people take medication. Here we want to explore these factors, whilst widening the scope of our inquiry to take in healing and recovery. What is it about human nature that helps us to understand how the placebo effect heals? And what does it mean to say that you have recovered from psychosis? Indeed, we shall argue that using the word recovery in this way is problematic. It implies a naive acceptance of medical explanations for psychosis. This is not the case; recovery is a complex phenomenon with many meanings. Personal and descriptive accounts of recovery share a great deal in common with the non-pharmacological factors that characterize the placebo response. The commonality is the social and cultural processes that constitute healing. Postpsychiatry involves an approach to human experience that transcends dualisms. We believe that this is essential if we are to make recovery a possibility. This means adopting a form of psychiatric practice that is grounded as much in culture and history as it is in biology and psychology. It is when we encounter survivors' personal accounts of recovery that we can really grasp the true significance and value of the hermeneutic phenomenology that we outlined in Chapter 6.

To begin with, we return to aspects of the origins of medicine to discover features that were important in those distant origins are just as relevant and important today in terms of healing. We then return to Daniel Moerman's work on the placebo, or meaning, response, which we considered briefly in Chapter 6. His work is helpful because it enables us to suspend our understanding of the placebo response between body and mind, and mind and society. In other words, it is possible to approach healing and recovery without having to come down on one side or another of these dualisms. His work also demonstrates the value of narrative in healing and recovery. Stories, whether about the power of the Gods or molecular genetics, underpin recovery. In the last chapter, we critically examined the role of narrative in medicine. In this chapter, we grasp the full significance of this, for we shall see that recovery only becomes possible when survivors are able and allowed to speak their own stories in their own words. It is vital that they are in control of the telling, and the meanings, of their stories. This ties in with the relationship between power and subjectivity that we developed in Chapter 3. So, another way of thinking about recovery is in terms of resistance and a struggle against the domination of subjectivity by what Nikolas Rose (1979) has called the 'psy' complex. We end the chapter by considering the moral implications of recovery through the work of the philosopher Susan Brison.

Medicine, magic, and meaning

To practise medicine is to dwell in that crepuscular region between the all-revealing light of science, and the dark ambiguous realm of human experience. It is to bestride C.P. Snow's two cultures. Since the dawn of civilization, healing has consisted of an uneasy mix of religious rite and empirical treatment. According to Roy Porter (1997), the Egyptian *Book of Wounds* contains 48 case histories showing that 4000 years ago Egyptian healing involved both empirical and religious elements. Cuneiform tablets from the library of Assurbinapal in Sumeria in the 7th century BC refer to seers who healed by divination, priests who healed through ceremonies of witchcraft and exorcism, and physicians who used drugs and bandages. In Classical Greece, medical texts were secular, but Greek society regarded healing as sacred. One of the most important figures in the origins of Greek, and thus Western, medicine was Hippocrates of Cos.

Hippocrates was born in the 5th century BC. He left behind a large body of writing, so we have a good understanding of the theory and practice of Hippocratic medicine. According to Roy Porter, Hippocratic medicine drew a distinction between medicine and religion, and forged an empirical basis for understanding disease and the practice of medicine through a natural philosophy. Hippocrates' view was that man is a part of the cosmos and thus subject to the same general rules that govern the rest of the universe. This provided the basis for an empirical and rational practice of medicine, by studying the workings of the body in its natural environment. Hippocrates is best known for the humoral theory of disease, and it is of course arguable that there is an affinity between this and contemporary neurotransmitter theories of psychosis and depression. Disease was to be treated according to rational principles, with conservative regimens of diet, exercise and healthy living. Drugs were used but only as a last resort; surgery was looked down on. In Hippocrates' Greece, a split developed between religion, healing ceremonies and ritual on the one hand, and empirical medicine based in rational theories of the aetiology of disease on the other. Despite its rational and empirical underpinnings, it is worth remembering that the Hippocratic Oath begins with the invocation of the Gods Apollo, Asklepios and Hygeia.

Marketos (2000) and Rynearson (2003) suggest that the cult of Asklepios continued to expand and flourish long after the school of Hippocrates, and that 'incubation', the healing ritual of Asklepios, served an important function for Greek citizens. Rynearson has examined anatomical votives taken from the archaeological sites at Epidauros and Corinth to show that the cult's rituals held a deeply meaningful, symbolic view of the body that co-existed alongside Hippocratic medicine:

> Our own rationalist tendencies and our conception of 'scientific progress' should not obscure the fact that the cult was not replaced or overshadowed by Hippocratic medicine but in fact thrived and expanded in precisely the same period and continued to be an extremely popular and important cult into late antiquity. (Rynearson 2003: 4; quoted with the author's permission)

He suggests that each votive represented a successful healing narrative that encouraged the re-telling of the story that led to its dedication. His account is redolent of the Grotto at Lourdes. The margin of the cave where the French peasant girl Bernadette Soubirous had a vision of the Virgin Mary is fringed with hundreds of walking sticks, artificial legs and arms, crutches and wheel chairs, all left behind by pilgrims in search of healing and cure. The prominent display of such artefacts and their association with healing are potent symbols of hope for each new suppliant or pilgrim. Writing about Epidauros, Rynearson continues:

> ... each votive is both a fragment of biography, as a record of the momentous occasion of that divine contact in the life of a mortal, and a *tekmêrion*, a direct proof of the power of the god himself. (Rynearson 2003: 8)

The collection of votives thus becomes a powerful symbol of the meaning-fulness of the ritual of healing, and symbolic of the healing power of Asklepios embedded within the cult. This meaning is collective; it is shared by all those who have set out on their journeys in search of healing. There is another symbolic aspect to the votives, for in representing a particularly important and charged moment in each pilgrim's story, they also mark a transition, a turning point on a journey. Specifically, they mark the departure from the temple and return to the outside world. Thus we can see that in Greece two and a half thousand years ago, healing and recovery involved a set of shared narratives that were expressed metaphorically in the form of a journey or a quest for transformation. In symbolic terms, the presence of the votives suggests that these processes involved relinquishing something, having to give a part of oneself up.

Rynearson's work on Asklepios is important to our purpose because it suggests that rational and empirical approaches to healing (in this case Hippocratic medicine) are insufficient in themselves. Human beings have always had a need to interpret the experience of illness in ways that transcend the material body. In addition, the process of narrative is a social and collective activity. The votive offerings at the sanctuaries of Asklepios indicate that healing cannot take place without belief systems that are common to those in search of healing and those who deliver it. Social networks are necessary to sustain those in search of healing. Healing is mediated through the shared symbols of ritual and ceremony. In other words, cultural processes are at the heart of healing.

William Halse Rivers Rivers made a similar point almost 100 years ago. In *Medicine, Magic and Religion*[1], he (Rivers 1924) describes the close relationship between the origins of medicine and religion in the cultures of the Melanesian islands. He points out that there is considerable overlap between them. For example, to predict the course of disease, the islanders resort to divine intervention. The rituals involved in the interventions they use for epilepsy are almost indistinguishable from those used in religious ceremony. Yet at the same time, the Melanesian islanders had sophisticated understandings of disease, and were not restricted to supernatural accounts or divine intervention. Throughout his book, Rivers draws attention to the links between medicine, magic and ritual, particularly the use of religious and magical ritual in prognosticating and curing. He attaches particular importance to the relationship between religion and medicine. He points out that our predilection for science and rational accounts of ourselves should not blind us to the fact that psychical factors, or faith and belief, continue to play a major part in the practice of medicine:

> As medicine has progressed and has been differentiated from magic and religion, this play of psychical factors has not ceased. Few can now be found who will deny that the success which attended the complex prescriptions, and most of the dietetic remedies of the last generation, was due mainly, if not entirely, to the play of faith and suggestion... If medicine is to maintain its hold on certain aspects of disease which should come properly within its sphere, it must find that it has much to learn from the priest... (Rivers 1924: 106–107)

This extract is significant as we shall see shortly when we consider Moerman's work. The 'psychical' factors Rivers refers to are of course the cultural referents that attend the practice of medicine, and the faith that patients have in doctors. Rivers' argument is that medicine cannot progress at the expense of faith. It had (and still has) a great deal to learn from the priest. If medicine is to take into account the cultural and social contexts in which it is practised, physicians must:

> ...overlap the function of priest... teacher, the jurist, the moralist, the social reformer. (Rivers 1924: 107)

For healing to be possible, we must appreciate the context and meaning of illness. Rivers pointed out that for physicians to function as healers, they must be aware that they are emulating priestly activities. They must be engaged with

---

[1] Rivers was a member of the 1898 Cambridge University expedition to the Torres Straits, as was one of the first medical anthropologists. It is worth noting that he was writing about other cultures at a time when the British Empire and colonialism was at its apogee. Nevertheless, his writing is relatively enlightened. He vigorously disagreed with Lévy-Bruhl, who believed that so-called 'primitive' cultures were irrational, and incapable of logical thought. Rivers (p. 49) argues that although Europeans would not accept the premises upon which Melanesian cultures based their healing practices, they contain an impeccable logic that ties their rituals to their understanding of disease.

their cultures. This holds an important truth about our role as doctors, and we concur with Rivers as far as psychiatry is concerned. He implies that we must reach out and engage with culture in its widest sense, in recognition of the complex relationship between illness, human life and culture. Many will disagree with this. They will argue that we have moved on from the dark days of ignorance and superstition. In the 21st century, modern scientific medicine grounded in molecular biology and genetics promises real *cure* based on rational explanations of disease processes, not *healing*. They may concede that ritual and meaning may have been important in days gone by, before the advent of modern science, but recent developments render such superstition redundant. We disagree. We take nothing away from the potential of science to cure, and the hope this brings, but meaning and narrative remain every bit as important in healing as scientific medicine. Today they stand alongside science and technology, just as the votives at Asklepios stood alongside the practice of Hippocratic medicine. Rynearson's point is well made; we should not allow science and technology to overshadow the importance of healing. Moerman's work on the placebo response shows just how important non-material influences are in healing.

The meaning response

These days, the use of placebos is frowned upon. Their effects are too unpredictable; they are difficult to justify ethically because their use depends upon deception (De Deyn & d'Hooge 1996). For these reasons, it has been suggested that their use should be banned (Hill 2003). Despite this, they continue to be used. Nitzan & Lichtenberg (2004) found that 60% of the doctors and nurses they surveyed in two large hospitals in Jerusalem admitted using placebos on at least one occasion a year. The great majority (94%) found their use to be generally or occasionally effective. They were given in a variety of forms, saline infusions or injections, vitamin C or sugar tablets, and for a variety of conditions, including pain and anxiety, insomnia, asthma, angina and labour pains. Most (two-thirds) of those who used placebos did so telling patients they were receiving real medicine. Commenting on this paper, Spiegel (2004) points out that most placebos are harmless, and that for many patients their use may represent a welcome, holistic alternative to the powerful toxic drugs used widely in medicine. He goes on to say 'That an idea, feeling, or relationship can have a real effect on the body is now well established.' (p. 927). This effect has been described in detail by the medical anthropologist Daniel Moerman.

In his book, *Meaning, Medicine and the 'Placebo Effect'*, Moerman (2002) describes how values, feelings and relationships are important in healing. He deals with the cultural significance of treatment, especially the meanings that are embedded in this for us, and the interaction between these meanings and the physiological properties of drugs. We overlook the fact that all our interventions, making a diagnosis, measuring blood pressure, giving medication, psychotherapy, even surgery, are laden with meaning and significance. These meanings are mediated by the rituals and symbols of treatment, for example the appearance of medication, whether it is given in the form of pills, capsules or injections, the colour of tablets, the dose schedule, the space and timing of psychotherapy sessions, and, perhaps most important of all, the personal characteristics of doctors as healers. Moerman shows how powerful the influence of such factors is on the outcome of treatment, indeed as powerful as their physiological or pharmacological properties.

He considers the medical act of making a diagnosis. Normally we think of treatment and diagnosis as being distinct, but logically related processes. In reality, the situation is more complex. Brody & Waters (1980; quoted in Moerman 2002: 25) report the case of a man who presented with recent onset of ulcer symptoms after his wife had returned to work. At first he denied a link between the two events, but when seen 2 weeks later he reported a reduction in the severity of pain. He had discussed the situation with his wife, who had not realized how lonely he felt. Discussing it drew them closer together, improving the quality of their relationship. Thus making a diagnosis was therapeutic because it provided the man with an acceptable way of understanding his experiences, despite the fact that he initially disagreed with his doctor's diagnosis. It made his pain understandable, and pointed a way forward. There is nothing new here. Perceptive physicians see this and recognize its importance every day of their lives.

If we place ourselves in the position of this man, we can surmise that what took place must have been complex. The doctor's diagnosis was not well received at first; the patient was 'very unhappy with it' (Moerman 2002: 26). But it appears to us that this must have triggered off a series of human processes involving the telling of stories. The healing arose out of the conflict between the diagnosis, the patient's response to this and the discussion that he had with his wife. In other words, it emerged out of the processes of story telling, the changing and shifting processes of negotiating meaning, especially with those in our lives who are most important to us. It seems to us that the processes of story telling and negotiation between the man and his wife were every bit as important as the making of the diagnosis. The point is that what is salient in healing is not simply the physiological action of a medical intervention, but the *meaning* of the intervention[2] and how we interpret this.

---

[2]In this case, making a diagnosis had a positive outcome, but the opposite can apply. Consider the cultural significance of the word schizophrenia. For most people to whom the word is applied, the privileged, rational meaning that the word has for psychiatrists is simply not relevant. In the spaces of popular culture in which we all dwell (psychiatrists included), the word is saturated with negative significations (Philo *et al.* 1994). It conveys no hope. Paradoxically, the privileged meaning of the word for psychiatrists deems that there is no meaning in the experiences that lead to the diagnosis being made. Diagnosis can work both ways; it may create the possibility for recovery and healing, or it may serve only to imprison a life in pain and suffering.

For this reason, Moerman prefers to call the placebo response the meaning response. The way he puts it resonates with Rynearson's account of the Cult of Asklepios:

> Much of the meaning of medicine, of the meaning response (and in the narrowest sense, the placebo effect), is a cultural phenomenon engaged in a complex interplay on the meanings of disease and illness. The modern triumph of a universalist biology tends to blind us to the dramatic variations in the ways that people experience their own physiology based on who or what they are. (Moerman 2002: 70)

The point here is that culture plays a far more important role in treatment and healing than we think. In psychiatry, so-called 'eclectic' approaches to assessment, such as the biopsychosocial model, tend to regard culture as an epiphenomenon, of little more than peripheral interest. Cultural differences tend to be seen as mere local variations, like the different spices in a curry, underneath which lurk the universal 'meat' of biologically determined conditions such as schizophrenia (Fig. 8.1). We disagree profoundly with this view of the relationship between culture and biology. Culture lies at the heart of those human activities that concern how we know, understand and make sense of things. We made this point in Chapter 4, where we considered the philosophy of Heidegger and hermeneutic phenomenology. Across the world, differences in language, history, religion, social and family structures, all these cultural differences, impose different meanings on our knowledge about ourselves and the world. As a result '... comparing one place to another we find significantly different fabrics of meaning woven from these different strands' (Moerman 2002: 72).

Moerman's work introduces some important ideas about the nature of healing, and the relationship between narrative and healing in particular. Treatment in

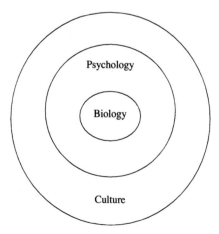

Fig. 8.1 The 'hard' biomedical model.

Western biomedicine tends to be seen as a passive process in which disencultured human bodies are acted on by powerful drugs that shape and change physiology. It assumes that biology and physiology ultimately determine outcome. There is no space for human agency and culture, all of which shape meaning and in doing so create the possibility of healing. Moerman expresses it this way:

> There is more to biology than biology. This isn't always the case (leaping from a sixteenth-story window ledge will not much be affected by desire, will, or culture). But far more often than we realize, what appears to be an 'obvious' biological matter is richly freighted with meaning, history, tradition, or the like; or requires consciousness to do its thing. Indeed, it is probably wise to assume that this is the case until it's proven otherwise. (Moerman 2002: 84)

His point has implications for how we think of the relationship between biology, psychology and culture, and the role played by all three in shaping human experience. In effect, this is a restatement of one of the key issues we dealt with in Chapters 4 and 5, the problems of dualism. So-called eclectic ways of thinking and working in psychiatry such as the biopsychosocial model (Fig. 8.2) recognize that experience is constituted through the biological,

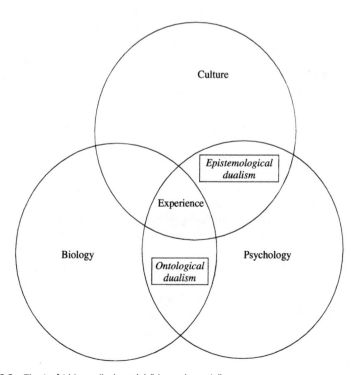

Fig. 8.2 The 'soft' biomedical model (biopsychosocial).

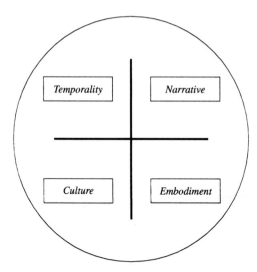

Fig. 8.3 Hermeneutic phenomenology.

psychological and cultural. The weakness of this model from our perspective is that it still posits separate mental, biological and cultural realms. The problems of dualisms remain, however, with the result that it is all too easy to become sidelined into reductionist and deterministic arguments about the nature of experience. The hermeneutic phenomenology (Fig. 8.3) that we proposed in Chapter 4 sees human experience as being indissolubly tied to culture and narrative, with temporality and embodiment. In this view, there are no separate biological, psychological or cultural worlds that exist outside human experience.

This view of illness transcends the dualism implicit in Fig. 8.2, and acknowledges the complexity and integrity of human experience. It recognizes the embodied, encultured and historically contingent nature of human experience, and at the same time places experience at the centre of our attention. This view has major implications for the education of doctors and psychiatrists, especially in appreciating the important contribution of the humanities and cultural studies in medicine and science.

Moerman shows that the narrative processes involved in telling stories are essential components of healing. He describes two features of narrative that are important here. The first is the ability to tell the story from different perspectives (polysemy), telling it from my own perspective, from that of my partner, from friends' perspectives, and so on. These new perspectives do not change the story, but from these re-tellings new meanings emerge. Secondly, many of the things that happen to us in our lives are beyond the abilities of simple causal explanations to account for. Consider William's story. His best friend, his father and grandmother all died within a matter of weeks. There is no way of explaining these events; they were purely stochastic. But in the face of events of such enormity, events that shake our basic assumptions about who we are and the purpose and meaning of our lives, we are forced to search for meaning in them. We shall return to the effect that trauma has on our grounded-ness towards the end of this chapter. William needs to tell his story to himself and to others, and to repeat this process over and over again, as part of his search for meaning. Each time he tells the story he has choices to make concerning what to leave out or what to include. Moerman points out that these factual omissions and inclusions are unimportant; telling the story is what really matters. At this point, we want to take forward these insights in relation to recovery and psychosis.

Recovery and schizophrenia?

Professional attitudes to psychosis in general and schizophrenia in particular are unremittingly negative. 'Abandon hope all ye who enter' were the words written above the entrance to Hell according to Dante in the *Divine Comedy*. They might just as well have been found inscribed on the title page of the National Institute for Clinical Excellence's (NICE 2002) clinical guidelines for schizophrenia. If we assume that biology (or psychology) is all that matters in helping people to recover from schizophrenia, then we are missing out on something really important, the transformative power of stories in our lives. We believe that nowhere in medicine is this more true than in psychiatry, and particularly when it comes to grasping the significance of recovery. To begin with, though, we must consider the various meanings of 'recovery', specifically in the context of schizophrenia. The word is nuanced. It has many shades of meaning. We want to stress that the psychiatric literature speaks of the unlikelihood of *restitutio ad integrum*, or a return to a state that pre-existed the ravages of a condition such as schizophrenia.

In Chapter 7 of his book *The Psychiatric Team and the Social Definition of Schizophrenia*, Robert Barrett (1996) examines the origins of the concept of schizophrenia in asylums and the first academic departments of psychiatry. He locates these origins within 19th century cultural preoccupations that shaped the concept. One is a literary–clinical concern with the contrast between the integrated/disintegrated individual. The other is a politico-clinical concern with progress and its obverse, degeneration. These preoccupations had a great influence on the emerging discourse about schizophrenia, and this is apparent today. It is found in the belief that schizophrenia is a condition that inevitably has a poor prognosis, and from which the chances of recovery (in the sense of *restitutio ad integrum*) are slim[3]. It is also found in words such as 'deterioration', 'deficits' and 'defect state', and instantiated in services whose purpose is to ensure the rapid and early drug treatment of young people in their first

---

[3] The evidence for this is contested. See Thomas (1997) Chapter 5, and, more recently (and more comprehensively) Alain Topor (2001), especially Chapter 3.

episode of psychosis to prevent deterioration. The problem here, as Glenn Roberts and Paul Wolfson (2004) have pointed out, is that these assumptions lead to low expectations for people who experience psychosis, and to '...erode hope and collude with chronicity' (Roberts & Wolfson 2004: 37).

We concur fully with Peter Barham's (1997) call for a debate about the nature of 'chronicity'. Are so-called negative symptoms and poor outcome an integral feature of the condition, or are they associated with the use of long-term neuroleptic medication and institutionalization? Are they, to use Barham's expression, fact or artefact? He describes the consequences of this for the 'schizophrenic' person as follows:

> In the traditional framework, schizophrenia is not so much an 'I have' illness, as an 'I am' illness, a condition which the person can be said to 'become'. If we ask 'who and what existed *before* the illness' and who and what persists *during* and *after*, one answer is that there is no 'after' with schizophrenia, only a 'before'. (Barham 1997: 93; emphases in the original[4])

This draws out the conflict in psychiatry between the person's subjective experiences of psychosis on the one hand, and the way this is dismissed by psychiatry. It is, in very real terms, a manifestation of the baleful impact that Jaspersian phenomenology has upon the lives of a great many psychiatric patients. In our view, we can best respond to the questions that Peter Barham poses through the Heideggerian framework we outlined in Chapter 4. Indeed, his questions have no value when posed strictly within the restricted phenomenological framework that has dominated psychiatry throughout the 20th century, and which seeks only to describe and categorize experience. But to take our argument further, we must consider the different meanings of the word recovery in everyday parlance.

Meaning *and* recovery

The *Shorter Oxford Dictionary* gives several meanings for the word recovery, three of which are currently in use. The most commonly accepted meaning is the restoration or bringing back of a person to a healthy or normal condition. This makes two assumptions, first that the state from which the person is recovering is not normal, and that the state of abnormality was brought about by illness. This raises the first problem. Throughout this book, we have repeatedly drawn attention to the contested nature of madness; not all those who experience madness accept that they have been ill, or that their experiences are to be accounted for in terms of disease models. So, if you do not believe that you have been suffering from an illness, it is not possible to talk of recovery in the sense of having recovered health after an illness. But there is more to it than that, because many

---

[4]Barham acknowledges the influence of Susan Estroff's (1989) paper on self and subjectivity in a themed issue of *Schizophrenia Bulletin*.

people who experience madness challenge the distinctions that are made between experiences that are considered 'normal' and those that are considered 'abnormal'. For example, in Chapter 2, we referred to Louise Pembroke's (1996) powerful account of how she understood and interpreted her experiences. In society, her experiences would be regarded as not 'normal', but she does not see it that way. She lives her life to the full, and is accepted by her many friends despite her experiences. Neither she nor her friends regard her as 'abnormal'. So, however psychiatrists might understand recovery, when survivors and service users talk about it they are not necessarily using the word to mean the restoration of a person to healthy or normal conditions.

This brings us to the two other meanings—the recovery of something lost or taken away, and a third, legal meaning—the fact or procedure of gaining possession of some property or right by a verdict or judgement of court. In our view, these two meanings bring us closer to the meaning of recovery in the sense used by survivors, and especially when used in connection with the recovery movement. Recovery from illness (in the medical sense) is an individual process. Illnesses affect individuals. But if we recover something that is lost or taken away, the meaning of this expression is thrown into the social domain. The questions that must be asked are what is it that was lost or taken away and, if taken away, who took it? Recovery in this sense involves something recovered from or through others. There is a powerful moral sense to this meaning of recovery. By virtue of the fact that something was taken away without justification, an injustice has been committed, one that must be acknowledged and rectified by others. The dictionary definition of this legal sense is that this may possibly be through a court judgement. In psychiatry, that which has been taken away is the right to talk about one's experiences in one's own way. It seems to us that it is this that is being reclaimed and recovered. There is a very powerful moral dimension to this meaning for survivors of psychiatric systems, one that is echoed by the voices that we encounter in survivor networks all over the world[5]. As we shall see, recovery as a moral project emerges as a powerful theme in Susan Brison's work on trauma.

For the survivor movement, recovery involves speaking out, the act of reclaiming language, or, as Ron Coleman has put it, having a voice. Without a language to speak and a voice to speak with and with which to make yourself heard, there can be no story and no recovery. Through social action, the survivor movement has created safe spaces in which individuals can start the process of telling their own stories. We shall return to this theme in the next chapter. The point we want to emphasize here is that the meaning of recovery in Britain (Coleman 1999; Faulkner & Layzell 2000; May 2000) and America (Chamberlin 1978; Deegan 1996) is very closely tied to the struggle of survivors to have the right to tell their own stories in their own way.

---

[5] 'We have the right!' and 'It is allowed to be different!' are the words written on the banners of the supporters of the European Network of (ex) Users and Survivors of Psychiatry (ENUSP; see http://www.enusp.org/ accessed November 3, 2004).

Personal accounts of recovery

Several survivors have written from the perspective of personal experience about the importance of finding or having a voice in the process of recovery (see, for example, Coleman 1999; Dillon & May 2002; O'Hagan 2002). Rufus May has described his recovery (May 2004) in terms of social and psychological elements. Social recovery involved re-establishing old and developing new valued social relationships. Psychological recovery involved integrating the experiences of psychosis back into his life, developing ways of coping with psychosis and distress, and perhaps most important of all establishing meanings and understandings of the experiences of psychosis. He points out that social and psychological recovery are independent of clinical recovery, and that recovery without professional help is perfectly feasible (he hasn't used mental health services since his early twenties). He also describes the importance of hope in recovery. Staff attitudes related to his diagnosis of schizophrenia had a devastatingly negative impact on his view of himself as an 18-year-old with his life stretching ahead of him:

> The belief held by hospital staff was that I would be powerless to influence the return of psychotic symptoms that could at any moment strike again. For me to escape this prophecy, it felt like wading through miles and miles of swamp. This was an incredibly lonely journey. I had no guides, no specialist support, no stories of success. (May 2004: 246)

He also describes (May 2000) how access to alternative positive stories about his past, present and future was important in his recovery. He recounts an incident in which he was playing pool with a nurse, who sang the words 'Maybe some day you will be a star'. He remembers the different ways in which he tried to interpret this seemingly innocent incident. Was the nurse being sincere? Was it a message that Rufus was a secret agent (a prominent aspect of his beliefs when psychotic)? Was the nurse trying to wind him up? Was it a message from the Cosmos that he could achieve anything he wanted? On reflection, he decided that it meant that no matter how bad things might seem, one day he would shine: 'I think that music must reach parts mere words cannot' (May 2000: 7). At that moment, he needed hope and something positive to believe in about himself and his future, and he found it in this serendipitous incident. Related to this is the importance of optimism in people's potential and abilities. He recalls an incident from his childhood where a teacher had said to his parents 'This boy will do well.'

Personal stories of recovery are revealing, but it can be difficult to draw out more general conclusions from them. Over the last 5 years, there have been five well-executed descriptive studies of recovery from psychosis (Topor 2001; Lapsley *et al.* 2002; Onken *et al.* 2002; Tooth *et al.* 2003; Thornhill *et al.* 2004). Table 8.1 summarizes the main features and findings of these studies. They were undertaken in different contexts, in Sweden, the USA, New Zealand,

Table 8.1 Summary of principal findings of five major studies of recovery

Study	Number of subjects	Subject identification	Methods	Main factors identified
Topor (2001)	16; 29–63 years; 'schizophrenia' = 9; 'paranoid psychosis' = 1; 'affective disorder' = 2; 'personality disorder' = 2; 'schizoid' = 2. Ethnicity not specified	Subjects self-defined recovery, and self-identified and included on the basis that they also met external criteria for recovery based on professional assessment of social functioning	Literature review. Depth interview by A.T., open-ended guide questions to elicit subjects' stories	Personal struggle with symptoms/existential problems. Maintaining relationships. Diversity of relationships (family, friends, professionals). Material circumstances (money, work, structure, medicine). Shared meanings (medical, therapeutic, spiritual, interactional)
Lapsley et al. (2002)	11 Maori; 10 Maori; 10 non-Maori; 9 non-Maori. Diagnoses not given	Subjects self-defined recovery from 'disabling mental health problems'. Not on medication. No service use for 2 years	Consultation with service user reference group. Pilot interviews. Unstructured interviews by psychology graduates (some of whom were mental health service users) to elicit subjects' stories	Learning from others, Emotional growth. Material circumstances (housing, work, education). Relationships (family, friends, professionals) and social supports. Virtues (self-management, spiritual belief, medication). Hope, Esteem, Agency, Transition in identity Several themes. Material resources (adequate income, housing).
Onken et al. (2002)	Interviews with 115 subjects in 10 focus groups from nine US States. Self-identified diagnoses: bipolar = 37%; depression = 36%; schizophrenia = 13%; PTSD = 12%; schizoaffective disorder = 11%; anxiety = 7%	Subjects recruited from nine State Mental Health Agencies to '...involve people who were at different stages of awareness and involvement in recovery...' using a purposive sampling strategy to reflect diverse experiences of services, gender, ethnicity, etc.	Exploratory, phenomenological approach using Grounded Theory in structured focus group interviews. Questions devised by research group with survivor experience.	Self/whole person. Hope, meaning, purpose. Choice. Independence. Social relationships. Meaningful activities (help and hinders). Peer support. Formal services (help and hinders). Staff attitudes (help and hinders)

Table 8.1 (Continued)

Study	Number of subjects	Subject identification	Methods	Main factors identified
Tooth et al. (2003)	57; 21–60 years. Duration of illness 2–42 years; 82% on medication. Diagnosis 'schizophrenia'. Ethnicity not specified	Adverts in local press. Recovery self-defined. Subjects only excluded if they were unwell, and if they had not met DSM-III-R criteria for schizophrenia in the past	Two service user focus groups. Discussions about recovery. Four-part interview open ended and semi-structured, in which subjects were encouraged to talk about their 'journey of recovery'.	Personal determination/struggle to get better. Finding own ways of managing illness. Recognizing need to help self. Accepting friends. Negative impact of medication. Negative impact of professionals
Thornhill et al. (2004)	15; 30–70 years; 'schizophrenia' = 7; 'schizoaffective disorder' = 2; 'affective disorder' = 2; 'psychosis' (n.o.s.) = 4; 'depression' = 2	Adverts/word of mouth. Self-identification and self-definition of recovery	Research team had personal experience of recovery/mental health service use. Open ended interviews to elicit 'narrative account'. Narrative analysis for genre, tone and core narrative. Subjects invited to comment on analysis	Escape narratives (e.g. hospital), tone of *anger* and *protest*. Enlightenment narrative (e.g. conversion, spiritual insight) tone of *protest* at imposition of medical view. Endurance narrative (struggle with the negative and loss of the positive) tone of *resignation*, *angry protest*

Australia and England, respectively, with a culturally diverse group of subjects. In total, 243 people have been interviewed in these studies, most of whom identified themselves as having recovered, although in two of the studies (Topor 2001; Tooth *et al.* 2003), additional independent criteria were used to establish whether subjects had recovered, in terms of either social function (Topor) or presence of psychotic experiences (Tooth *et al.*). Despite the heterogeneity of subjects in terms of culture and geographical location, we can see the emergence of common themes in these subjects' stories, these include meaning, struggle, supportive relationships and material circumstances.

Meaning is perhaps the most important feature to emerge in all five studies. Alain Topor's study provides the most comprehensive account of meaning, so we shall consider what his subjects had to say about this in detail. They used a rich variety of metaphors to describe recovery. These include journey metaphors such as a descent to the depths, travelling through a cold, isolated, desolate landscape, returning to places of warmth and fellowship. Other metaphors included a 'turn for the worse' and 'downward spirals', in which previously ordinary lives became extraordinary and problematic, eventually hitting 'rock bottom'. Then followed turning points, recovery and a journey back up. But there is more to meaning than metaphorical accounts of journeys, descents and turning points. Alain Topor describes how his subjects were active agents in seeking out meaning against a variety of contexts. He is at pains here to avoid imposing his own meaning on his subjects' stories (and thus falling into one of the traps that we described in Chapter 7) by using the categories his subjects use without reorganizing them. His subjects experimented with four explanatory models in their search for meaning; life history, medical, spiritual and social.

Not surprisingly, those who had been in psychotherapy interpreted their experiences in the category of life history. This involved telling a story in which difficult childhood experiences led to problems in adolescence, culminating in psychosis. Recovery took place over a lengthy period, and was realized through psychotherapy. Medical explanations were complex and shot through with ambiguity and ambivalence. For some, the medical model was important in their attempts to find meaning in their experiences, but none of his subjects used the medical model to explain what had happened to them. People described complex, ambivalent relationships with medication[6]. Some spoke of it as a 'necessary evil'; recovery was associated with the feeling that your life was no longer dominated by drugs, that medication had ceased to be an issue, even though some continued to use it. It was important to get the 'right dose' (i.e. minimal side effects), so being able to negotiate the dose with your psychiatrist was important. Most people in the study indicated that there was much more to the role of medication besides dose and side effects. What

---

[6]It is worth recalling here the ambiguities towards the role of medication expressed by subjects in the *Strategies for Living* project that we considered in Chapter 2.

emerges here ties in with Moerman's point about the symbolic role played by medication in a human interaction (or ritual). Alain Topor puts it this way:

> Many of the interview subjects who report that the right medication in the right dose has been an important factor in their recovery regard medication in a social–psychological context, as an occasion for human interaction . . . Other respondents raise the question of medication in connection with other important factors in their recovery process; primarily that of having a social network consisting of both family and professionals, but also medication as a complement to their own abilities. (Topor 2001: 216–217)

Again, this indicates that there is much more to medication than its physiological properties. The contexts in which medication is discussed, prescribed and monitored are just as important. The rituals of attendance at the out-patient clinic, greeting, expressing mutual respect, the communicative rituals of solicitations of progress, questioning, acknowledging, listening, agreeing, disagreeing, compromising and concluding are laden with meaning for both participants. We say 'ideally' because sadly there is evidence that the reality of psychiatrist–patient communication in out-patient clinics falls far short of this (McCabe *et al.* 2002). However, this should not detract from the value of properly negotiated approaches to medication in recovery. When it occurs thoughtfully and considerately, it allows doctor and patient to participate in an ancient ceremony of care-giving rich in symbolic meaning, and whose roots we described at the start of this chapter. Although spiritual meaning featured prominently in the recovery stories of many of Alain Topor's subjects, it was not important in providing explanations for people's experiences. However, in the New Zealand study (Lapsley *et al.* 2002), spiritual belief and practices were clearly important in subjects' recovery stories.

The fourth element in these recovery stories is a social one of interactions with others, something we have already encountered in the symbolic importance of negotiation around medication. In Alain Topor's study, people spoke of the importance of telling one's story to others, especially the processes of negotiation and give and take when listeners either accept or reject the story. One woman, who had been hospitalized for many years with psychosis, describes how her understanding of her experiences changed. At first she believed she heard voices because she had read a book about the experience, and that the voices had somehow become absorbed into her head. Later she had a brain scan. She believed the scan would reveal the person whose voice she could hear, thus proving her belief correct. When the scan was performed, there was no evidence for the existence of such a person, so she reappraised her situation and began to accept that the staff who had told her that her belief was mistaken were correct. Cognitive therapists will argue that this change in her belief simply demonstrates the importance of reality testing. But her account of the change in her beliefs defies such glib explanations. The change for her is not a logical, rational process. Her new understanding acquires an almost poetic, positive new meaning for her, in which the logic and rationality of psychiatric or psychological thought are superfluous:

> You've told me how your appearance has changed in the last two or three years. Have you changed in any other way?
>
> Yes. I have. My soul is red now. It used to be black. Everything is easier now. I can breathe. I can't explain it, but I feel happy. I'm satisfied with myself.
>
> Red is an intensive colour . . .
>
> I'm burning with a love for life. I accept life now. (Topor 2001: 198)

The simple beauty of this extract is that it reveals the complexity of recovery in relation to what might be called 'insight'. Although some will hold that the attainment of insight, or the recognition of the erroneousness and falsity of delusional beliefs and hallucinations, is all there is to recovery, this extract indicates that personal meaning, setting your experiences in the wider context of your life story, and an existential acceptance of self are infinitely more important, and transcend such narrow interpretations.

There is a drawback or limitation of looking at recovery as a narrative process. By focusing attention on personal testimony, we tend to overlook the role that other people have to play in recovery. We have seen, for example, that the empirical studies of recovery show that mental health professionals can either help or hinder recovery (see Table 8.1). At this point, we want to place the narrative approach to recovery in context, and the reality of that context for the great majority of people who use mental health services is one that is shaped by psychiatrists and psychiatric interpretations of madness. This raises for us important moral and ethical questions that can only be addressed by thinking of recovery as a moral project.

Recovery as a moral project

In her book *Aftermath: Violence and the Remaking of the Self*, the philosopher Susan Brison (2002) points out that most of us share in common the belief that we live in a just world. We want to believe that nothing that is either terrible or undeserved will happen to us. Yet our personal experiences of life, and our work as psychiatrists, certainly suggests this is not the case. Still, we struggle upstream against the current in maintaining this belief. In the face of trauma, abuse and random tragedies not authored through human agency, we cling to the belief that the world is a just place. But it isn't, and it is for this reason that some have argued that the acknowledgment of injustice should lie at the heart of recovery, and following on from that the possibility of bearing witness and of reparation. We argue that this has to be so if recovery, in the second and third senses of the word we discussed earlier, is to be possible.

To begin with, we argue that there are several parallels between recovery from trauma and recovery from psychosis. First, empirical work suggests that many people who experience psychosis have also experienced trauma. For example, vivid visual hallucinations are known to be associated with life-threatening stress (Siegel 1984). More pertinently, there is an association between sexual abuse and so-called borderline personality (Bryer *et al.* 1987; Westen 1990), as well as psychosis (Greenfield *et al.* 1994). Bernadine Ensink (1992) found that 28% of 97 Dutch women who had been sexually abused in childhood heard voices. Most of the women had had these experiences for years, and most of these experiences (85%) were indistinguishable from Schneiderian First Rank Symptoms. A review by Goodman *et al.* (1997) found that women with a diagnosis of schizophrenia had high rates of sexual abuse in both childhood and adulthood. More recently, a community survey of over 8500 households by Bebbington *et al.* (2004) showed that people suffering from psychoses were particularly likely to report the experience of sexual abuse in childhood compared with those suffering from depression or no psychiatric disorder. The point we want to make here is that there is a considerable overlap between the experiences and sequelae of trauma and abuse, and major psychoses such as schizophrenia.

In addition to this, many survivors of mental health services experience psychiatric interventions such as detention in hospital, restraint and forced treatment as abusive (see Chapter 7). Our colleague Joanna Moncrieff (1999, 2002) has described the barbaric and abusive nature of the physical interventions meted out in the past, in the name of psychiatric treatment. Even today, beneath the lab-coated garb of science and evidence-based medicine, we imprison psychiatric patients; we lock them up in hospitals, physically restrain them and remove their freedom. We inject their bodies with drugs against their wishes. We force them to undergo electro-convulsive therpay (ECT) and psychosurgery. Thus we breach the integrity of patients' bodies. We force into their bodies things and substances they do not wish to be inside their bodies in ways that ape the way the rapist breaches the integrity of his victim's body. Service users and survivors often talk of their experiences of restraint and forced medication as 'rape'. Of course, rape and madness are not the same. But rape often drives women mad (and some men). The purpose of our analogy is to draw attention to similarities between the two that can help us to understand the important processes in recovery, especially victims' ability to talk about their experiences, and the response of others. Both events mark out the person from the rest of society. The person is stigmatized. This is crucially important for the narrative processes of recovery.

In her book, Susan Brison interweaves her account of her experience of a brutal, murderous sexual assault in which she was left for dead, with her reflections on these life-shattering events from a philosophical perspective. She writes as follows about the importance of narrative and story telling in her recovery:

> By constructing and telling a narrative of the trauma endured, and with the help of understanding listeners, the survivor begins not only to integrate

the traumatic episode into a life with a before and an after, but also to gain control over the occurrence of intrusive memories. (Brison 2002: 53–54)

and

Piecing together a dismembered self requires a process of remembering and working through in which speech and affect converge to form a narrative. (Brison 2002: 56)

There are three themes in her book that are pertinent to recovery from psychosis: the importance of social networks, the struggle for justice, and the reconstructive and reconstitutive aspects of narrative. She draws attention to the limitations of language in speaking of trauma and suffering, in speaking the unspeakable when it comes to conveying to others what it is like to have survived trauma. This difficulty, of being able to name one's experiences, has much in common with the social position of someone going through or recovering from psychosis. It is only when we can attach words to our experiences that we can communicate with others, to make meaning possible for self and others[7]. She describes vividly the failure of those around her, family and friends, to acknowledge the horror of what she went through. This added to her inability to talk through her experiences. For the first few months following her assault, she received no letters or get well cards. Yet her friends and relatives were all kind, compassionate people who would have written to her had she had her appendix removed. The most important people in her life found it extremely difficult to share her pain and suffering. In this sense, she was socially ostracized in much the same way that people who use psychiatric services are.

In her book, she also talks about the struggle of fighting back. Social networks and social action were vital in her recovery. She joined a women's self-defence class to learn, literally, how to fight back. She points out that some feminist critics argue that one of the drawbacks of counselling and therapy for victims of abuse and rape is that they focus too much attention on the individual at the expense of justice, and the wider political and cultural environments that are responsible for injustice in the first place. Thus moral action was particularly important in her recovery. She became actively involved in political action with other women, by campaigning to promote the Violence Against Women act in

---

[7] We can understand the nature and implications of this namelessness through Heidegger's philosophy. One of us (Bracken 2002; see particularly Chapter 7) has drawn attention to the importance of Heidegger's distinction between fear (which is present in the world), and anxiety in which the question of being, or *Dasein*, has become threatening. Anxiety is the mood that reveals the groundlessness of the world, and the nothingness that lies at the heart of being. In addition, life-threatening situations throw us into confrontation with the indefinite inevitability of death. Anxiety draws us into relationship with our own death, highlighting the fragility and transience of the world and our solitariness and isolation in it. Our meaningful connections with the social world, wrought through narrative, are ruptured.

the USA. The point here concerns the importance of re-establishing a sense of meaning through a common cause and a struggle for justice shared with others. She may have been forced to endure the most horrific circumstances, but she took every action possible to ensure that no one else had to go through what she went through. This is part of a powerful moral quest for justice that resonates strongly with the psychiatric survivor movement across the world. One implication of this is that in order to help people to recover, we must engage with the wider society by standing alongside those who are oppressed and abused. We must bear witness to their suffering and use our position to draw attention to it.

There are more deeply felt personal moral aspects to recovery from trauma. Rape, and psychiatric assaults such as restraint and forced medication, remove the person's physical and emotional freedom, and the freedom to think about oneself in a particular way, or to believe in one's existence as a particular type of person (i.e. as one who has not been raped, or forced to take medication against one's wishes because of one's beliefs or experiences). In other words, we lose the right to define ourselves as human beings in quite specific ways. All this constitutes loss of autonomy. Susan Brison describes how the self that survives rape is different from that which existed before. Narrative plays an important reconstitutive role in recovery. Although she describes her life as being in fragments, she points out that being fragmented placed her in a position in which she had choices about the parts of her life that she could throw (or had to throw) away. This meant that she was able to rework, and create something new and better from the bits that were left over. This casts a slightly different light on Moerman's point about the role played by telling and re-telling in recovery.

Our work is centred on the stories that patients tell us. We are continually caught up in a skein of listening, story telling, narration and re-narration. But we stand on fragile ground, and in trying to help others we always run the risk of making things worse and causing harm. The danger is that we misappropriate the stories people tell us, that we deface them by ripping from them that which suits our purpose. How easy it is to obliterate the other when we do this, even though we consider that our intentions are for the best. We speak for you. We silence you (Brison 2002: 55). When we write in your case notes that you have schizophrenia, and we name you a 'schizophrenic', we take away your speech and your ability to name yourself, we obliterate you. The moral position that we must adopt is one in which we bear witness and resistance. To bear witness means accepting the reality of lives harmed and damaged by many things, including psychiatry. We can no longer deny this, as has commonly happened. It is through resistance that we foreswear the possibility that it might ever happen again.

9 Citizenship and the politics of identity

As we draw towards the end of this book, we want to describe how our ideas have influenced our work as psychiatrists. We believe we can best do so by looking not only at our involvement in the development of services, and in our work as members of multidisciplinary teams, but also at our engagement with the communities in which we work and live. In this chapter, we will focus on services. Again, we must emphasize that we do not claim to have the right answers. Postpsychiatry is nothing more than a way of orienting ourselves. It is a tool for probing and problematizing our engagement with madness, of questioning the assumptions and authority with which we speak. The only claim we make for postpsychiatry is that it helps to clarify the implications of the decisions we make in our work. One of the main purposes of our critique of psychiatry is to create a silence in which it is possible to hear voices that are usually drowned out. For this reason, the emphasis in much of our work concerns the legitimacy of those who may speak about madness, not on what we might have to say about it. Thus we attach much significance to service user and community involvement, both inside and outside the boundaries defined by mainstream mental health services.

Our account of our work has to begin by attending to the social and cultural contexts in which we are situated, so we start this chapter with a brief description of the City of Bradford. The most aspect feature of our work is the process of reaching out to engage actively with those who traditionally have no voice in discussions about mental health. There are two elements to this, although we do not claim ownership of either of them. Both have at their core what we consider to be the Foucauldian project of creating ethical spaces in which people can explore alternative realities, spiritualities and perspectives on madness. These two projects work within quite different communities, but have broadly similar objectives. They are Sharing Voices Bradford, a community development project set up 4 years ago to engage with Bradford's Black and minority ethnic (BME) communities; and the work of Rufus May and his colleagues in Evolving Minds in the West Yorkshire town of Hebden Bridge. Much of our work would not have been possible without the support of Bradford District Care Trust (BDCT). Recently, the Trust has devoted a great deal of energy to developing what it has called a Citizenship Agenda. Again, this project is independent of our own work and 'postpsychiatry', although there is a resonance between the two. Both reach out beyond the clinic to engage with the world outside. For reasons that we have already examined in great detail back in Chapter 7, we are not attempting to describe in formal terms our clinical work. We will try to convey something of what it is like at the end of this book.

Bradford: a city and its people

Like many industrial Pennine towns, Bradford's population reflects the multicultural nature of modern English identity. Historically, the city has strong links to the textile industry, particularly the spinning, weaving and dyeing of wool. By the middle ages, it was a small market town, and at the turn of the 19th century its population was about 16 000. Until then, wool manufacture took place in cottages and farms. Industrialization changed this. From the end of the 18th century, the growth of the canal network, then the introduction of the steam power, the introduction of new machines and technology and the growth of the rail network transformed the domestic processes of wool carding and yarn spinning into heavy industry in large mills. By the mid 1840s, there were about 40 woollen mills in the town, and 10 years later Bradford was the wool capital of the world with a large engineering industry to service the mills. Its population reached 180 000, and the town changed from a small rural market town nestling on the banks of the river Aire, to a large industrial sprawl up the sides of the valley. The fictional *Coketown* in Charles Dickens's novel *Hard Times* vividly evokes what it must have been like to have lived in such a large industrial town 150 years ago (although *Coketown* was almost certainly in the south of England).

The demand for labour marked Bradford out as a culturally diverse city from the early years of industrialization. As the need for mill workers grew, workers moved in to the town from the neighbouring rural areas of Yorkshire and Lancashire, but the growth of industry fuelled a drive for migrant workers from further afield. The Great Famine of 1845 resulted in the first wave of Irish Diaspora arriving in the town. In the census of 1851, about 10% of Bradford's population originated from central and western Ireland. German wool merchants had also settled in the town in the early 19th century, building the town's fine architectural heritage known today as Little Germany. The composer Fredric Delius, born in the town in 1862, had German ancestors, and there is still a German Evangelical Church opposite the former site of Bradford Home Treatment Service. At the end of the 19th century, most of Bradford's wool merchants were German, and upheavals in the middle of the 20th century in central and eastern Europe resulted in Jewish, Italian, Polish, Latvian, Ukrainian, Estonian, Lithuanian, Byelorussian, Hungarian and Yugoslavian émigrés arriving. After 1945, a shortage of labour driven by the need to rebuild following the war resulted in successive governments encouraging people from the New Commonwealth to relocate to Britain. The pattern of migration changed, with the arrival of people from Asia, especially Pakistan, Bangladesh and India, and from the Caribbean and Africa. The years following the unrest in the Middle East, the Balkans and Africa have seen the arrival in the city of people seeking refuge from conflict in those countries as asylum seekers.

The population of the city in the 2001 census was just under 468 000, of whom 14.5% described themselves as Pakistani, 2.7% Indian and 1.1% Bangladeshi[1]. The city has a significant Muslim community; at 16.1% this is the fourth highest figure in the country. The demography of the city's BME community is evolving, with growing numbers of British-born Muslims, Hindus and Sikhs. These figures fail to reveal the way in which the city's BME communities are concentrated in the inner city areas. Figure 9.1, taken from the 2001 census based on Bradford District Local Authority Wards (the local government administrative divisions), shows that the two wards, City (the area around the city centre and university, population 18 579) and Manningham (to the north of the city centre, population 16 863) have the highest proportion of people of Pakistani origin.

People living in these areas face high levels of social adversity, in terms of overcrowding, high levels of long-term illnesses, and lower levels of economic activity (Fig. 9.2).

Local government and health service boundaries are not co-terminous, so it is difficult to be clear about the geographical relationship between the two, but Bradford City teaching Primary Care Trust (tPCT) is responsible for commissioning health services, including mental health services, for most of the people resident in these two local authority wards. It also commissions services for residents in other inner city areas, corresponding roughly to Little

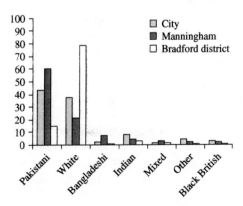

Fig. 9.1 Ethnic origin as a percentage of the population of two Bradford Local Authority Wards compared with the city as a whole.

---

[1] These, and all subsequent figures describing Bradford are taken from the Research and Consultation Service, City of Bradford Metropolitan District Council, accessed at http://www.bradfordinfo.com/census/WardProfiles.cfm on November 30, 2004.

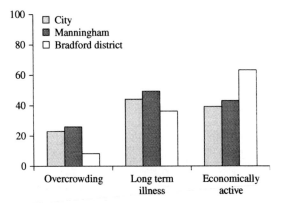

Fig. 9.2 Indices of social adversity in two Bradford Local Authority Wards compared with the city as a whole.

Horton (south and southwest inner city area, population 17 368) and Bowling and Barkerend (southeast and east of inner city, population 18 226). These two wards are broadly similar to the City and Manningham, with high levels of poverty and social adversity. This has important implications for the health of the residents in these areas. Figures from the National Database for Primary Care Trusts indicate that Bradford City tPCT ranks fifth in England in terms of having Super Output Areas[2] (SOAs) that are in the 20% most deprived in England. In other words, the health of the residents of inner city Bradford is more likely to be adversely affected by socio-economic factors such as poor housing, overcrowding and unemployment than that of the residents of more prosperous parts of the city, or for that matter most other parts of the country. Social adversity and poverty disproportionately affect people from BME communities, and this is reflected in their experiences and use of mental health services, as the recently published NIMHE/Department of Health report *Inside Outside* has shown (2003*b*).

But we do not intend to dwell on the negatives. All too often, life in inner city areas is portrayed in terms of fear and dread. Whilst it is true that many of the complex problems associated with inner city life are experienced by the people who live in such areas, these communities are resilient, have vision and political awareness. Bradford is no exception. It is a truly diverse, multicultural and international city. Its diverse communities are reflected in its cultural and business activities. There is a strong and successful business and

---

[2]SOAs have recently been introduced in an attempt to find a standardized way of comparing the socio-economic and demographic characteristics of different localities and neighbourhoods, in recognition of the problems of using local government boundaries. They were generated by computer using data gathered in the 2001 population census. The difficulty with electoral wards is that they vary greatly in size, and are subject to regular boundary changes. SOAs provide a useful way of comparing the characteristics of the populations served by Primary Care Trusts (the main health commissioning agencies in England).

entrepreneurial community, exemplified by the Bombay Stores[3] and Mumtaz Restaurant[4]. Over the last 30 years or so, both of these businesses have become nationally well known, having started from extremely humble origins. Mumtaz products are to be found on sale in Harrods in London. Both symbolize the strength and creativity of some aspects of British Muslim and British Asian culture. At a time of rampant Islamophobia, the city is increasingly seen in Britain as a platform Muslim and Asian politics. This is reflected in the activities of one of the city's best known cultural products, the band Fun-Da-Mental. Their music is a fusion of rap, punk, Asian qawwali singing (deeply rooted in the Sufi tradition), and sampled extracts from the speeches of Malcolm X and other Black leaders. Aki Nawaz, one of the group's founders, has spoken of how his experiences of racism in his Bradford childhood shaped his political, cultural and Islamic identity, which in turn has found an outlet in his music. He puts it this way:

> Islam for me was more punk than punk! I can't understand why people say it is restrictive...It was the demonisation of the Afro-Caribbean community, then it became demonisation of the Indians, or the Asians or the Pakistanis or the Muslims. I'm not willing to fight ignorance anymore. (Nawaz 2004)

Sharing Voices Bradford[5]

This community development project was established in 2002 in response to concern about the relationship between Britain's BME communities and statutory mental health services. We will not revisit the evidence here. It has been thoroughly covered by the publications we reviewed in Chapter 1. Health inequalities disproportionately affect members of our BME communities in all health areas, particularly in mental health. This is the reality in Britain today. In 1999, a small group in Bradford[6] wrote a proposal for a community development project which was unsuccessfully submitted for Department of

---

[3]See http://www.bombaystoresonline.com/Bombay/About%Us.asp
[4]See http://www.mumtaz.co.uk/main.htm, the first thing that strikes you as you leave immigration control in Islamabad International Airport and enter the main arrivals area is a large advertisement for Mumtaz of Pakistan and Bradford, welcoming you to Islamabad/Rawalpindi. The same signs appear on the outskirts of the town of Mirpur in Kashmir. Many members of England's Pakistani community come from this area. We live in a shrinking world with increasingly porous cultural identities (Bibeau 1997).
[5]We are particularly grateful to Paul Henderson of the Community Development Foundation for his permission to rely substantially on the Evaluation Report (2003–2004) produced by the CDF, and to Patience Seebohm from the Sainsbury Centre for Mental Health, Carole Munn-Giddings University of East Anglia, and other members of the evaluation team for their permission to use material from the Early Findings of the Evaluation of Sharing Voices Bradford in this chapter, particularly Glenis Ritchie, Jeff Dawkins, Nazreen Akhtal, Amjid Hussain, Jean Williams, Khabir Ahmed, and Mamuna Bibi, all of whom worked as community researchers.
[6]The group consisted of Dr Hasan Daudjee, until recently consultant psychiatrist in transcultural psychiatry, and Maureen Goddard, business manager with Bradford Community Health Trust as it was then, and the present authors.

Health funding as part of the Health Action Zone Initiative. This occurred at about the same time that the city's Transcultural Psychiatry Service closed, and a health service reorganization resulted in the formation of Bradford City tPCT. Thus there was a need to reformulate statutory services' response to the mental health needs of Bradford's BME communities. The City tPCT recognized that it had to respond to the needs of its BME communities, and agreed to fund the *Sharing Voices Initiative*, for a period of 3 years. The project is supported by the Community Development Foundation, England's main community development organization, and the Centre for Citizenship and Community Mental Health (CCCMH). In March 2002, the project coordinator was appointed, two community development workers recruited, and it became operational 5 months later. For the first 2 years of its life, it was positioned outside the statutory sector, under the aegis of one of Bradford's main local voluntary sector organizations, *Asian Disability Network*. In 2004, the project reconstituted itself as a company limited by guarantee as *Sharing Voices Bradford* (SVB) in order to become independent. The SVB coordinator is a member of BDCTs Citizenship Group, and is a core member of CCCMH. Thus it has close links to the School of Health Studies in the University of Bradford, and the main mental health service provider. At the time of writing, SVB is being evaluated by the Sainsbury Centre for Mental Health (SCMH).

SVB uses community development as a means of reaching out to and engaging with Bradford's BME communities. Community development in health works on the assumption that social exclusion and adversity brought about by the experiences of poverty, racism, unemployment, family difficulties, sexual abuse, domestic violence and spiritual conflict have a profound impact on mental health. For most people who use, or who are at risk of using, mental health services, these issues are central to their problems. Community development prioritizes the understandings that ordinary people have of their difficulties, by facilitating and fostering the growth of networks of support around particular issues. It draws together groups and individuals who share in common experiences of distress, and helps them to exercise more autonomy. It strengthens group and individual self-esteem; it fosters empowerment. Community development recognizes that statutory mental health services have an important role to play in responding to the needs of BME communities, but it also stresses the importance of choice. This is important given the failure of mental health services to meet the needs of BME communities. A great deal of mental health practice is based on theoretical assumptions about the nature of the self, and the relationship between self, family and community that are alien to people from non-European cultures. Community development tries to find ways around this by helping people to establish support networks and shared understandings of distress within particular communities of interest and cultural traditions. The project's work falls into five main areas; the Mutual Interest Group (MIG), volunteers, activities, partnership projects and policy work. The MIG meets every 6 weeks or so, attended on average by around

12 people. It is a forum for discussion and for sharing different perspectives. It draws together people who have experienced distress and have used services, those who have recovered from distress with the help of alternative forms of support, carers, community activists and professionals interested in culture and mental health. It is variously seen as the 'bedrock' or 'sounding board' of the project. The work of the MIG is a good example of how grass roots community development can help foster community cohesion and build capacity within communities. Without the enthusiasm and commitment of the volunteers, SVB would flounder. By March 2004, there were eight or nine active volunteers, and a further 20 registered with the project, some of whom have had personal experience of distress and used mental health services. They contact and support people in the community who are in distress, and participate in group and self-help activities. The community development workers support them in their activities. The volunteers and community development workers are at the heart of SVB, from individual work, planning meetings for self-help groups, helping groups with funding applications, and training.

SVB has established partnerships with a wide range of organizations that are concerned about mental health. Most of these work with specific communities, such as Bradford's Bangladeshi Youth Organization, Kushboo Women's Group and COFRAB (a self-help group established by French-speaking African people, many of whom are refugees). SVB's partnership with COFRAB helped the group gain funding for their own premises and to become independent. SVB participates in wider, multi-agency activities aimed at breaking down hostility, mistrust and suspicion between different communities in the city. It is a partner organization in the Programme for a Peaceful City established by the School of International and Social Studies in the University of Bradford, which was set up by the University following the Ousley Report into the 2002 riots. The project is organizing a series of workshops 'Participation—Why Bother?' jointly with the International Centre for Participation Studies (in the university) to explore the barriers to participation in the design and delivery of mental health services, jointly between service users from the city's BME communities and service providers. There are close links between SVB and CCCMH; the community researchers evaluating SVB are based in CCCMH, and have access to university resources. Finally, SVB is contributing to policy development and implementation, both locally and nationally.

SVB evaluation

In October 2004, the SCMH started a 6 month evaluation of SVB, using participatory action research methodology (Meyer 2000; Winter & Munn-Giddings 2001). Community researchers, many of whom were volunteers with the project, were trained in qualitative research methods. The first stage of the evaluation audited all those in contact with the project in November 2004

(Seebohm *et al.* 2004). Of the 125 people who completed audit forms, 41% were involved in one of the six self-help groups, 14% received support on a one to one basis, and 14% were volunteers. The rest had participated in work-shops or other activities. The majority of people (about three-fifths of the total) identified themselves as Pakistani. It is worth noting that about a third of those in contact with the project were aged less than 25 years, and about 60% were women with childcare responsibilities. Only two-fifths of participants had used specialist mental health services, whereas two-thirds had consulted a GP in connection with a mental health problem. Everyone was invited to complete a series of visual analogue rating scales describing how they felt before and after their involvement with SVB, on a scale from –5 (much worse) to +5 (much better). There were statistically significant improvements in 'ability to do things that are important to me' and 'sadness' (Figs 9.3 and 9.4).

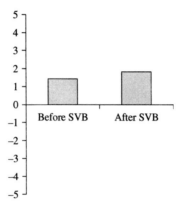

Fig. 9.3 Changes in mean score for 'unable to do things' on as a visual analogue rating scale before and after SVB ($P < 0.001$ by Wilcoxon matched pairs signed ranks test).

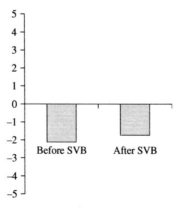

Fig. 9.4 Changes in mean score for sadness' on as a visual analogue rating scale before and after SVB ($P < 0.001$ by Wilcoxon matched pairs signed ranks test).

These quantitative findings are borne out by the qualitative study. For example, a woman attending the Ham Dard women's group spoke of how she felt empowered through her involvement with the group and SVB, and how her mood improved as a result:

> It's made me a lot stronger to fight for my rights and everything. And I feel that if [problems] do happen at home, I can be a lot stronger about it. And I can get it off my chest and I can talk about it. . . . I don't have to get depressed and put myself down. (Ham Dard group member[7])

These are early results from a continuing evaluation, so there must be a great deal of caution in their interpretation. Nevertheless, they do suggest that the project is effective in engaging with people from BME communities, and supporting them in addressing their emotional well-being in ways that they define for themselves. The project appears to bring significant benefit to the lives of those who have been involved with it, through the provision of a supportive and empowering network.

Before moving on, we want briefly to consider how the work of SVB relates to postpsychiatry. It should be clear that the project is rooted in the community, and that it works hard to represent the interests and concerns of those sections of Bradford's BME communities with which it is in contact. In our view, the self-help and support networks sustained by SVB create safe spaces in which people can explore their experiences unconditionally. The powerful languages of psychiatry, psychology and therapy are absent and excluded; they have no place in shaping the experiences of the participants, who are free to commence the narrative processes of exploring and negotiating their experiences for themselves. This is related to the Foucauldian view of power in constituting subjectivity, which, as we have seen, is not to be seen in an entirely negative light. Some aspects of SVB's work demonstrate the positive aspects of this relationship. In SVB, ordinary people are free to talk about their lives and experiences in their own terms, rather than in terms given to them by psychiatrists, psychologists, or for that matter the pharmaceutical industry.

This leads to the second point. The evaluation interviews suggest that when people are encouraged to say how they understand their lives and difficulties, they do so in non-medical ways that express the need for hope and meaning in life. The following extract is taken from an interview with the Community Development Worker who set up the Men's Fitness group together with a young man who had been using mental health services for a few years:

> An individual who came to us about a year ago—who was down, feeling low, who was on medication. He also suffers from dyslexia. . . . He was withdrawn, he wouldn't leave the house. . . . So I went to see him at home. And then I started working with him you know, got to know him, he started to trust me, so he started to come out with me. . . .

---

[7] All quotations here are taken from Seebohm *et al.* (2004), with permission. The final report has since been published by the Sainsbury Centre for Mental Health (Seebohm *et al.* 2005).

> He says 'I wish I could do something related to fitness'. . . I said 'Let's set up
> a group for you, so you can have experience and then, you know, you can
> help people that have been in a similar situation to yourself' . . . We set up a
> group at Manningham—he's the group fitness co-ordinator now there. . . .
> And then he's actually gone on to do a degree—at university, at Bradford, so
> within a twelve months period we've seen, you know, dramatic changes.
> (from Seebohm *et al.* 2004)

This clearly shows the importance of meaning brought about through
supportive human relationships, of a sense of purpose and hope for the future,
all issues that we raised in Chapter 4 and in Chapter 8.

Evolving Minds

Evolving Minds is a group established by the psychologist and survivor
activist Rufus May in the Pennine town of Hebden Bridge[8], in West Yorkshire.
Neither of the current writers is directly involved with the group, but its
activities have a strong bearing on issues that we have raised here, and we are
grateful to Rufus May for his permission to refer to the group's work. It was
set up in April 2004, following a public showing of the film *Evolving Minds*[9]
in the town's Trades Club, which was attended by over 70 people. The group
provides a public forum to discuss different understandings of and approaches
to mental health problems, including spiritual, social and personal understandings. Evolving Minds, which meets monthly in a function room in a local
pub, aims to create a public space in which different understandings of distress
can be explored, with the purpose of increasing public acceptance of those
who experience it. The group is also concerned with social justice and human
rights issues in relation to mental health. On average, between 20 and 40 people
attend meetings, which usually begin with a creative session such as poetry,
story telling or music. The group's activities also include social action such as
campaigns against coercion in psychiatry, personal stories of recovery from
madness, forum theatre, surviving a mad world, spiritual healing, reclaiming
languages of selfhood, and creativity and mental health. These issues are usually
covered in small group discussion, with the emphasis on non-technological ways
of coping with distress, based in the values of hope, respect for different ways
of understanding experience, and subjective wisdom. Alongside these regular
activities is a series of theatre workshops using the ideas of Augusto Boal
(2000). Many people have described how attending the group has increased

---

[8]Hebden Bridge is a small, former cotton town between Bradford and Manchester, population
about 8600 including outlying rural areas. It is a relatively prosperous, almost exclusively White
(97.9%) community. It is the self-proclaimed 'Lesbian hub of the north' (see http://www.
guardian.co.uk/gayrights/story/0,12592,1179316,00.html accessed December 13 2004), and since
the 1970s the town has developed a strong 'counter-culture'.

[9]For details see http://www.undercurrents.org/minds/.

their understanding of unusual experiences and distress, and given them the confidence to get involved in community action in a positive way.

The group exists through social capital; its contributors receive no payment. It has no funding. A collection is made at the end of each meeting to pay for the hire of the room. It has raised the profile of madness and psychosis, and the responses of the local community to it, in a positive way. It campaigns actively around the town, its posters prominently displayed. One asked the question 'How sane is it to be well-adapted to a sick society?' The group has good relationships with the local newspaper, which carries regular reports on its activities. It also participated in the local arts festival through *Culture and Madness*, readings of poetry, short stories and autobiography involving the writer Sarah Maitland, and poet Clare Shaw. The group is also supporting the foundations of a northern branch of the survivor organization Mad Pride. Although these activities are focused on a local community, it is also working with CCCMH in fostering a recovery approach being developed in the acute admission wards at Lynfield Mount Hospital in Bradford. Rufus May and a member of Evolving Minds, Adam Jhugroo who is also a nurse in the hospital, have started a 'Road to Recovery' group on Oakburn ward[10]. The group is open to any resident on the ward. Subjects nominated for discussion have included spirituality, reclaiming power in your life, rights during hospital admission and interviewing the psychiatrist. In this session, the group reversed the power relationships that symbolize the power relationships on acute psychiatric admissions units by interviewing the Trust's medical director.

This brief overview of Sharing Voices Bradford and Evolving Minds demonstrates that social action and community development cover a wide range of activities[11]. Although these projects work with very different communities, they share in a common approach that is rooted in local practices and beliefs. Both are collective and accountable, and assume that madness is of concern to everybody. The Great Confinement was physical, ideological and political. Evolving Minds and Sharing Voices challenge this by taking madness back into the heart of the community. They refuse to accept that madness is the exclusive domain of the psychiatrist and mental health expert. Both propose that we have a collective responsibility to engage with madness and distress, and to see such states as part of a range of understandable responses to conflict, abuse and trauma.

---

[10]Five years earlier, this ward was also the site of an innovative approach which focused nursing staff activity away from 'observations' to active engagement with residents aimed at helping them to resolve social crisis and problems and thus getting them out of hospital much more rapidly (Dodds and Bowles 2001).

[11]There are of course many other groups in England, and in other countries engaged in broadly similar activities. It is in their nature that they are not organized, but they are very active within local communities. Examples include the work of the Hearing Voices Network across Europe, and in England (http://www.hearing-voices.org/), and the activities of some of their local groups and organizations, such as the Joan of Arc Room in Exeter.

Citizenship and mental health services

In Chapter 3, we examined the value of the concept of citizenship as applied to mental health in some detail. In recent years, the idea of citizenship has also gained favour with survivors of mental health services. In England, the Centre for Citizen Participation at Brunel University is directed by Peter Beresford, a prominent survivor of mental health services. In America, Judi Chamberlin, another prominent survivor, has written of the value of a citizenship rights approach in the field of mental health. She points out that all too commonly the rights of the mentally ill are discussed from a narrow perspective of people's 'right to treatment'. She proposes that rights (and thus citizenship) refer much more widely to fundamental aspects of the relationship between the individual and society. As we described earlier, this relationship originates in democracy and autonomy. She questions the way in which the supposedly medical diagnosis of mental illness curtails people's rights and impugns their autonomy, through detention, restraint and the compulsory administration of medical treatment. She asks the following question:

> Is it ethically justifiable to confine people against their will, to subject them to procedures against their will, or to overrule their life choices, on the basis of an ostensibly medical diagnosis? I believe that until we frame this question properly, *as a human rights question*, we will continue to make the simple complicated. (Chamberlin 1998: 406; emphasis added)

In Chapter 3, we examined citizenship in terms of human rights, not simply in terms of equitable access to the rights that all citizens enjoy in society, full employment, decent housing, freedom from oppression (i.e. in terms of passive citizenship), but also in terms of the right to be able to define oneself, to understand oneself in a particular way (e.g. as a Black person, or a gay person or as just 'crazy' or mad). The question then arises as to whether it is possible to take these political and cultural perspectives on citizenship and bring them to bear in very practical ways in mental health work. Is it possible to adapt these ideas so that they can influence the way mental health services work? This for us is a really important question. Throughout the book, we have tried to create bridges between the world of ideas and the world of mental health practice. So far, a great deal of this has focused specifically on what takes place between individual patients and psychiatrists or mental health practitioners. At this stage, we want to consider the implications of our ideas for a mental health service. We will describe how one service provider organization, BDCT, has tried to develop a citizenship model of care. Achieving change in large organizations like the NHS is rather akin to watching a river in flow. Some parts move faster than others. Sometimes the middle flows more quickly than the outside. The speed of flow varies with the depth of the river. Deep pools fill reluctantly and sluggishly; the water flow cascades enthusiastically down rocky outcrops. This metaphor for change applies well to the NHS. Some parts want change yesterday. Others resist until the last moment and are dragged into the new order, resisting until the final moments. Whilst we believe that real change will only be achieved through social, political and cultural action, we recognize that this must be complemented by changes in services. Citizenship, as we shall see at the end of this chapter, has its drawbacks. Nevertheless, our view is that it does have the potential to move mental health services and professional practice forward.

In the NHS Plan, the government announced its intention to set up integrated Health and Social Care Trusts in an attempt to overcome the problematic division between health and social care that has bedevilled Britain since the introduction of the NHS in 1948. Social care trusts (SCTs) are statutory NHS bodies based on Primary Care and NHS Trusts. As single organizations, the intention is that they should deliver integrated health and social care services. NHS and Local Authority health-related functions are delegated to them, not transferred. The government had a number of objectives in setting up SCTs, such as improving the quality of care by delivering seamless services, providing services that were centred on the needs of patients and carers, and built on a single strategic approach. In the government's view, the introduction of SCTs offered a pragmatic way of broadening the range and nature of health and social services, and delivering integrated care in a way that improved quality. These are major changes. They build on the agenda set out in the NHS Plan, but in doing so SCTs take us to the core of an ideological split between health and social services in Britain. We express it crudely in this way; health services are dominated by ideology of illness, pathology, treatment and cure; social services are dominated by the ideology of disability and adaptation. The question is how the new SCTs will navigate their way around these deep-rooted differences.

BDCT came into being in April 2002. It was one of the first four SCTs in the country, and the only one to encompass both mental health and learning disabilities. Its first task was to consult with stakeholders to find out what difference people thought being an SCT should make to the values and work of the organization. It organized a series of focus groups attended by about 300 people. The emphasis was on a 'bottom-up' approach to ensure both that the process was democratic and that all interested parties felt they had ownership of the outcome[12]. Those consulted included representatives from different service sectors or directorates, the unions, service users and representatives from different communities. The main outcome of this process was the mission statement and values in Table 9.1.

---

[12]The process of consultation used by BDCT described here is reminiscent of the process the government used to draw up the NHS Plan which we described in Chapter 1.

Table 9.1   Mission statement
• Putting you at the heart of everything we do
• Our purpose is to provide mental health and learning disability services that meet the assessed needs of our diverse communities
Values
• Everyone has a voice
• Effective and honest communication by listening and showing that we have heard
• Respecting individuals, celebrating diversity
• Making people feel valued whoever they are
• Providing services which are accessible, informative, flexible and appropriate
• Working together, sharing ideas to make services better
• Promoting learning, developing potential
• Moving towards excellence by learning from ideas and good practice

It was important that the organization as a whole should adopt the mission statement and values. In June 2003, one of the present authors (P.B.) addressed the Trust Board on the subject of Citizenship, and 3 months later the Trust formally agreed to develop a citizenship framework of care over a 5 year period. The board and senior management were clear about the enormous challenge of trying to get the workforce to accept ownership of a framework that would almost certainly have major implications for its work. To start this process, the Trust initiated a two-stage consultation process. The first stage involved 18 workshops and focus groups, involving service users, staff (from across all directorates), local statutory organizations and community groups. One of the focus groups was organized on behalf of BDCT by SVB, in an attempt to gain the participation of as many BME community groups in the process. We will return to this later. The groups were asked to consider a series of questions—what does being a citizen mean, what matters in making you feel more or less of a citizen, and what would the organization look like in the future if it successfully implemented a citizenship framework? Notes and records of these workshops were taken and analysed into main themes which informed the second stage of consultation. This involved a further seven workshops in which participants were invited to choose and discuss five of the 10 most frequently cited themes. Again, participants came from diverse backgrounds, this time with more people from outside the Trust. Again, the records of these discussions were analysed thematically, and in January 2004 the Trust set up two bodies to assume the corporate responsibility of implementing its citizenship framework. The Citizenship Group consisted of senior managers responsible for different directorates (e.g. learning disability, child and family, adult mental health, personnel, and so on), together with service user, community (SVB) and academic representation. The Group is responsible for the strategic implementation and development of the citizenship framework, and is chaired by the Trust's

Chief Executive. The Citizenship Committee provides an external yardstick to monitor the work of the Citizenship Group. The Citizenship Group condensed the 10 themes that emerged from the second series of focus groups into the six work groups with a lead director responsible for each (Table 9.2).

This ambitious project is still in its infancy. The five workgroups were only agreed towards the end of 2004, and it is too early to say what impact they will have on the experience of people who use Bradford's mental health services. We would make the following points. For over 20 years there has been a strong tradition in Bradford of service user empowerment and activism, going back to the pioneering work of a small group of radical survivor activists in the city who worked with Peter Barham and Robert Hayward[13]. In some ways, the Trust's citizenship agenda can be seen to emerge out of this tradition. It is an attempt to take forward the values of that pioneering work, and place it at the heart of statutory mental health services. It is important to point out that the Trust's citizenship framework arose largely independently of 'postpsychiatry', although it would be disingenuous to say that our work has had no influence on it. The main driving force has been the enthusiasm of the Chair of the Trust Board, the Chief Executive, the Medical Director and a small number of committed service directors.

Although we fully support the Trust's work in this area, the organization is entering a complex terrain riven with fissures and sink-holes. There are internal barriers to change. The citizenship agenda represents a potential challenge to professional roles and expertise. This is because it prioritizes the concerns of the people who use the service, their families and communities, not those of the professionals who work in it. It is perfectly clear, therefore, that one of the main practical obstacles to the successful implementation of citizenship will be the resistance of professional interests. Another important area concerns the involvement of external partners in the community, such as local employers, schools, Jobcentre Plus and the media. The health service has little if any experience in working with local communities in this way. The difficulty here is that for 150 years our culture has sequestered the mad in institutions and services. The community at large no longer sees itself as having any duty or responsibility for the mad. This applies even before we come to consider the issue of stigma. The public might be excused for saying—'Madness? That's a psychiatrist's job'[14]. Yet it is beyond the ability of

---

[13]Their book *From the Mental Patient to the Person* (Barham and Hayward 1991) describes in detail this work, and the lives and experiences of some of the survivor activists in Bradford. Peter Relton, service user development worker with Bradford Home Treatment and more recently the Trust's senior user worker, was involved in this pioneering work in Bradford in the 1980s. Two large user-run non-statutory sector organizations, Bradford and Airedale Mental Health Advocacy Group and Bradford Mind, arose out of the work of the survivor activists included in Barham and Hayward's book.

[14]That this is a genuine concern is well demonstrated by the infamous spat between the late Dr Robert Kendell, then President of the Royal College of Psychiatrists, and the then Home Secretary Jack Straw. This took place on BBC Radio Four's *Today* programme (one of the UK's most highly regarded news and current affairs programmes), and was subsequently reported in the *British Medical Journal* (Warden 1998). The Home Secretary criticized the profession for failing

Table 9.2 Work groups arising from citizenship workshops. Bradford District Care-Trust

Work group	Priorities identified	Lead director
Employment and education	Increase number of service users and BME staff working for Trust Robust performance monitoring down to service level Influence external partners Review support for potential applicants Education programmes to support staff/managers recruit from hard to reach groups	Director of Personnel
Carers and families	Explore option of opening up access to Trust childcare services for service users working for other employers Explore option of providing service users seeking employment access to BDCT childcare team for advice Respite care/associated activities to support families to enable them to stay out of services	Director of Nursing and Director of CAMS
Attitudes and stigma	Service user survey of attitudes and behaviour encountered whilst using services Increase number of service users on recruitment panels Use service users in staff induction programmes Raise awareness of advocacy and service user groups to new inductees Proactively promote core competencies, e.g. by including in recruitment packs	Director of Personnel
Information, rights, responsibilities	Information for service users, carers and families about Trust services to facilitate informed choice Standard quality information for service users and carers about treatment and medication Promoting 'userbility' and other initiatives to enhance service users' access to information about their rights and responsibilities	Director of Personnel
Service user involvement, having a choice and being heard	Develop framework of support for service user reps on Trust Board Monitor support and engagement of service users across Trust in Trust activities Explore opportunities for service users to access non-statutory services, e.g. commissioning community and voluntary organizations to provide day care services	Citizenship Lead
Independence and social involvement	Work with stakeholders to create inclusive environments for service users Work with stakeholders to help service users retain/become independent	Citizenship Lead

health or social services alone to effect the sort of social and cultural shifts necessary to impact in a positive way on the lives of those who use mental health services. Unless the Trust is able to break through such attitudes, the citizenship agenda is unlikely to have much of an impact on the lives of those who use services. Finally, there are the conceptual problems of citizenship, and we shall end this chapter by considering these in some detail.

Citizenship and the politics of identity

One of the most active user organizations in the UK in recent years has been the group Mad Pride. In Chapter 3, we saw that Mad Pride and a growing number of other user-led organizations (such as Mad Chicks, launched in November 2004) argue that a great deal of the suffering they endure arises not from their mental illness as such but from the different ways that society responds to people who are identified, or who identify themselves, as mad. There are clear parallels here with the Gay Rights movement and, indeed, Mad Pride grew out of the 1997 Gay Pride festival in London[15]. Early on in its history, the Gay Rights movement challenged the idea that homosexuality was an illness. The fight against discrimination and oppression combined with a positive campaign in which gay people struggled to 'define' themselves and develop their own agendas for the future. Alongside arguments against the medical framing of homosexuality as some sort of disease was a move to celebrate gay culture. The Mad Pride movement is now international. On Bastille Day (July 14) 2004, Mad Pride events were held in Paris, Toronto, London, and in several cities in the USA, from Washington to Eugene, Oregon.

Earlier, we referred to a paper by Judi Chamberlin, who makes the following point in arguing the case for a citizenship rights approach in mental health:

> The ethical system . . . that drives the involuntary treatment system is paternalism, the idea that one group (the one in power, not oddly) knows what is best for another group (which lacks power). The history of civilisation is, in part, the struggle against paternalism and for self-determination. People in power are always saying that they know what is best for those they rule over, even if those poor unfortunate individuals think they know best what they

---

to deal effectively with people like Michael Stone, who was convicted of the double murder of a mother and daughter, when he was under treatment for a 'psychopathic disorder'. Dr Kendell's point was that psychopathy was not a mental disorder and so was not treatable under the Mental Health Act. Jack Straw claimed that it was extraordinary that the profession should only take on patients it regarded as 'treatable'. He attacked the profession for its 'narrow interpretation of the law', and a trend towards a narrower interpretation of the law over the last . In other words, he was berating the profession for moving towards a more limited role in society.

[15]See http://www.madpride.org.uk accessed December 21, 2004. Mad Pride recognizes that many survivor and service user groups find its position disquieting, but they point out that the purpose of the group is to reclaim the meaning of the word 'Mad', in much the same way that Gay and Black groups have done.

want. The powerful seldom cast their own motives in anything but benevolent terms. Rulers and slave masters like to think (or to pretend) that their subjects love them and are grateful to them, often having to ignore much evidence to the contrary. The struggle for freedom has always been seen by the powerful as a denial of the obvious truth of the superiority of the rulers. (Chamberlin 1998: 406)

We want to reflect on this powerful statement in which Judi Chamberlin is asking us to consider the issue of power relationships in the context of citizenship. One implication is that insofar as citizenship in inextricably tied to democracy and human rights, it is not within the 'gift' of professionals. It is, perhaps, just as paternalistic for mental health professionals to say to service users 'Look! Here is citizenship. Take it! It is good for you. It will liberate you' as it is for them to say, 'Look! Here is Prozac. Take it. It will make you feel better.' Chamberlin is urging us to be cautious about the effects of power relationships in so-called liberatory discourses[16]. This is why it is important that we end this chapter by subjecting the idea of citizenship to a critical gaze.

The idea of active citizenship can be traced back to ancient Greece but, according to Marinetto (2003), it has only very recently re-emerged as a prominent feature of the political discourse of advanced liberal democracies. Nikolas Rose (1996) has developed a Foucauldian critique of the way in which society is governed in advanced liberal democracies, and the structural changes associated with this form of political governance. Foucault (1991) coined the term 'governmentality' to describe a particular type of mentality that characterizes state activity in liberal democracies. Its main feature is that the state can, should and must manage and regulate all aspects of society and individual behaviour. Foucault's ideas about governmentality are of great importance in relation to citizenship. What we understand to be citizenship, the rights we enjoy such as the right to work, to be housed, to participate in democracy, the right to be autonomous self-determining beings, all these privileges stand in a complex relationship to governmentality. This is because advanced liberal democracies require their citizens to be free, in order that the apparatus of state can divest itself of the burden of control to the individual. They no longer rely on centralized institutions to foster and maintain the state's power and control of its citizens. But this freedom comes at a price. It means that we are expected to internalize forms of morality and notions of normality, especially in terms of our sexuality and rationality, that is to say in terms of how we are permitted to think and experience the world. Nikolas Rose (1996) sees the government's emphasis on community as part of these processes. 'Community' has become incorporated into professional and expert discourses and programmes of knowledge. The same can be said of citizenship,

---

[16]In this respect, her position is broadly similar to that of the Brazilian pedagogue and political reformer Paulo Freire, who writes as follows: 'This, then, is the great humanistic and historical task of the oppressed: to liberate themselves and their oppressors as well . . . Only power that stems from the weakness of the oppressed will be sufficiently strong to free both.' (Freire 1996: 26).

which has become a focus for government attempts to deal with complex social phenomena such as crime and drug misuse. As a result, a new sector of government has appeared which develops policy programmes which rely on the capabilities of communities. This, according to Rose, is how we may understand active citizenship, where:

> ... new modes of neighbourhood participation, local empowerment and engagement of residents in decisions over their own lives will, it is thought, reactivate self-motivation, self-responsibility and self-reliance. (Rose 1996: 335; cited in Marinetto 2003: 109)

Seen in this light, community participation and involvement may be seen as a form of government. As Marinetto puts it:

> Encouraging active citizenship promotes a particular type of personal morality and positive form of life for communities, individuals and governments. (Marinetto 2003: 109)

Halperin, writing from the perspective of queer politics puts governmentality this way:

> The state no longer needs to frighten or coerce its subjects into proper behavior: it can safely leave them to make their own choices in the allegedly sacrosanct private sphere of personal freedom which they now inhabit, because within that sphere they *freely and spontaneously* police both their own conduct and the conduct of others—and so 'earn' by demonstrating a capacity to exercise them, the various rights assigned by the state's civil institutions exclusively to law-abiding citizens possessed of sound minds and bodies. (Halperin 1995: 18–19)

Active citizenship can be understood as a government strategy for regulating the population, which, by virtue of the fact that it appears not to be centralized, conveys the impression of decentred government. Marinetto, though, questions whether this is actually the case. He points out that central government, and other public authorities have immense power and control, through writing policies and gate-keeping resources that control and influence citizenship and community participation.

This is really important in relation to citizenship and madness. The caveat is that expressed by Halperin, that the right assigned by the state are granted '... exclusively to law-abiding citizens possessed of sound minds and bodies.' Citizenship is thus tied to a particular view of reality, one that excludes madness. This privileges subjectivities and ways of experiencing the world that are tied to Cartesian and rationalist assumption. The borderlands that are patrolled and policed by psychology and psychiatry are an excellent example of this. Foucault's analysis of power and governmentality suggests that citizenship in advanced liberal democracies is tightly bound up with hegemonic judgements about what is and what is not rational. In our view, citizenship should be inclusive; people should not be excluded simply because they do not experience reality in the way that the majority do.

So, for us, the really important question raised here concerns the type of values, morality and 'positive form(s) of life' (to quote Marinetto) promoted by active citizenship and the 'decentred' government. It may appear that there is no longer an authoritative state telling us how to lead our lives, or how we should interpret and makes sense of our lives and our relationships. Indeed in Chapter 6 we described how the global interests of the pharmaceutical industry are flooding the world with the view that we should interpret ourselves not as sad or demoralized, but as depressed. This is but one example of how we are encouraged to think about ourselves in ways that are not necessarily in our best interests. But we are also concerned that Nikolas Rose's account of this decentred approach to power and government may be misleading. Marinetto is right to point out that the state continues to exercise power and control in other ways. This is particularly the case in regard to the subjectivities of madness. Take, for example, the British government's highly contentious plans to change the 1984 Mental Health Act. Sitting alongside the rhetoric of democracy, citizenship, community engagement and participation, the government is planning to introduce proposals for compulsory treatment in the community based on wider legal definitions of mental disorder. In other words, it relinquishes power with one hand only to rein it back in with the other. Widening the legal definition of mental disorder will open up new realms of human subjectivity to be labelled, constrained and controlled by psychiatrists and mental health professionals acting as proxies for the state.

Of course it is essential that mental health service users are included and not excluded from society. Like other excluded groups, they must be free from the stigmatization and discrimination which in their case arises through their status as people who have used mental health services. But *inclusion* does not mean *incorporation*. Incorporation implies uniformity. There is a real danger that the political ideal of citizenship becomes a means of stifling and obliterating difference. These fears were expressed by members of Bradford's BME communities at the focus group organized by SVB as part of the development of BDCT's citizenship agenda. This group was organized and attended by Salma Yasmeen, manager of SVB, who reports[17] that the group was wary of citizenship. The group expressed concerns that the word reflected attempts to get Black and Asian people to become better citizens by relinquishing their own values, beliefs and traditions for White British values. In other words, people were concerned that citizenship was conditional, that it meant having to relinquish important part of one's identity as a Black British or Asian British person. If citizenship is to be unconditional and inclusive, it requires a sophisticated understanding of cultural and personal identity.

This point is vital for people from BME communities, for people who use mental health services, and all other marginalized, powerless and excluded

---

[17]Salma Yasmeen, personal communication, December 20, 2004.

groups. We must do everything possible to overcome and end their social exclusion and loss of citizenship but not at the expense of their identities. This is exactly the point made by Mad Pride. There must be no penalties for acquiring citizenship. There must be space for the difference of madness. On Bastille Day 2004, the Mad Pride activities in Eugene Oregon benefited the anti-war organizations Committee for Countering Military Recruitment and Justice Not War. These events celebrated madness and the actions of those opposing America's involvement in the Iraq War. Madness is a mirror to us all. It reflects back to us ourselves through art, poetry, literature, humour and political action, the insanity of the world we have created.

10 Are you local?

Responding to the challenge of globalization in mental health

We are conscious that throughout this book we have raised more questions than we have provided answers. No doubt we will be criticized because of this. However, our aim has never been to provide a model or a blueprint for how to move forward. Lots of people are doing this already. Our job, as we see it, is simply to challenge the authority of traditional psychiatry. Hopefully, this will be of support to those who are creating alternatives. We seek no authority. Ambiguity, uncertainty and doubt are no threat to the field of mental health; they represent an *opportunity*; an opportunity for debate, dialogue and democracy.

However, we are hopeful that postpsychiatry can help us to position ourselves more thoughtfully in the difficult land in which we dwell. The metaphor of the signpost is perhaps best suited to describe how we think of our critique: postpsychiatry is a set of directions telling us how we can leave the place where we are now, but not telling us where we should go.

In this last chapter, we want to examine some of the looming issues facing mental health in the coming years. Despite the strength of our criticism of positivism in psychiatry, we still believe that there is a strong case for the involvement of the medical profession in helping those who experience states of madness and distress. We agree strongly with our colleague Duncan Double who maintains that we do not need to postulate a biological basis for madness in order to justify the involvement of the medical profession (Double 2002). He points out that over the last 25 years the number of consultant psychiatrists has more than doubled in the UK and that as more resources have been allocated to mental health services, more resources are perceived to be needed. The factors that have driven the increase in these numbers are complex, but he draws attention to the common nature of mental health problems, coupled to an expansion of the boundaries of psychiatric disorder. He points out that diagnosis does not have to be couched in biomedical terms; it can also reflect an understanding of why it is that the patient has presented to the psychiatric services. These are issues we explored in depth in Chapter 8.

The point we want to consider here, though, concerns the expansion of psychiatry to which Duncan Double refers. The direction in which our ideas have progressed is driven as much by the reality of the world we live in, as it is by our philosophical critique. The growth of psychiatry in part reflects the enormous expansion of the NHS in Britain. There are many reasons for this, but one central theme is a relentless modernist quest to develop more and better technology. Technology has brought great benefits in health, but not as many as have resulted from the various social, political and economic developments of the past century. When it comes to mental health, we are sceptical of many of the claims made for medical science. Positive change has not been the result of developments in the *science* of psychiatry. It has been driven more by factors such as changes in social policy, changes in the legal framework around mental illness, improved welfare rights, a more vocal and active voluntary sector, special housing provision and political decisions about ending the role of large institutions

Postpsychiatry insists on an examination of these issues and argues that we interrogate the simple equation of progress with more technology. It demands that we put 'ethics before technology': raising questions about the seemingly limitless growth of psychiatry and the benefits that accrue from technology when set against the increasing costs of health care. Here, we want to explore the possibility that there might be more ethical and sustainable ways of responding to madness and distress. The problem of the harm caused by technology has featured prominently throughout this book, but so far we have not considered the implications of the burgeoning fiscal costs of health care. This is closely tied to the notion of progress, and thus the future role of psychiatrists. The question that arises concerns the sustainability of growth in mental health services and the NHS.

Progress through technology is expensive, whether we understand technology to be new drugs, or new therapeutic procedures in which mental health professionals have to be trained. We shall consider the implications for the future direction of mental health services, of the British government's recently published review of the funding of the NHS. We shall then consider the evidence that good outcomes in psychosis can be achieved in services that do not rely on expensive technology such as medication or therapy. In addition, there are important lessons to be learnt from the way in which mental health services have evolved, *faute de mieux*[1], in the economically disadvantaged (ED) countries of the world. In our view, we are witnessing a struggle between local and global approaches to distress.

Spend, Spend, Spend?

When it came to power in 1997, the British Labour government pledged a sustained increase in spending on the NHS, over and above inflation, until 2008. Nearly 10 years into this enormous programme of expansion, it is clear

---

[1]Not in the sense of 'for the want of something better', but 'out of necessity'.

that the NHS cannot go on growing endlessly. In March 2001, the Chancellor of the Exchequer appointed Derek Wanless, former chief executive of the NatWest Bank, to review the long-term growth and finance of the NHS. His brief was to consider the financial and other resources required over the following 20 years to ensure that the NHS could provide a publicly funded, comprehensive, high quality service available on the basis of clinical need and not on ability to pay[2]. In setting out the scope of his review, Wanless included the costs of social care because they are inextricably linked to health care. The final report, published in February 2004, made a number of recommendations (HMSO 2004) with a government promise of further consultation followed by a white paper. Its first recommendation is immensely important given the arguments we have developed in this book. We cite it in full:

> After many years of reviews and government policy documents, with little change on the ground, the key challenge now is delivery and implementation, not further discussion. A NHS capable of facilitating a 'fully engaged' population will need to shift its focus from a national sickness service, which treats disease, to a national health service which focuses on preventing it. The key threats to our future health such as smoking, obesity and health inequalities need to be tackled now. Where the evidence exists on how to do this cost-effectively, it should be used; where it does not, promising ideas should be piloted, evaluated and stopped if the evidence shows that to be appropriate. (Recommendation 9.1; HMSO 2004: 183)

In other words, the report proposes that a fundamental shift in ethos is necessary if the NHS is to continue to impact on the nation's health, maintain quality and be free at the point of delivery. The recommendation proposes a move away from the ideology of disease to the ideology of public health. It represents a shift from the current focus on the treatment of disease to the prevention of ill health. This is because a health service that prioritizes disease and biomedical models of illness, and the associated 'high-tech' drugs and treatments, is not sustainable, given the likely resource base over the next 20 years. Instead, it proposes a public health model that recognizes the importance of dealing with health inequalities and other environmental factors such as smoking and obesity, as well as engaging actively with patients and communities to involve them in decisions about health priorities. The summary of the report paints a wide definition of public health as:

> ...the science and art of preventing disease, prolonging life and promoting health through the organised efforts and informed choices of society, organisations, public and private, communities and individuals. (HMSO 2004: 3)

---

[2]The review also stressed the value of setting out a long-term plan for funding the NHS as a means of trying to establish some stability in the service, given the uncertainties that had characterized much of the institution's financial and organizational arrangements in the previous 25 years.

Furthermore, the report acknowledges the importance (indeed, necessity) of piloting and evaluating innovative approaches to tackling these problems, even in the absence of established evidence. It highlights the role of Primary Care Trusts, local authorities and other partners in modifying national objectives in the light of local need to establish shared local objectives, and it attaches particular importance to the 'full engagement' of the population in order to improve 'health literacy' especially in chronic conditions:

> The forthcoming consultation ahead of the White Paper is a good opportunity to engage the population on the issue of their own health and the balance between an individual's 'right to choose' and the impact that individual behaviour has on the wellbeing of others. (Recommendation 9.18; HMSO 2004: 186)

Apart from financial considerations, the report points out that there is a moral justification for adopting a public health approach. Ultimately it is the aggregate actions of individuals that influence the health of the nation overall, but individuals are ultimately responsible for their own health. We do not accept the inevitable libertarian implications of such a view, but report it here in order to draw attention to the growing belief that science alone will not improve the nation's health.

The Wanless Report draws many conclusions, most of which are concerned with the future arrangements for funding the NHS. However, we want to stress the shift from the ideology of biomedicine and disease to that of public health and prevention. One way of interpreting the report's recommendations is that the public must temper its expectation that progress in health can only be achieved through the endless growth of science and technology. It is simply not sustainable. However, we want to set this view against the wider, global context, which the Wanless Report does not attempt. Instead, it adopts a limited international perspective, only referring to other economically advantaged (EA) countries, Australia, Denmark, France, Germany, The Netherlands, New Zealand and Sweden. The issue of sustainability of health care in rich countries must be set against a global context characterized by gross inequalities in wealth, and where interpretations of distress are dominated largely by the interests of the global pharmaceutical industry (Chapters 1 and 6). In this respect, it is worth noting that the Wanless Report is dominated by a preoccupation with technological evidence. There is no attempt to foreground values and ethics. No attempt is made to question what we understand by health or what we consider to be important in maintaining it. We will return to these themes shortly, but first we want to explore the evidence that it is possible to help people through psychosis without recourse to high technology therapies and drugs.

The message of Loren Mosher

Although the psychiatric profession has played a key role in helping the pharmaceutical industry to dominate the way we interpret our lives and feelings, this has not always been the case. The tradition of helping people through acute psychoses with minimal use of medication has lived on in the work of the late Loren Mosher[3]. In the mid-1960s, he spent a year working with R.D. Laing at Kingsley Hall in London and, on his return to America, whilst working with the National Institute of Mental Health (NIMH), he became collaborating investigator and then research director of the Soteria Project.

The name Soteria is taken from the Greek word for salvation or deliverance. The original Soteria House was a medium sized family home that helped to support between six and eight residents through acute psychotic episodes, with no or minimum drug interventions. This work was partly influenced by the therapeutic community movement and partly by the view that the milieu shared by a small group of people living together for an extended period of time could be an agent for personal growth and change. With regard to psychosis, the main idea behind Soteria is that a first episode of psychosis is a critical period, and the nature of any intervention made in this period has a great influence on the subsequent course and outcome. In Soteria, neuroleptic medication was not used during the first 6 weeks, partly in order to give an adequate trial of psychological and social interventions, but also because of concerns over the risk of tardive dyskinesia, a clinical syndrome associated with a largely irreversible form of brain damage strongly associated with the long-term use of this class of drugs. Consequently the role of the psychiatrist became largely marginal:

> The program's psychiatrist, for example, was a consultant who did initial client interviews and staff training, but had no ongoing contact with the clients. As the programme matured, the psychiatrists came to be seen, and to see themselves, as mostly peripheral to it.[4] (Mosher & Burti 1994: 128)

Particular importance was attached to the personal qualities of the staff and their relationships with residents, with the emphasis on a protective and tolerant social environment. Ideally, staff had no fixed preconceptions about the best way of understanding psychosis, and functioned within a non-hierarchical structure. Staff who had dealt with personal problems, or lived with people who had experienced psychosis and who were also engaged with their local communities, were found to be particularly well adapted to work in Soteria. In

---

[3]When we were writing this book, we were immensely saddened to hear of Loren Mosher's death in Berlin in July 2004. Only a few weeks earlier he had visited Britain, speaking in London, Birmingham and Bradford. In November 2004, the first meeting of INTAR, an international group with participants from the USA, Ireland, Germany, Austria, Finland, Canada and England, reaffirmed the core values of Soteria (see http://intar.org/participants.html). It is a measure of the shift that has taken place in American psychiatry over the last 25 years that Loren Mosher was once the lead researcher for NIMH's schizophrenia research programme, and the founding editor of the journal *Schizophrenia Bulletin*.

[4]This accords well with our own experiences of work as consultant psychiatrists in Bradford Home Treatment Service (see Bracken 2001) and Dryll-y-Car, a crisis house in Gwynedd, North Wales (see Williams *et al.* 1999).

addition, personal experience of psychosis was a particularly valued staff attribute. A significant number of former residents subsequently went on to work in Soteria as members of staff (Loren Mosher, personal communication). Personal qualities of staff were discovered to be much more important than their professional training or expertise.

Before his death, Loren Mosher published a number of papers describing the outcomes for people treated in Soteria compared with standard hospital treatment. Subjects were selected on the basis that their demographic characteristics suggested that they would be more likely to have poor outcomes, and thus likely to make heavy use of psychiatric services over the coming years (single status, age under 32). At 2-year follow-up, people admitted to Soteria with a diagnosis of schizophrenia had significantly better outcomes in terms of psychotic experiences, work and social function than the control group (Bola & Mosher 2003). These outcomes were achieved with much lower levels of medication. At 2-year follow-up, only 58% of Soteria subjects had received neuroleptic medication at any point during the 2 years, and only 19% were on medication continually. In another study from McAuliffe House, a similar project along the lines of Soteria, overall treatment costs in a residential crisis programme were found to be 44% lower compared with an acute admissions ward, with no differences in clinical or social outcomes (Fenton *et al.* 2002)[5].

Soteria also relied on a form of interpersonal phenomenology, partly based on the earlier psychoanalytic work of Harry Stack Sullivan and Freda Fromm-Reichman, and influenced by the work of Medard Boss, John-Paul Sartre and Paul Tillich. Mosher & Burti (1994) emphasized that this was not therapy. There were no fixed 'therapeutic' sessions in Soteria. Interpersonal phenomenology (IP) is a form of intensive interpersonal support described as follows[6]:

> The core practice of interpersonal phenomenology focuses on the development of a non-intrusive, noncontrolling but actively empathetic relationship with the psychotic person without having *to do* anything explicitly therapeutic or controlling. In shorthand, it can be characetrised as 'being with', . . . The aim is to develop, over time, a shared experience of the meaningfulness of the client's individual social context—current and historical. (Mosher 1999: 144)

In his book, *Community Mental Health*, co-authored with Lorenzo Burti, Loren Mosher illustrated the use of IP with three examples taken from a manual, of disturbing unusual beliefs and regression. This was published in German

---

[5]It is worth pointing out that the success of Soteria is not dependent on the personal characteristics of the charismatic, committed clinician who set up the original project in the heady days of late 1960s California. The model has been replicated in Switzerland (Ciompi *et al.* 1992), Germany and Hungary. Community-based services using Soteria principles have been set up in Sweden (Cullberg *et al.* 2002) and Finland (Tuori *et al.* 1998).

[6]IP shares some features in common with Prouty's Pretherapy (Prouty 2001). Both are heavily influenced by hermeneutic phenomenology and the work of Medard philosopher Boss, and that of the existential psychotherapist Ludwig Binswanger and philosopher Martin Buber.

(Mosher *et al.* 1994). IP encourages staff to see the world through the client's eyes in a flexible and non-judgemental manner. Mosher and Burti stress how important it is that staff respond to clients' needs in deference to their own sense of what is right or wrong. It is for this reason that they preferred to have staff who had no commitment to a particular model.

It is important to point out that patients in Soteria were not refused neuroleptic medication. The approach pioneered by Loren Mosher is not 'antimedication', nor for that matter is it antipsychiatry. Medication was carefully negotiated with residents. They were given choices. Consequently, less than one in five of them was on medication continually over the 2 year evaluation. Again, this reflects our own experiences in the Bradford Home Treatment Service and Dryll-y-Car.

Loren Mosher famously resigned from the American Psychiatric Association in 1998, pointing out that one might be excused for believing that its acronym (APA) stood for the American Psychopharmacological Association[7]! He did so in order to draw attention to the domination of psychiatry and psychiatric treatment by the pharmaceutical industry and medication. We share his view that the current emphasis on medication in psychosis is unnecessary. There is a great deal to be gained by reducing our reliance on medication as the main intervention in psychosis, depression and other states of suffering. There are three benefits that accrue from this. First, it reduces the baleful hold of the pharmaceutical industry on the profession (Chapter 6). Secondly, it reduces the potential harm that medication may wreak[8]. Thirdly, people experiencing psychosis may actually fare better if they are helped and supported through the experience without the use of medication (recovery, Chapter 8).

It is important to consider the implications of Soteria for mental health practice today. Soteria was set up in the days before community care had really gathered momentum, inspired by residential facilities such as Kingsley Hall and Chestnut Lodge which were set up as alternatives to the asylums that dominated care 40 years ago. Nevertheless, there are core values enshrined in Soteria that are just as relevant today. Mosher and Burti are explicit about the personal values they expect workers to adopt:

- Do no harm
- Do unto other as you would have done unto yourself
- Be flexible and responsive
- In general the user knows best
- Valuing choice, self-determination, the right to refuse and informed consent

---

[7]A copy of this letter is available at http://www.critpsynet.freeuk.com/Mosher.htm accessed March 8, 2005.
[8]See Robert Whitaker's paper 'The case against antipsychotic drugs' for a well argued antimedication statement (Whitaker 2004).

- Anger, dependency, sexuality and personal growth are acceptable and expected
- Where possible, legitimate needs should be met
- Take risks
- Make power relationships explicit

(Adapted from Mosher & Burti 1994: 101).

Table 10.1 presents the values their therapeutic programmes adopted. It is clear that respect for patients, especially approaching their experiences non-judgementally and seeing the potential for meaning in them, lies at the heart of these values. Soteria helped to create ethical spaces where people could arrive at their own understandings of their experiences. These values are just as relevant today, and they resonate strongly with those we have endeavoured to promote at the Centre for Citizenship and Community Mental Health in Bradford[9]. In a post-community care context, with the British Government seriously considering the adoption of mental health legislation that will enable mental health professionals to force people to take medication against their wishes in the community, it is important to reaffirm these values. In addition, it is important to recognize the negative effect that noxious social environments have on mental health. This means that we have an obligation, as doctors working with people whose lives have been damaged and harmed by these environments, to do whatever we can to mollify them[10]. This is why we believe that Rufus May's work with Evolving Minds and that of Sharing Voices Bradford (Chapter 9) is so important. Both recognize the importance of creating peaceful and sustainable communities of interest around spirituality, creativity and health. They also highlight what, in our view, is an important overlap between such work and community action aimed at increasing social cohesion, building on social capital, and struggling against inequity and oppression. In other words, it reinforces the view that social justice and mental health are inseparable (Chapter 8).

---

[9]See http://www.brad.ac.uk/acad/health/research/cccmh/index.php and follow the links to the Business Plan.

[10]There is nothing new in this. In Amsterdam, in the middle of the 20th century, the Dutch social psychiatrist Arie Querido developed a community-based mental health service that worked with people in acute distress, and engaged directly with the social contexts that were implicated in the individual's breakdown (see for example, Querido 1966). Querido worked for a short period with the American physiologist W.B. Cannon in Harvard, who in turn was interested in Claude Bernard's work on the *milieu intérieur*. Cannon coined the word homeostasis to describe the internal processes that ensured the internal environment of the body was strictly regulated within fixed parameters. Querido adapted this idea, using the expression social homeostasis, to describe how acute mental health crises could be understood in terms of disturbances in the social environment. This work in turn had a great influence on the work of Marius Romme (personal communication).

Table 10.1   Service values

Community responsiveness	Stresses the importance of socio-political and clinical contexts, and participatory processes that include all stakeholders, especially service users and advocacy groups.
Accountability	The service is primarily accountable to the general public and to people who use the service.
Equality and diversity (service environment)	Recognizing the importance of shaping service delivery delivery in recognition of the cultural and socio-economic diversity of the people who use the service.
Client-focused	Mutually respectful, collaborative problem-solving effort involving client, staff, family and other services. Respecting the right of clients to decline particular service interventions (e.g. medication).
Treatment diversity	Many interventions are therapeutic. Every interaction between client and staff is potentially therapeutic. Therapy is not restricted to psychotherapy or medication.
Family involvement	Valuing the strengths and resourcefulness of families, and supporting them in the difficulties they may encounter with a member in distress. Holding families accountable when involved in treatment.
Ecological view	Recognizing the importance of taking the whole context in which the person is embedded into account, including family, work, educational, accommodation, cultural, ethnic and socio-economic factors.
Normalization	The importance of enabling people who use services to lead the most normal possible, e.g. where they live, how they spend their time, and so on.
Medication	Medication is only used within the context of a collaborative, mutually respectful therapeutic alliance.
Professional standards	All staff employed are expected to adhere to the highest standards of professional conduct in their particular field.

From Mosher & Burti (1994: 100). These values are those adapted from the Montgomery County Department of Addiction, Victim and Mental Health Services.

Local developments in a global context

At this point, we want to cast these arguments into a wider arena. There are several themes running through our discussion so far. One questions the sustainability of mental health systems that depend on the unfettered growth of technology, employing more psychiatrists and mental health professionals and using ever greater quantities of drugs. This is specifically a feature of mental health systems in the EA countries.

Another concerns the form and structure of services, their values and philosophy. We have seen that mental health services such as Soteria can function effectively and more economically because they are not reliant upon expensive technological interventions in the form of medication, 'therapy' or other forms of professional expertise. Yet a third theme, one we identified earlier in this book, counters the tendency of science and technology to become a hegemonic, universal discourse, driven by the interests of the pharmaceutical industry (Chapters 3 and 6). It is important now to set these issues in a global context. This is because there is growing evidence that EA countries have much to learn from the ways that ED countries have had to adapt Western models in the light of their economic and political circumstances.

Kwame McKenzie and colleagues (McKenzie *et al.* 2004) have pointed out that although services in low income countries are under-resourced, it has been possible to develop these into creative and adaptable services through ingenuity and the application of local knowledge[11]. One example of this is the work of a community-based rehabilitation (CBR) project, Ashagram, in one of the poorest districts of Madhya Pradesh in India which had no 'biomedical mental health facility'. The authors (Chatterjee *et al.* 2003) are clear about the values base of the project: accessibility, cultural sensitivity and community participation. They describe it as follows:

> Community-based rehabilitation is a model of community care based on the active participation of people with physical disabilities and their families in rehabilitation that takes specific cognisance of prevailing social, economic and cultural issues. (Chatterjee *et al.* 2003: 59)

CBR consists of three tiers, with out-patient care at the top, followed by a second tier of mental health workers drawn from the local community, who

---

[11]Richard Warner's book *Recovery from Schizophrenia: Psychiatry & Political Economy* (Warner 1994) makes the point that social and cultural factors have an enormous influence on the outcome of schizophrenia, much more so than treatment and other therapeutic interventions grounded in science and technology. He examined the results of dozens of studies which looked at outcome and recovery in people given a diagnosis of schizophrenia, over five different periods in the last 100 years, each of which had different socio-economic characteristics. Some studies were performed in times of relative economic prosperity with high levels of employment (e.g. 1941–1955, unemployment rates USA = 4.1%, UK = 1.5%). Others were performed in recessions with high levels of unemployment (e.g. 1921–1940, USA = 11.9%, UK = 14.0%). Warner found a very high correlation between unemployment rates and the extent to which people suffering from schizophrenia were able to make a full recovery. In other words, more people recovered when employment levels are high and their chances of getting back to work were good. He also draws attention to the constant finding from the WHO and other studies of the outcome of schizophrenia in different cultures. He points out that a likely explanation of this is to be found in the greater ease with which people who have experienced psychosis can be reintegrated back into non-industrialized communities, and found meaningful roles in those societies.

were given a 60 day training programme. They each covered five or six villages, with a case load of 25–30 patients. The third tier consisted of family members and the *samitis*: local village health groups which planned culturally relevant rehabilitation measures as well as measures to reduce social exclusion. These included a variety of interventions such as fortnightly user group meetings, monthly community group meetings, access to social benefits, enhancing social networks and vocational rehabilitation. In addition, medication and family counselling were included and links with traditional healers were strongly encouraged.

The hierarchical description of the service in the paper in terms of 'tiers', with mainstream out-patient care at the top and community activities at the bottom, seems misleading, and downplays the importance of CBR. In Table 1 of their paper (Chatterjee *et al.* 2003: 58), the authors compare the main features of CBR with out-patient care. In the latter, people were seen once a month for between 20 and 30 min. In CBR, they were seen weekly for between 60 and 90 min by the mental health workers. When the user groups and community groups are taken into account, it is clear that CBR represents a much more substantial and significant investment of time and effort in clients' care than out-patient care. The paper describes a longitudinal comparison of outcome at 12 months in two groups (not randomly assigned), one of whom received standard out-patient care and the other CBR. The CBR group had significantly better clinical (as measured by the Positive and Negative Symptom Scale) and disability (WHO Disability Assessment Schedule) outcomes. Engagement was significantly better in the CBR group.

This suggests that an approach that is committed to engaging families and local communities, was more effective in responding to economic and cultural barriers. The authors write:

> (CBR) relies on the engagement of communities in the management of disability. Patients and their families were empowered to become informed partners in the planning and implementation of rehabilitation strategies that were ecologically feasible. The village *samitis* provided broad-based local community support for the programme and made a significant impact by generating a positive social milieu that facilitated recovery. (Chatterjee *et al.* 2003: 60)

McKenzie *et al.* (2004) make the important point that the objective of traditional forms of care is not to transfer social responsibilities from the state to under-resourced families and communities, but to recognize the important contribution that social capital makes to a nation's wealth. This point is of vital importance, and it applies with equal force to EA countries. It means that we should see traditional forms of care and approaches rooted in community development (like Sharing Voices Bradford, Chapter 9) as being dependent upon natural human resources that must be invested in, nurtured and developed in a sustainable manner. They must not be seen as 'cheap' alternatives to technological psychiatry. In other words, within the economic constraints that apply in particular cases, all countries have choices to make about the extent to which they invest in local resources such as traditional forms of care, or in high cost technological resources.

A balance has to be struck between central or state control and responsibility, and the empowerment of local communities to take the lead in responding to their health and mental health needs. Our analysis of citizenship at the end of Chapter 9 drew attention to the fear that in advanced liberal democracies, citizenship is becoming a system of governmentality. Discourses of local empowerment are becoming a means for governments to shape subjectivity in particular ways. But this is not a reason to excuse central government's responsibilities for safeguarding the well-being and health of the most vulnerable members of the community. On the other hand, we agree with Kwame McKenzie's analysis that investment in social capital must be exactly that—the investment of resources that support and encourage grass-roots initiatives in mental health. There is now growing recognition that investment in social capital and the mobilization and involvement of local communities are key elements in the development of ethically based and culturally sensitive health and mental health services, notwithstanding the enormous economic inequities between EA and ED countries.

In England, the charity Interaction[12] and its sister organization, the Centre for Reflection on Mental Health Policy, are encouraging local groups of mental health service users and communities to question the tendency for large transnational organizations such as the WHO to impose the type of global initiatives that we described in Chapter 1 on ED countries, or those whose economies are in transition. Policy Paper Number 1 (Interaction 2005) argues that top-down approaches to mental health policy fulfil the interests of powerful groups such as the global pharmaceutical industry and transnational elites such as the WHO, governments, and professional groups such as psychiatrists. All this is at the expense of the local interests of ordinary people, families and communities. Global initiatives reproduce and maintain existing power relationships and support the *status quo*, therefore helping to sustain gross socio-economic disparities that have a particularly malign influence on people who experience mental health problems. Thus they help to perpetuate social exclusion. These power relationships are rooted in colonial and neo-colonial practices that are patriarchal, elitist and insensitive to cultural difference (see Table 10.2). Historically, top-down (or global) approaches to the development of mental health policy have consistently failed to meet the needs of local communities:

> Notwithstanding best intentions, neither governments nor most international agencies have achieved goals or expected results ... In transitional economies[13] and developing countries this presents an additional challenge in promoting and managing alternatives to old orthodoxies of capitalism or socialism and the need to promote culturally acceptable and relevant policies. (Interaction 2005: 2)

---

[12]See htp://www.interaction.uk.net/ accessed March 8, 2005.
[13]For example, countries in the former communist block, and the Balkan states.

Table 10.2 Local versus global knowledge and organizations

	Local	Global
Epistemology	Heterogeneous (heteroglossia —see Chapter 7)	Universal (monological —see Chapter 7)
Values	Participatory Democratic Social justice Negotiated Sustainable—human relationships, environment	Oligarchy Un- or pseudodemocratic Global capitalism Marketing Exploitation—human relationships, environment
Economy	Social capital, bartering (e.g. LETS) and other alternatives to money	Transnational capitalism
Interests served	Ordinary people, service users, individuals and groups Families Communities	Global corporations and organizations Governments Professional groups—psychiatry, psychology
Interpretive systems	Religious faith and spirituality Alternative belief systems Social and political struggles Political groupings	Science and biomedicine Psychiatry and psychology Sociology
Views of madness	Crisis, risk Inclusion Recovery	Mental illness, risk Exclusion 'Cure'
Accountability	Local communities	Unclear? oligarchs and shareholders

LETS, the Local Employment Trading Scheme, is a system of exchanging service without recourse to money.

Like Kwame McKenzie, we believe that EA countries have much to benefit from engaging with the ideas and creative developments that are beginning to emerge in the ED countries. The grass roots initiatives that we described in Chapter 9, Sharing Voices Bradford and Evolving Minds, share features in common with the local developments that are beginning to emerge in some of the ED countries. Table 10.2 attempts to summarize these shared features of local versus globalized forms of knowledge and organization structure. One of the problems in adapting lessons learnt from low income countries to high income ones is that, all too often, traditional beliefs and practices are belittled and looked down on. Such attitudes are found on both EA and ED sides of the fence, and result in traditional forms of care being regarded as 'second rate' and inferior. For example, our own experience in England indicates that there is enormous resistance on the part of mental health services to recognize the valuable contribution to be made by Hakims and other traditional healers.

Desjarlais *et al.* (1996: 265) point out that culture and local institutions assign different meanings to phenomena such as depression, suicide and violence against women. These issues are frequently the subject of lively debate and argument within local cultural, religious and political contexts. In addition, we must be aware that they may arise out of local power structures and patriarchal interests, and be highly oppressive. They point out that 'traditional' forms of healing may be just as oppressive as some traditional responses to new brides or widows. The values embodied by the best examples of traditional care apply to high and low income countries alike. They include:

- recognition of cultural diversity
- locally controlled and administered
- build on local strengths and resources
- repair local weaknesses
- attempt to mitigate economic and structural inequalities
- promote human rights
- recognize the fundamental connection between individual well-being and the well-being of communities (from Desjarlais *et al.* 1996: 266)

There is a strong resonance between these values and those described by Loren Mosher in the Montgomery County Service (Table 10.2).

Postpsychiatry: rethinking the role of science, technology, and expertise

In a paper published in 1988 in the journal *Social Science and Medicine*, Higginbotham and Marsella wrote about the export of Western mental health technologies and the problems engendered by this. They examined the way in which psychiatric care varied little in the capital cities of Southeast Asia, in spite of large social, cultural and linguistic differences between the peoples of these cities. This 'homogenization of psychiatry' was brought about through the inputs of Western (mainly British, American and Dutch) psychiatric experts. Via the mechanisms of international mental health education, consultation and collaboration, a form of psychiatric practice had been created in these different cities that looked to the West for its conceptual foundations and for ideas about innovation and progress. This created a homogenous system of mental health interventions with:

> (A) Common language uniting international and local levels (deriving) from shared assumptions about the shared nature of psychopathology, the use of

standardised assessment, and the efficacy of scientifically derived bio-medical or bio-behavioural interventions. (Higginbotham & Marsella 1988: 553)

While the anticipated effect of these developments was a better standard of patient care, these authors pointed to the unanticipated and very negative consequences which meant, in practice, an actual deterioration in the care received by many people with mental health problems. They stood back from the general approbation associated with the export of psychiatry and presented evidence for serious deleterious 'after-shocks' within local cultural systems. For example:

The inability of local centres to generate research and evaluate services, in combination with pervasive resource and personnel deficiencies, means that hospitals become custodial end-points for chronic cases. Drugs and electric shock treatment are overused and non-psychotic patients are drawn into hospital work forces. (Higginbotham & Marsella 1988: 557)

They were able to demonstrate how the diffusion of Western-based knowledge had promoted professional élitism, institutionalized responses to distress, and had undermined local indigenous healing systems and practices. They argued that in reality:

The net result of introducing a formal treatment system for psychological problems is less help for those in need (Higginbotham & Marsella 1988: 559)

Postpsychiatry is an attempt to take such evidence seriously. It tries to come to terms with the fact that framing distress as a technical problem can have serious negative consequences for individuals, families and communities. It is about facing up to the fact that science can obscure and silence as well as illuminate and liberate. But let us be clear: this is not a naïve or Luddite call for a return to the past, or an argument that all forms of traditional healing and interventions are to be valued. What we mean is that the answers to the problems of mental health across the world will not be met by the development and export of more and more technical interventions. Instead we are interested in promoting diversity even though we are aware that this will lead to increased complexity and contradictions.

A final metaphor

Questioning the legacy of the European Enlightenment has been at the heart of this book. This movement equated progress with the light of science. Perhaps we should think of psychological and psychiatric science in terms of light. And just as the light of the sun (in the form of daylight) reveals a world to us, a world of colour and complexity, so too does psychiatric science open up many aspects of the world of mental illness in a positive way. However, the sun's brilliance has another effect; it obscures the more delicate light of the stars and the planets. It is only when the sun sets that the glory of the night sky is revealed. Of course all the stars are there during the day but we cannot see them because daylight is too strong. Postpsychiatry is our attempt to subdue the bright light of medical science: not because we want to get rid of it or to deny its benefits, but because we believe that the insights of other approaches are equally important and valuable. These approaches lack the organization and funding of academic psychiatry. We hope that our critique of the central assumptions of the psychiatric canon will open up a space in which other voices will be heard and taken seriously. We believe that these voices hold the key to the future.

The veil

When you become one with the universe and meld with it, when all barriers cease to be and you are both light and darkness, when God is in your head, in your mouth, in your eyes, in your ears and in your heart, then madness has become you.

They told me that I was a schizophrenic.

And you realize that you are reviled and despised for what you are. You bear His stripes for what you are. So I became still, a frosted landscape draped in the cold white sameness that fell noiselessly from heaven. All difference must be obscured. I was frozen and dared not to move, for when I moved each and every atom in me stirred and radiated out my being, drawing the eyes of the world to my shame.

They showed me a scan of my brain after they had tried to persuade my mum to take the ring off me. They showed her, too. See here, they said pointing, the cortex is thinner than it should be, and these passages here, they are wider than they should be. These are the hallmarks of schizophrenia.

They told me that my experiences were caused by a serious illness.

She wouldn't listen. She ignored them and took me away from them. I swear that she saved my life the day she sprang me out of that hospital. It must have been so difficult for her. She was struggling too, I know, Juliette told me. But she wouldn't talk about it. Instead she smuggled me out. Then, when I was at home, they tried to drag me back down into purgatory again, this time with the police. We left the house minutes before they arrived; she drove me to Bradford to stay with my uncle. Then, back at home, she cared for me through months of drooling inactivity as I came off the drugs. She told me that I must come off them slowly. She had it all worked out; she must have had some advice from somewhere.

In the end, we were able to talk about things a bit, you know, how difficult she had found it. Just before I left, we were walking down by the river, where 2 years earlier I had last walked with dad. I told her what happened that hot August day after he died.

They told me that it was in my best interests not to dwell on my experience; they tried to persuade her to take the ring back.

I understand, she said. I understand because he speaks to me. He blames me too. We sat and watched the midges' Brownian dance in the morning sunlight over the water. We are so alike, you and I, she said squeezing my hand. I asked if I could go back to Bradford; my uncle was a lecturer in the university there. We went the next day. In Bradford I knew I could get away; up onto the moors and find some space for myself.

You see, although I am different from other people, that's not the real problem. The real problem is how other people see me and respond to me. There are times when my soul opens out to the world. Then I must think, and reflect. I feel the world passing through me, taking me over. That's when I must go out into the wide sky and a world that stretches out in every possible direction, space beyond imagination. I have to be by myself.

They told me that I would not make a full recovery, but that if I were fortunate and took my medication religiously, I might avoid a defect state.

So, I shout and talk to myself. I jabber and I hit them; yes, I hit words for six as they carouse out of me, shooting away at crazy angles. Mad words for which there is yet no use, like light rays whose task it is to find dark places in need of illumination. So I dive to my right and to my left to catch these words before they streak away into space and elude me completely, words that are deliciously slippery as they slide over each other in their rush out of me. The stolid others stop and gape. They gaze down on me and say to themselves how odd, how strange he is, how different he is from us. He is not rational. Unlike us he cannot keep his thoughts in check. When they see me beside myself do I offend them? Does my desire and my passion stir in them some deep forgotten longing for life? I would that it did.

Moving to Bradford took a great deal out of me. In the beginning I was weary and scared. For the first few weeks I kept my head below the parapet. I marked time, reading, listening to music. Gradually my energy and confidence started to come back. I felt a bit stronger. I started to go out and meet a few people.

They told me that I might just manage to hold down an unstressful job, but they strongly advised me against returning to my studies. They said it would over-tax me.

My uncle asked me what I thought about getting back to university. Eighteen months was a long time out, so I began an introductory course on comparative religion, nothing too heavy, but it did get me to think about things in ways that were more natural for me than the psychology I had been studying 2 years earlier. I decided that there was no way I was going back to that. Six months later I started a philosophy degree. For the first time in over 2 years I felt my life was getting back on course.

They told me that my condition was prone to relapse, and the severity of relapse would be likely to increase with time.

Thus my future was written away by a medical malediction, my life chained to a 19th century imprecation from the pen of the doctor on the banks of the Neckar. The more I resisted, the more it ate away inside. Kraepelin's curse fuelled a storm inside me. Whose life was it, mine or theirs? In the end, it was too much; it rose up irresistibly, carrying me away before it, spewing out my anger, rage and despair in a great torrent of madness that erupted on the day of the demonstration against the BNP march in the city centre. I was arrested. My mum rescued me again, this time with my uncle. The next Monday the doctor at student health referred me to Home Treatment. My heart was full of dread before they came. At that moment all I wanted was to leave creation.

I wanted no more of it and needed the white silence. I would give anything for peace and silence, anything, life itself even. The nurse from Home Treatment asked me had I thought of ending my life.

They told me that although the issue of risk was much exaggerated, a small number of schizophrenics posed significant risk to others. However, I was not to worry about this because most schizophrenics were at greater risk of harming themselves than others.

Maybe, I answered, knowing no inner doubt. You won't force me into hospital will you? I don't know, she said, adding that's up to you. I gave her the parac-etamol. She returned the next day. You won't force me to take medication will you? Again, that's up to you, she said. Speak to the doctor when she comes.

They told me that I would have to remain on medication for the rest of my life.

Whether or not you take medication is up to you, she said. It was the first time a doctor had spoken to me like that. You might find it helps for short periods; it can see you though a difficult time. It might even help you to find the peace and tranquillity you are looking for. But you don't have to think of it as a cure for an illness. She smiled at me. Then she asked what I thought the problem was. Why did I hear voices? Why was it my thoughts were some-times so mixed up that no one, not even I, could make sense of them? Why did I want to leave creation? I found all these questions impossible to answer. I fell silent. The next day the nurse introduced me to Ahmad who was to be my support worker. We hit it off right away. He told me that I must be mad because I supported Carlisle United. I asked him if rational beings supported Bradford City. We went for a coffee, and then up to Howarth for a walk on the moors. Over the following weeks those walks became very important. He told me that although he loved walking the smooth barren northern moors, this was nothing compared with Kashmir. There, he told me, the autumn mists hung in deep valleys, the trees bowed with great apples and apricots the size of oranges. He longed to return to see his uncle and nephews, but the troubles had drawn a line of steel between the two families.

One day, we stopped to rest at Top Withens, looking over the wide bowl of Airedale stretching out from West to East below. He asked me why I had said that I wanted to leave creation. I told him that there really was something inside me that was different from other people. This thing, whatever it might be, was at the same time indescribably beautiful and unbearably painful. Sometimes it took me over, and when it did I felt that every single nerve fibre in my body was connected to every particle in the universe. In those moments, I knew everything there was to know; I felt everything there was to feel. And when this happened, William was lost, I said. I didn't know who he was; William became a stranger swallowed up in this all-consuming light. It was too beautiful and too painful to bear. When it happened I had to seek release.

They told me that my experiences were meaningless.

You aren't alone, he replied. Do you know about the Sufis? They have struggled for hundreds of years to understand what you have described, through prayer, devotion, song, and dance.

> *The veil of creation I have made*
>
> *As a screen for the Truth, and in creation there lie*
>
> *Secrets which suddenly like springs gush forth.*

They are a few lines from a poem by a Sufi saint. It is one of my brother's favourites. He is always reciting it. If you like I can ask him to take you to one of their meetings. You would be very welcome.

My mum came along to the meeting they had organized in order to discharge me from Home Treatment. Ahmad was there too, and my doctor. I told them I was ready to go back to university, and that I didn't want to take the medication any more. They asked me if there was anything else they could do to help after I was discharged. There was only one thing I wanted. I told them about the meetings with Ahmad's brother. They meant a great deal to me. They brought me comfort and for the first time in years a sense of belonging and of purpose. Ahmad said that was fine and that his brother had said that with time my qawwali singing might even improve. Then mum asked the doctor what she thought the problem was. He's had a psychosis, came the reply, but he's fine now. But my mum wasn't satisfied. Two years ago in his first admission they told me that he was suffering from schizophrenia. She looked searchingly into the doctor's face. Well, they would say that wouldn't they. Look, it's just a label; it's just one way of trying to do something we all have to do; make sense of the world. There are other ways besides. She smiled and shrugged her shoulders. As we left, I smiled too, and I thought how does the sun shine? Does it matter if we can explain the secret inner workings of the sun? Does that knowledge really change what it means to see the earth's rim rise to swallow the reddening disc, plunging our world into darkness and suspense? Can't we cling to our innocence too? Can't we be allowed to live in hope, even though we may be uncertain of the return of light?

References

Abbasi, K. and Smith, R. (2003) No more free lunches. *British Medical Journal*, **326**, 1155–1156.

Abraham, J. (2002) Making regulation responsive to commercial interests: streamlining drug industry watchdogs. *British Medical Journal*, **325**, 1164–1167.

Amminger, G., Edwards, J., Brewer, W., Harrigan, S. and McGorry, P. (2002) Duration of untreated psychosis and cognitive deterioration in first-episode schizophrenia. *Schizophrenia Research*, **54**, 223–230.

Anderson, E.W. (1963) Foreword. In Jaspers, K. *General Psychopathology* (trans. J. Hoenig and M.W. Hamilton). Manchester: Manchester University Press, p. vi.

Angell, M. (2004) *The Truth About the Drug Companies. How they Deceive Us and What to do About it*. New York: Random House.

Bakhtin, M. (1981) *The Dialogic Imagination* (ed. M. Holquist, trans. C. Emerson and M. Holquist). Austin, University of Texas Press.

Bakhtin, M. (1984) *Problems of Dostoevsky's Poetics* (ed. and trans. C. Emerson). Minneapolis: University of Minneapolis Press.

Bardelay, D. and Kopp, C. (2002) Commentary: concern over drug industry's influence on regulatory policy in Europe. *British Medical Journal*, **325**, 1167–1168.

Barham, P. (1997) *Closing the Asylum: The Mental Patient in Modern Society*, 2nd edn. London: Penguin.

Barham, P. and Hayward, R. (1991) *From the Mental Patient to the Person*. London: Routledge.

Barrett, R. (1996) *The Psychiatric Team and the Social Definition of Schizophrenia*. Cambridge: Cambridge University Press.

Barrett, T.R. and Etheridge, J.B. (1992) Verbal hallucinations in normals. I: people who hear voices. *Applied Cognitive Psychology*, **6**, 379–387.

Beaumont, P.J.V. (1992) Phenomenology and the history of psychiatry. *Australian and New Zealand Journal of Psychiatry*, **26**, 532–545.

Bebbington, P., Bhugra, D., Brugha, T. *et al.* (2004) Psychosis, victimization and childhood disadvantage: evidence from the second British National Survey of Psychiatric Morbidity. *British Journal of Psychiatry*, **185**, 220–226.

Beck, A., Rush, A., Shaw, B. *et al.* (1979) *Cognitive Therapy of Depression*. New York: Guilford.

Bekelman, J., Li, Y. and Gross, C. (2003) Scope and impact of financial conflicts of interest in biomedical research. *Journal of the American Medical Association*, **289**, 454–465.

Bentall, R.P. (1990) The syndromes and symptoms of psychosis: or why you can't play 'twenty questions' with the concept of schizophrenia and hope to win. In *Reconstructing Schizophrenia* (ed. R.P. Bentall). London, Methuen.

Bentall, R.P. (2003) *Madness Explained: Psychosis and Human Nature*. London: Allen Lane.

Berrios, G.E. (1991) Delusions as 'wrong beliefs': a conceptual history. In Delusions and Awareness of Reality. Proceedings of the Fourth Leeds Psychopathology Symposium (ed. A. Sims). *British Journal of Psychiatry*, Supplement **14**, 6–13.

Berrios, G.E. (1993) Phenomenology and psychopathology: was there ever a relationship? *Comprehensive Psychiatry*, **34**, 213–220.

Berry, C. (1994) *A Bit on the Side: East–West Topographies of Desire*. Sydney: Empress, pp. 21–57.

Bhatia, V. (1993) *Analysing Genre: Language Use in Professional Settings*. London: Longman.

Bhui, K., McKenzie, K. and Gill, P. (2003) Delivering mental health services for a diverse society: We need to marry policy and practice. *British Medical Journal*, **329**, 363–364.

Bibeau, G. (1997) Cultural psychiatry in a creolizing world: questions for a new research agenda. *Transcultural Psychiatry*, **34**, 9–41.

Black, D., Morris, J.N., Smith, C. and Townsend, P. (1982) *Inequalities in Health: The Black Report*. Harmondsworth: Penguin.

Boal, A. (2000) *Theater of the Oppressed* (trans. C. McBride, M.-O. McBride and E. Fryer). London: Pluto Press.

Bodenheimer, T. (2000) Uneasy alliance—clinical investigators and the pharmaceutical industry. *New England Journal of Medicine*, **342**, 1539–1544.

Bola, J. and Mosher, L. (2003) Treatment of acute psychosis without neuroleptics: two-year outcomes from the Soteria Project. *Journal of Nervous and Mental Disease*, **191**, 219–229.

Bolton, D. and Hill, J. (1996) *Mind, Meaning and Mental Disorder: The Nature of Causal Explanation in Psychology and Psychiatry*. Oxford: Oxford University Press.

Bolton, G. (2003) Opening the word hoard: who's speaking. *Medical Humanities*, **29**, 97–102.

Borger, J. (2001) USA: the pharmaceutical industry stalks the corridors of power. *Guardian Unlimited*, February 13. Viewed at: http://www.guardian.co.uk/bush/story/0,7369,437338,00.html.

Boseley, S. (2001) Just say no to drug ads. *The Guardian*, December **10**, p. 17.

Boss, M. (1979) *Existential Foundations of Medicine and Psychology* (trans. S. Conway and A. Cleaves). New York: Jason Aronson.

Boyle, M. (1993) *Schizophrenia: A Scientific Delusion?* London: Routledge.

Bracken, P. and Cohen, B. (1999) Home treatment in Bradford. *Psychiatric Bulletin*, 23, 349–352.

Bracken, P. (2001) The radical possibilities of home treatment: postpsychiatry in action. In *Acute Mental Health Care in the Community. Intensive Home Treatment* (ed. N. Brimblecombe). London: Whurr Publishers, pp. 139–162.

Bracken, P. (2002) *Trauma: Culture, Meaning and Philosophy*. London: Whurr Publications.

Bracken, P. (2003) Postmodernism and psychiatry. *Current Opinion in Psychiatry*, **16**, 673–677.

Brison, S. (2002) *Aftermath: Violence and the Remaking of the Self*. Princeton, NJ: Princeton University Press.

Brody, H. (1994) 'My story is broken; can you help me fix it?' Medical ethics and the joint construction of narrative. *Literature and Medicine*, **13**, 79–92.

Brody, H. and Waters, D. (1980) Diagnosis is treatment. *Journal of Family Practice*, **10**, 445–449.

Brown, B., Nolan, P., Crawford, P. and Lewis, A. (1996) Interaction, language and the 'narrative turn' in psychotherapy and psychiatry. *Social Science and Medicine*, **43**, 1569–1578.

Brown, G. and Harris, T. (1978) *The Social Origins of Depression: A Study of Psychiatric Disorder in Women*. New York: Free Press.

Brunner, P. (1996) A survival story. In *Speaking Our Minds: An Anthology* (ed. J. Read and J. Reynolds). London: Macmillan, Open University, pp. 16–22.

Bryer, J.B., Nelson, B.A., Miller, J.B. *et al.* (1987) Childhood sexual and physical abuse as factors in adult psychiatric illness. *American Journal of Psychiatry*, **144**, 1426–1430.

Bullard, A. (2002) From vastation to Prozac nation. *Transcultural Psychiatry*, **39**, 267–294.

Button, G., Coulter, J., Lee, J. and Sharrock, W. (1995) *Computers, Minds and Conduct.* Cambridge, Polity Press.

Campbell, P. (1996) Challenging loss of power. In *Speaking Our Minds: An Anthology* (ed. J. Read and J. Reynolds). London: Macmillan, Open University, pp. 56–62.

Chadwick, P. and Birchwood, M. (1994) The omnipotence of voices: a cognitive approach to auditory hallucinations. *British Journal of Psychiatry*, **164**, 190–201.

Chaika, E. (1974) A linguist looks at 'schizophrenic' language. *Brain and Language*, **1**, 257–276.

Chamberlain, J. (1978) *On our Own: Patient Controlled Alternatives to the Mental Health System.* New York: McGraw-Hill.

Chamberlin, J. (1998) Citizenship rights and psychiatric disability. *Psychiatric Rehabilitation Journal*, **21**, 405–408.

Chatterjee, S., Patel, V., Chatterjee, A. and Weiss, H. (2003) Evaluation of a community-based rehabilitation model for chronic schizophrenia in rural India. *British Journal of Psychiatry*, **182**, 57–62.

Chomsky, N. (1959) Review of B.F. Skinner's *Verbal Behaviour. Language*, **35**, 26–58.

Chomsky, N. and Miller, G. (1963*a*) Introduction to the formal analysis of natural languages. In *Handbook of Mathematical Psychology II* (ed. R. Luce, R. Bush and E. Galanter). New York: Wiley, pp. 269–322.

Chomsky, N. and Miller, G. (1963*b*) Finitary models of language users. In *Handbook of Mathematical Psychology II* (ed. R. Luce, R. Bush and E. Galanter). New York: Wiley, pp. 419–491.

Choudhry, N., Stelfox, H. and Detsky, A. (2002) Relationships between authors of clinical practice guidelines and the pharmaceutical industry. *Journal of the American Medical Association*, 287, 612–617.

Choudhry, N.K., Stelfox, H.T. and Detsky, A.S. (2002) Relationships between authors of clinical practice guidelines and the pharmaceutical industry. *Journal of the American Medical Association*, **287**, 612–617.

Ciompi, L., Dauwalder, H.P., Maier, C., Aebi, E., Trutsch, K., Kupper, Z. *et al.* (1992) The pilot project 'Soteria Berne'. Clinical experiences and results. *British Journal of Psychiatry*, Supplement **18**, 145–153.

Clifford, J. (1984) *Introduction: Partial Truths* in *Writing Culture: The Poetics and Politics of Ethnography* (ed. J. Clifford and G. Marcus). Berkeley: University of California Press.

Clifford, J. (1988) *The Predicament of Culture: Twentieth Century, Ethnography, Lliterature, and Art.* Cambridge, MA: Harvard University Press.

Cohen, J.D. and Servan-Schreiber, D. (1992) Context, cortex and dopamine: a connectionist approach to behaviour and biology in schizophrenia. *Psychological Review*, **99**, 45–77.

Coleman, R. (1999) *Recovery: An Alien Concept.* Gloucester: Handsell Publishing.

Craddock, N., Owen, M., Kurian, B., Thomas, P. and McGuffin, P. (1994). Familial cosegregation of major affective disorder and Darier's disease (keratosis follicularis). *British Journal of Psychiatry*, **164**, 355–358.

Cullberg, J., Levander, S., Holmqvist, R., Mattsson, M. and Wieselgren, I.-M. (2002) One-year outcome in first episode psychosis patients in the Swedish Parachute project. *Acta Psychiatrica Scandinavica*, **106**, 276–285.

Davies, P., Leudar, I. and Thomas, P. (1999) Dialogical engagement with voices: a single case study. *British Journal of Medical Psychology*, **72**, 179–187.

Davies, P., Thomas, P. and Leudar, I. (1999) Dialogical engagement and verbal hallucinations: a single case study. *British Journal of Medical Psychology*, **72**, 179–187.

De Deyn, P. and d'Hooge, R. (1996) Placebos in clinical practice and research. *Journal of Medical Ethics*, **22**, 140–146.

Deegan, P. (1996) Recovery as a journey of the heart. *Psychiatric Rehabilitation Journal*, **19**, 91–97.

Dentith, S. (1995) *Bakhtinian Thought: An Introductory Reader*. London: Routledge.

Department of Health (1995) *Variations in Health: What Can the Department of Health and the NHS Do?* London: Department of Health.

Department of Health (1998*a*) *Modernising Mental Health Services: Safe, Sound and Supportive*. London: Department of Health. (http://www.DH.gov.uk/nsf/mentalh.htm)

Department of Health (1998*b*) Press release *Strategy launched to modernise mental health services*. December **8**, 1998.

Department of Health (1999) *Modern Standards and Service Models: Mental Health National Service Frameworks*. London: Department of Health.

Department of Health (2002) *Prescription Cost Analysis 2001*. London, HMSO.

Department of Health (2003) Delivering Race Equality: A Framework for Action 1/10/2003 http://www.dh.gov.uk/Consultations/ClosedConsultations/ClosedConsultations Article/fs/en?CONTENT_ID=4067441&chk=vZZvm%2B accessed January **25**, 2005.

Department of Health (2004) *Delivering Race Equality in Mental Health Care: An Action Plan for Reform Inside and Outside Services*. London: DoH.

Department of Health (2005) Delivering race equality in mental health care: an action plan for reform inside and outside services and the Government's response to the Independent inquiry into the death of David Bennett http://www.dh.gov.uk/ PublicationsAndStatistics/Publications/PublicationsPolicyAndGuidance/ PublicationsPolicyAndGuidanceArticle/fs/en?CONTENT_ID=4100773&chk= grJd1N accessed January **25**, 2005.

Descartes, R. (1968) *Discourse on Method and the Meditations* (ed. F.E. Sutcliffe). London: Penguin Books.

Desjarlais, R., Eisenberg, L., Good, B. and Kleinman, A. (1996) *World Mental Health: Problems and Priorities in Low Income Countries*. Oxford: Oxford University Press.

Dewan, V. (1996) The pressure of being a human chameleon. In *Speaking Our Minds: An Anthology* (ed. J. Read and J. Reynolds). London: Macmillan, Open University, pp. 23–27.

Dillon, J. and May, R. (2002) Reclaiming experience. *Clinical Psychology*, **17**, 25–28.

Dobson, F. (1998) *Foreword in Modernising Mental Health Services: Safe, Sound and Supportive*. London: Department of Health.

Dodds, P. and Bowles, N. (2001) Dismantling formal observation and refocusing nursing activity in acute inpatient psychiatry: a case study. *Journal of Mental Health and Psychiatric Nursing*, **8**, 183–188.

Doerner, K. (1981) *Madness and the Bourgeoisie: A Social History of Insanity and Psychiatry*. Oxford: Basil Blackwell.

Dostoyevsky, F. (1955) *The Idiot* (trans D. Margashack). London: Penguin Books.

Double, D. (2002) The limits of psychiatry. *British Medical Journal*, **324**, 900–904.

Dreyfus, H. (1991) *Being-in-the-World. A Commentary on Heidegger's Being and Time*. Cambridge, MA: MIT Press.

Eagleton, T. (1983) *Literary Theory*. Oxford: Oxford University Press.

Edwards, J., Maude, D., McGorry, P., Harrigan, S. and Cocks, J. (1998) Prolonged recovery in first-episode psychosis. *British Journal of Psychiatry*, **172** (Supplement 33), 107–116.

Ellett, L., Lopes, B. and Chadwick, P. (2003) Paranoia in a non-clinical population of college students. *Journal of Nervous & Mental Disease*, **191**, 425–430.

Ensink, B. (1992) *Confusing Realities: A Study on Child Sexual Abuse and Psychiatric Symptoms*. Amsterdam: VU University Press.

Ensink, B. (1993) Trauma: a study of child abuse and hallucinations. In *Accepting Voices* (ed. M. Romme and S. Escher). London: MIND.

Escher, S., Romme, M., Buiks, A., Delespaul, P. and Van Os, J. (2002) Independent course of childhood auditory hallucinations: a sequential 3-year follow up study. *British Journal of Psychiatry*, **181** (Supplement 43), 10–18.

Estroff, S. (1989) Self, identity and the subjective experiences of schizophrenia. *Schizophrenia Bulletin*, **15**, 189–196.

Faulconer, J.E. and Williams, R.N. (1985) Temporality in human action. An alternative to positivism and historicism. *American Psychologist*, **40**, 1179–1188.

Faulkner, A. and Layzell, S. (2000) *Strategies for Living: A Report of User-led Research into People's Strategies for Living with Mental Distress*. London: Mental Health Foundation.

Faulkner, A. and Thomas, P. (2002) User-led research and evidence based medicine. *British Journal of Psychiatry*, **180**, 1–3.

Fenigstein, A. and Vanable, P. (1992) Persecutory ideation and self-consciousness. *Journal of Personality and Social Psychology*, **62**, 129–138.

Fenton, W., Hoch, J., Herrell, Mosher, L. and Dixon, L. (2002) Cost and cost-effectiveness of hospital vs. residential crisis care for patients who have serious mental illness. *Archives of General Psychiatry*, **59**, 357–364.

Fernando, S. (1991) *Mental Health, Race and Culture*. London: Macmillan/MIND.

Fisher, J. (1987) Object of fetishism. In *Framing Feminism: Art and the Women's Movement 1970–1985* (ed. R. Parker and G. Pollock). London: Pandora Press, pp. 322–323.

Foucault, M. (1970) *The Order of Things. An Archaeology of the Human Sciences*. London: Tavistock Publications.

Foucault, M. (1971) *Madness and Civilization: A History of Insanity in the Age of Reason*. London: Tavistock.

Foucault, M. (1977*a*) *Discipline and Punish* (trans. Sheridan, A. London: Allen Lane).

Foucault, M. (1977*b*) *Language, Counter-Memory, Practice* (ed. D.F. Bouchard). Ithaca, NY: Cornell University Press.

Foucault, M. (1980) Truth and Power. In *Power/Knowledge: Selected Interviews and Other Writings 1972–1977* (ed. C. Gordon). Brighton: Harvester.

Foucault, M. (1981) *The History of Sexuality, Volume 1*. London: Penguin.

Foucault, M. (1991) Governmentality. In *The Foucault Effect: Studies in Governmentality* (ed. G. Burchell, C. Gordon and P. Miller). Chicago: University of Chicago Press, pp. 87–104.

Frank, J. (1961) *Persuasion and Healing: A Comparative Study of Psychotherapy*. Baltimore: Johns Hopkins Press.

Freemantle, N., Anderson, I.M. and Young, P. (2000) Predictive value of pharmacological activity for the relative efficacy of antidepressant drugs: meta-regression analysis. *British Journal of Psychiatry*, **177**, 292–302.

Freire, P. (1996) Pedagogy of the oppressed. (Trans. Myra Ramos.) Harmondsworth: Penguin.

Frith, C. (1992) *The Cognitive Neuropsychology of Schizophrenia*. Hove: Lawrence Erlbaum Associates.

Fulford, K.W.M. (1989) *Moral Theory and Medicine Practice*. Cambridge: Cambridge University Press.

Fulford, K.W.M. (1994) Closet logics: hidden conceptual elements in the DSM and ICD classifications of mental disorders. In *Philosophical Perspectives on Psychiatric Diagnostic Classification* (ed. J.Z. Sadler, O.P. Wiggins and M.A. Schwartz). Baltimore: The Johns, Hopkins University Press.

Fulford, K.W.M. (2004) Ten principles of values-based medicine. In *The Philosophy of Psychiatry: A Companion* (ed. J. Radden). New York: Oxford University Press, pp. 205–234.

Fuller-Torrey, E. (2002) The going rate on shinks. *The American Prospect*, Vol. **13**, no. **13**, July 15. Viewed at: http://www.prospect.org/print/V13/13/torrey-e.html

Gaines, A. (1992) Ethnopsychiatry: the cultural construction of psychiatries. In *Ethnopsychiatry: The Cultural Construction of Professional and Folk Psychiatries.* (ed. A. Gaines). Albany, NY: State University of New York Press, pp. 3–49.

Geddes, J. and Wessely, S. (2000) Clinical standards in psychiatry: how much evidence is required and how good is the evidence base? *Psychiatric Bulletin*, **24**, 83–84.

Geddes, J., Freemantle, N., Harrison, P. and Bebbington, P. (2000) Atypical antipsychotics in the treatment of schizophrenia: systematic overview and meta-regression analysis. *British Medical Journal*, **321**, 1371–1376.

Gillon, R. (1985) *Philosophical Medical Ethics*. Chichester: Wiley.

Goldberg, E.M. and Morrison, S.L. (1963) Schizophrenia and social class. *British Journal of Psychiatry*, **109**, 785–802.

Goodman, L., Rosenberg, S., Mueser, K. *et al.* (1997) Physical and sexual assault history in women with serious mental illness: prevalence, correlates, treatment, and future research directions. *Schizophrenia Bulletin*, **23**, 685–696.

Gordon, C. (1990) Histoire de la Folie: an unknown book by Michel Foucault. *History of the Human Sciences*, **3**, 3–26.

Greenfield, S.F., Strakowski, S.M., Tohen, M. *et al.* (1994) Childhood abuse in first-episode psychosis. *British Journal of Psychiatry*, **164**, 831–834.

Greenhalgh, T. (1999) Narrative based medicine: narrative based medicine is an evidence based world. *British Medical Journal*, **318**, 323–325.

Greenhalgh, T. and Hurwitz, B. (1999) Narrative based medicine: why study narrative? *British Medical Journal*, **318**, 48–50.

Guardian (2003) Minister bars asylum seekers from surgery. February 26. http://www.guardian.co.uk/uk_news/story/0,3604,903216,00.html

Guardian (2004) Comment by Naomi Klein. October 2004. http://www.guardian.co.uk/comment/story/0,,13228664,00.html

Gupta, M. and Kay, L.R. (2003) Phenomenological methods in psychiatry: a necessary first step. *Philosophy, Psychiatry and Psychology*, **9**, 93–96.

Hacking, I. (1982) Language, truth and reason. In *Rationality and Relativism* (ed. R. Hollis and S. Lukes). Cambridge MA: Cambridge University Press, pp. 185–203.

Haddock, G., Bentall, R.P. and Slade, P.D. (1993) Psychological treatment of chronic auditory hallucinations: two case studies, *Behavioural and Cognitive Psychotherapy*, **21**, 335–346.

Halperin, D. (1995) *Saint Foucault: Towards a Gay Hagiography*. Oxford: Oxford University Press.

Haraway, D. (1988) Situated knowledge. *Feminist Studies*, **14**, 575.

Hardt, M. and Negri, A. (2000) *Empire*. Cambridge, MA: Harvard University Press.

Haynes, B. and Devereaux, P. (2002) Physicians' and patients' choices in evidence based practice: evidence does not make decisions, people do. *British Medical Journal*, **324**, 1350.

Heidegger, M. (1962) *Being and Time* (trans. J. Macquarrie and E. Robinson). Oxford: Blackwell.

Heixheimer, A. (2003) Relationships between the pharmaceutical industry and patient's organisations. *British Medical Journal*, **326**, 1208–1210.

Higginbotham, N. and Marsella, A. (1988) International consultation and the homogenization of psychiatry in Southeast Asia. *Social Science and Medicine*, **27**, 553–561.

Hill, J. (2003) Placebos in clinical care: for whose pleasure? *Lancet*, **362**, 254.

HMSO (1989) *Caring for People*. Cm **849**, London: HMSO.

HMSO (1992) *The Health of the Nation*. Cm 1986, London: HMSO.

HMSO (2000) *The NHS Plan: A Plan for Investment, A Plan for Reform*. Cm 4818-I, London: HMSO.

HMSO (2004) *Securing Good Health for the Whole Population*. London: HMSO. Available at http://www.hm-treasury.gov.uk/Consultations_and_Legislation/wanless/consult_wanless_final.cfm accessed March 7, 2005.

Hobart, M. (1985) Anthropos through the looking glass: or how to teach the Balinese to bark. In *Reason and Morality* (ed. J. Overing). London: Tavistock, pp. 104–134.

Hoeller, K. (1988) Phenomenology, psychology, and science. In: *Heidegger and Psychology* (ed. K. Hoeller). Seattle, Review of Existential Psychology and Psychiatry.

Hoffman, R.E. (1986) Verbal hallucinations and language production processes in schizophrenia. *Behavioural and Brain Sciences*, **9**, 503–548.

Holmes, J. (2000) Narrative in psychiatry and psychotherapy: the evidence? *Journal of Medical Ethics and Medical Humanities*, **26**, 92–96.

Holquist, M. (1981) *Introduction*. In Bakhtin, M. *The Dialogic Imagination* (ed. M. Holquist, trans. C. Emerson and M. Holquist). Austin: University of Texas Press, pp. xv–xxxiii.

Holquist, M. (1990) *Dialogism Bakhtin and his World*. London: Routledge, pp. xv–xxxviii.

Home Office (1998) *Speaking Up for Justice*. Report of the Inter-departmental Working Group on the Treatment of Vulnerable or Intimidated Witnesses in the Criminal Justice System. London: Home Office.

Husserl, E. (1970) *Logical Investigations*, 2 vols. (trans J.N. Findlay). New York: Humanities Press.

Huxley, P. and Thornicroft, G. (2003) Social inclusion, social quality and mental illness. *British Journal of Psychiatry*, **182**, 289–290.

Ignatieff, M. (1989) Citizenship and moral narcissism. *Political Quarterly*, **60**, 63–74.

Illich, I. (1976) *Medical Nemesis*. New York: Bantum Books.

Ingleby, D. (1981) Understanding 'mental illness'. In *Critical Psychiatry: The Politics of Mental Health* (ed. D. Ingleby). Harmondsworth: Penguin.

Interaction (2005) *Policy Position Paper 1: Involving All Stakeholders in Mental Health Policy—A Challenge for the Intergovernmental Organisations*. Available at http://www.interaction.uk.net/pdf/policy_position.pdf accessed March 8, 2005.

Jackson, T. (2001) Are you being duped? How drug companies use opinion leaders. *British Medical Journal*, **322**, 1312.

Jameson, R. (1996) Schizophrenia from the inside. In *Speaking Our Minds: An Anthology* (ed. J. Read and J. Reynolds). London: Macmillan, Open University, pp. 54–55.

Jamous, H. and Peloille, B. (1970) Professions or self-perpetuating systems? Changes in the French university-hospital system. In *Professions and Professionalization* (ed. J.A. Jackson). London: Cambridge University Press, pp. 109–152.

Jaspers, K. (1963) *General Psychopathology* (trans. J. Hoenig and M.W. Hamilton). Manchester: Manchester University Press.

Jenkins, J. and Karno, M. (1992) The meaning of expressed emotion: theoretical issues raised by cross-cultural research. *American Journal of Psychiatry*, **149**, 9–21.

Johns, L., Nazroo, J., Bebbington, P. and Kuipers, E. (2002) Occurrence of hallucinatory experiences in a community sample and ethnic variations. *British Journal of Psychiatry*, **180**, 174–178.

Johnstone, L. (2000) *Users and Abusers of Psychiatry: A Critical Look at Traditional Psychiatric Practice*. London: Routledge.

Jones, A. (1996) Literature and medicine: an evolving canon. *Lancet*, **348**, 1360–1362.

Jones, A. (1997) Literature and medicine: narrative ethics. *Lancet*, **349**, 1243–1246.

Jones, A. (1999) Narrative based medicine: narrative in medical ethics. *British Medical Journal*, **318**, 253–256.

Jones, K. (1988) *Experience in Mental Health*. London: Sage.

Kelly, M. (1987) Beyond the purloined image. In *Framing Feminism: Art and the Women's Movement 1970–1985* (ed. R. Parker and G. Pollock). London: Pandora Press, 249–253.

Kendell, R. and Jablensky, A. (2003) Distinguishing between the validity and utility of psychiatric diagnoses. *American Journal of Psychiatry*, **160**, 4–12.

Kennedy, I. (1981) *The Unmasking of Medicine*. London: George Allen & Unwin.

Kerwin, R. (2004) e-Interview with Dominic Fannon. *Psychiatric Bulletin*, **28**, 313.

Khan, A., Warner, H.A. and Brown, W.A. (2000) Symptom reduction and suicide risk in patients treated with placebo in antidepressant trials: an analysis of the Food and Drug Administration database. *Archives of General Psychiatry*, **57**, 311–317.

Kirsch, I., Moore, T.J., Scoboria, A. and Nicholls, S.S. (2002) The Emperor's new drugs: an analysis of antidepressant medication data submitted to the U.S. Food and Drug Administration. *Prevention and Treatment*, Vol. 5, article 23, posted July 15. Viewed at: http://www.journals.apa.org/prevention/volume5/pre0050023a.html

Klein, N. (2001) No Logo. London: Flamingo.

Kleinman, A. and Cohen, A. (1997) Psychiatry's global challenge. *Scientific American*, **276**, 86–91.

Kottow, M. and Kottow, A. (2002) Literary narrative in clinical practice. *Medical Humanities*, **28**, 41–44.

Kovel, J. (1988) *The Radical Spirit. Essays on Psychoanalysis and Society*. London: Free Association Books.

Kramer, P.D. (1993) *Listening to Prozac*. New York: Viking.

Kuhn, T. (1962) *The Structure of Scientific Revolutions*. Chicago: University of Chicago Press.

Kundera, M. (1996) *The Book of Laughter and Forgetting*. New York: Harper Collins.

Kutchins, H. and Kirk, S. (1999) *Making Us Crazy. DSM: The Psychiatric Bible and the Creation of Mental Disorders*. London: Constable.

Laing, R.D. (1965) *The Divided Self*. London: Pelican Books.

Lancet (2002a) Europe on the brink of direct-to-consumer drug advertising. *Lancet*, **359**, 1709.

Lancet (2002b) Just how tainted has medicine become? *Lancet*, **359**, 1167.

Langenbach, M. (1995) Phenomenology, intentionality, and mental experiences: Edmund Husserl's *Logische Untersuchungen* and the first edition of Kaarl Jaspers's *Allgemeine Psychopathologie*. *History of Psychiatry*, **6**, 209–224.

Langer, M. (1989) *Merleau-Ponty's Phenomenology of Perception: A Guide and Commentary*. London: Macmillan.

Lapsley, H., Nikora, L. and Black, R. (2002) *Kia Mauri Tau!: Narratives of Recovery from Disabling Mental Health Problems*. Report of the University of Waikito Mental Health Narratives Project. Mental Health Commission, Wellington NZ. Available on http://www.mhc.govt.nz/publications/2002/Kia_Mauri_Tau.pdf accessed October **28**, 2004.

Laugharne, R. (2004) Psychiatry in the future. The next 15 years: postmodern challenges and opportunities. *Psychiatric Bulletin*, 28, 317–318.

Launer, J. (1999) A narrative approach to mental health in general practice. *British Medical Journal*, **318**, 117–119.

Lenzer, J. (2004) Bush plans to screen whole US population for mental illness. *British Medical Journal*, **328**, 1458.

Leudar, I. and Thomas, P. (2000) *Voices of Reason, Voices of Insanity*. London: Brunner Routledge.

Leudar, I., Thomas, P., McNally, D. and Glinki, A. (1996) What can voices do with words? Pragmatics of verbal hallucinations. *Psychological Medicine*, **27**, 885–989.

Lewis, B. (2000) Psychiatry and postmodern theory. *Journal of Medical Humanities*, **21**, 71–84.

Lewis, B.E. (2003) Prozac and the post-human politics of cyborgs. *Journal of Medical Humanities*, **24**, 49–63.

Lexchin, J., Bero, L., Djulbegovic, B. and Clark, O. (2003) Pharmaceutical industry sponsorship and research outcome and quality: systematic review. *British Medical Journal*, **326**, 1167–1170.

Lièvre, M. (2002) Alosetron for irritable bowel syndrome. Some patients may pay a high price for the FDA's decision to put the drug back on the market. *British Medical Journal*, 555–556.

Lombardo, P. (1983) Involuntary sterilisation in Virginia: from Buck v. Bell to Poe v. Lynchburg. *Developments in Mental Health Law*, **3**, 17–21.

Luborsky, L.B., Singer, B. and Luborsky, L. (1975) Comparative studies of psychotherapy. Is it true that 'everyone has won and all must have prizes?' *Archives of General Psychiatry*, **32**, 995–1008.

Lyons, J. (1991) *Chomsky*. London: Fontana Press.

Magee, B. (1978) *Men of Ideas: Some Creators of Contemporary Philosophy*. Oxford: Oxford University Press.

Marinetto, M. (2003) Who wants to be an active citizen? The politics and practice of community involvement. *Sociology*, **37**, 103–120.

Marketos, S. (2000) Medicine and humanities. *Archives of Hellenic Medicine*, **17**, 446–449.

Martin, J. and Penn, D. (2001) Social cognition and subclinical paranoid ideation. *British Journal of Clinical Psychology*, **40**, 261–267.

Matthews, E. (2002) *The Philosophy of Merleau-Ponty*. Chesham: Acumen.

May, R. (2000) Routes to recovery from psychosis: the roots of a clinical psychologist. *Clinical Psychology Forum*, **146**, 6–10.

May, R. (2004) Making sense of psychotic experience and working towards recovery. In *Psychological Interventions in Early Psychosis: A Treatment Handbook* (ed. J. Gleeson and P. McGorry). Chichester: Wiley, 245–260.

McCabe, R., Heath, C., Burns, T. and Priebe, S. (2002) Engagement of patients with psychosis in the consultation: conversation analytic study. *British Medical Journal*, **325**, 1148–1151.

McCrone, P. and Thornicroft, G. (1997) Credit where credit's due. *Community Care*, September, 18–24.

McCumber, J. (1999) *Metaphysics and Oppression: Heidegger's Challenge to Western Philosophy*. Bloomington: Indiana University Press.

McIntosh, C. (1996) The right to be informed. In *Speaking Our Minds: An Anthology* (ed. J. Read and J. Reynolds). London: Macmillan, Open University, pp. 7–72.

McKenzie, K. (1999) Something borrowed from the blues? We can use the Lawrence inquiry findings to help eradicate racial discrimination in the NHS. *British Medical Journal*, **318**, 616–617.

McKenzie, K., Patel, V. and Araya, R. (2004) Learning from low income countries: mental health. *British Medical Journal*, **329**, 1138–1140.

McLellan, M. (1997) Literature and medicine: physician writers. *Lancet*, **349**, 564–567.

Meehl, P. (1962) Schizotaxia, schizotypy, schizophrenia. *American Psychologist*, **17**, 827–838.

Melander, H., Ahlquist-Rastad, J., Meijer, G. and Beermann, B. (2003) Evidence b(i)ased medicine—selective reporting from studies sponsored by pharmaceutical industry: a review of studies in new drug applications. *British Medical Journal*, **326**, 1171–1173.

Mental Health Foundation (1997) *Knowing our Own Minds: A Survey of How People in Emotional Distress Take Control of Their Lives*. London: MHF.

Mercer, K. (1992) Skin head sex thing: racial difference and the homoerotic imaginary. *New Formations* **16**, 1–23. Republished in *How Do I Look: Queer Films and Video*. Bad-Object Choices. Seattle: Bay Press, pp. 169–210.

Messer, S.B. and Warren, C.S. (2001) Understanding and treating the postmodern self. In *Self-Relations in the Psychotherapy Process* (ed. J.C. Murran). Washington, DC: American Psychological Association.

Meyer, J. (2000) Using qualitative methods in health related action research. *British Medical Journal*, **320**, 178–181.

Mezzich, J.E. (1995) Classification of mental disorders: International perspectives on psychiatric diagnosis. In *Comprehensive Textbook of Psychiatry VI*, 6th edn, 2 vols. (ed. H.I. Kaplan and B.J. Sadock). Baltimore: Williams and Wilkins, pp. 692–702.

Miller, G. (1974) *Psychology, The Science of Mental Life*. Penguin: Harmondsworth.

Miller, P. (1986) Critiques of psychiatry and critical sociologies of madness. In *The Power of Psychiatry*. (P. Miller and N. Rose). Cambridge: Polity Press, pp. 12–42.

Miller, P. and Rose, N. (1986) *The Power of Psychiatry*. Cambridge: Polity Press.

MIND (2003) Evidence to The Independent Panel of Inquiry into the events leading to the death of David Bennett http://www.mind.org.uk/NR/rdonlyres/7ADC1B4D-1142-4BB5-81F2-6B82008F2341/1151/03bennettevidence.doc accessed January **25**, 2005.

Mishler, E. (1984) *The Discourse of Medicine: Dialectics of Medical Interviews*. Norwood, NJ: Ablex, p. 128.

Mishra, A.L. (1994) A phenomenological critique of commonsensical assumptions in DSM-III-R. The avoidance of the patient's subjectivity. In *Philosophical Perspectives on Psychiatric Diagnostic Classification* (ed. J.S. Sadler, O.P. Wiggins and M.A. Schwartz). Baltimore: The Johns Hopkins University Press, pp. 129–147.

Mitchell, W. (1915) The case of George Dedlow. In: *The Autobiography of a Quack and Other Stories*. New York: The Century, pp. 83–109.

Moerman, D. (2002) *Meaning, Medicine and the 'Placebo Effect'*. Cambridge Studies in Medical Anthropology. Cambridge: Cambridge University Press.

Moncrieff, J. (1999) An investigation into the precedents of modern drug treatment in psychiatry. *History of Psychiatry*, **10**, 475–490.

Moncrieff, J. (2002) *Drug Treatment in Modern Psychiatry: The History of a Delusion*. Talk given at Critical Psychiatry Network conference, 'Beyond drugs and custody: renewing mental health practice', April **26**, 2002. Available on http://www.critpsynet.freeuk.com/Moncrieff.htm accessed November 23, 2004.

Moncrieff, J. (2003) *Is Psychiatry for Sale? An Examination of the Influence of the pharmaceutical industry on academic and practical psychiatry*. Maudsley Discussion Paper. London: Institute of Psychiatry.

Moran, D. (2000) *Introduction to Phenomenology*. London: Routledge.

Mortimer, A. (1992) Phenomenology: its place in schizophrenia research. *British Journal of Psychiatry*, **161**, 293–297.

Mosher, L. (1999) Soteria and other alternatives to acute psychiatric hospitalisation: a personal and professional review. *Journal of Nervous and Mental Disease*, **187**, 142–149.

Mosher, L. and Burti, L. (1994) *Community Mental Health: A Practical Guide*. New York: W.W. Norton.

Mosher, L., Menn, A., Vallone, R. and Fort, D. (1994) *Dabeisein—Das Manual zur Praxis in der Soteria*. Bonn: Psychiatrie–Verlug.

Mowbray, C.T., Oyersman, D., Zemencuk, J.K. and Ross, S.R. (1995) Motherhood for women with serious mental illness. *American Journal of Orthopsychiatry*, **65**, 21–38.

Moynihan, R. (2002) Alosetron: a case study in regulatory capture, or a victory for patients' rights? *British Medical Journal*, **325**, 592–595.

Moynihan, R. (2003) Who pays for the pizza? Redefining the relationships between doctors and drug companies. 1: Entanglement. *British Medical Journal*, **326**, 1189–1192.

Muran, J.C. (ed.) (2001) *Self-Relations in the Psychotherapy Process*. Washington, DC: American Psychological Association.

Nawaz, A. (2004) Islam for me was more punk than punk. Aki Nawaz interviewed by Angela Saini in *Open Democracy*. October 7, 2004, available at http://www.opendemocracy.net/debates/article.jsp?id=6&debateId=91&articleId=2138 accessed December 2, 2004.

NICE (2002) Schizophrenia: Core Interventions in the Treatment and Management of Schizophrenia in Primary and Secondary Care. National Collaborating Centre for Mental Health, commissioned by the National Institute for Clinical Excellence. Available on http://www.nice.org.uk/page.aspx?o=42424, accessed October 8, 2004.

NICE (2002a) Technology appraisal No. 43: Guidance on the use of newer (atypical) antipsychotic drugs for the treatment of schizophrenia. London: National Institute for Clinical Excellence.

NICE (2002b) *Clinical Guideline 1: Schizophrenia. Core Interventions in the Treatment and Management of Schizophrenia in Primary and Secondary Care*. London: National Institute for Clinical Excellence.

NIMHE (2000) *Meeting of Minds*. London: Department of Health/National Institute for Mental Health in England.

NIMHE (2003) *Inside outside* 1/3/03 http://www.nimhe.org.uk/whatshapp/item_display_publications.asp?id=330 accessed January 25, 2005.

NIMHE (2003a) *Delivering Race Equality: A Framework for Action*. Leeds, National Institute for Mental Health in England.

NIMHE (2003b) *Inside Outside Improving Mental Health Services for Black and Minority Ethnic Communities in England*. Leeds: National Institute for Mental Health in England.

NIMHE (2003c) *Real Voices: Survey Findings from a Series of Community Consultation Events Involving Black and Minority Ethnic Groups in England*. Leeds: National Institute for Mental Health in England.

Nitzan, U. and Lichtenberg, P. (2004) Questionnaire survey on use of placebo. *British Medical Journal*, **329**, 944–946.

NSCNHS Strategic Health Authority (2003) Independent Inquiry into the death of David Bennett: An Independent Inquiry set up under HSG (94)27. http://www.nscha.nhs.uk/scripts/default.asp?site_id=117&id=11516 accessed on January 22, 2005.

Obeyesekere, G. (1985) Depression, Buddhism, and the work of culture in Sri Lanka. In *Culture and Depression: Studies in the Anthropology and Cross-Cultural Psychiatry of Affect and Disorder* (ed. A. Kleinman and B. Good). Berkeley: University of California Press.

O'Hagan, M. (1996) Two accounts of mental distress. In *Speaking Our Minds: An Anthology*. (ed. J. Read and J. Reynolds). London: Macmillan, Open University, pp. 44–50.

O'Hagan, M. (2002) Living well. Open mind, **118**, 16–17.

Olafson, F. (1987) *Heidegger and the Philosophy of Mind*. New Haven: Yale University Press.

Onken, S., Dumont, J., Ridgway, P., Dornan, D. and Ralph, R. (2002) *Mental Health Recovery: What Helps and What Hinders? A National Research Project for the Development of Recovery Facilitating System Performance Indicators*. Prepared for National Technical Assistance Center for State Mental Health Planning, National Association of State Mental Health Programme Directors, USA. Available on http://www.nasmhpd.org/general_files/publications/ntac_pubs/reports/MHSIPReport.pdf accessed November 4, 2003.

Page, S. (1977) Effects of the mental illness label in attempts to obtain accommodation. *Canadian Journal of Behavioral Sciences*, **9**, 85–90.

Pembroke, L. (1996) It helped me that someone believed me. In *Speaking Our Minds: An Anthology* (ed. J. Read and J. Reynolds). London: Macmillan, Open University, pp. 168–172.

Perkins, R. (1996) Choosing ECT. In *Speaking Our Minds: An Anthology* (ed. J. Read and J. Reynolds). London: Macmillan, Open University, pp. 66–70.

Perkins, R. (2001) What constitutes success? The relative priority of service users' and clinicians' views of mental health services. *British Journal of Psychiatry*, **179**, 9–10.

Phillips, J. (1996) Hermeneutics. *Philosophy, Psychiatry, and Psychology*, 3, 61–69.

Philo, G., Henderson, L. and McLaughlin, G. (1994) *Mass Media Representations of Mental Health/Illness*. Report For Health Education Board of Scotland by Glasgow University Media Group.

Pilgrim, D. and Rogers, A. (1999) *A Sociology of Mental Health and Illness*, 2nd edn. Buckingham: Open University Press.

Porter, R. (1987) *A Social History of Madness: Stories of the Insane*. London: Weidenfeld and Nicolson.

Porter, R. (1997) *The greatest benefit to mankind: A medical history of humanity from antiquity to the present*. London: Harper Collins.

Posey, T.B. and Losch, M.E. (1983) Auditory hallucinations of hearing voices in 375 normal subjects. *Imagination, Cognition and Personality*, **3**, 99–113.

Proctor, G. (2002) *The Dynamics of Power in Therapy: Ethics, Politics and Practice*. PCCS Books, Ross-on-Wye.

Prouty, G. (2001) The practice of pretherapy. *Journal of Contemporary Psychotherapy*, **31**, 31–40.

Puustinen, R. (2000) Voices to be heard—the many

Querido, A. (1966) The shaping of community mental health care. *British Journal of Psychiatry*, **114**, 293–302.

Rabinow, P. (1984) Representations are social facts: modernity and postmodernity in anthropology. In *Writing Culture: The Poetics and Politics of Ethnography* (ed. J. Clifford and G. Marcus). Berkeley: University of California Press, pp. 234–261.

Rabkin, J.G., Markowitz, J.S., Stewart, J.W., McGrath, P.J., Harrison, W., Quitkin, F.J. *et al.* (1986) How blind is blind? Assessment of patient and doctor medication guesses in a placebo-controlled trial of imipramine and phenelzine. *Psychiatry Research*, **19**, 75–86.

Raftery, M. and O'Sullivan, E. (1999) *Suffer the Little Children: The Inside Story of Ireland's Industrial Schools*. New Island: Dublin.

Ravetz, J. (1996) *Scientific Knowledge and its Social Problems*. New Brunswick, NJ: Transaction Publishers.

Ravetz, J. (1999) What is post normal science? *Futures*, 31, 647–654.

Read, J. (1996) What we want from mental health services. In *Speaking Our Minds: An Anthology* (eds. J. Read and J. Reynolds). London: Macmillan, Open University, pp. 175–179.

Read, J. and Baker, S. (1996) *Not Just Sticks and Stones. A Survey of the Stigma, Taboos and Discrimination Experienced by People with Mental Health Problems*. London: MIND.

Read, J. and Reynolds, J. (ed.) (1996) *Speaking Our Minds: An Anthology*. London: Macmillan, Open University.

Reis, S., Hermoni, D., Livingstone, P. and Borkan, J. (2002) Integrated narrative and evidence based case report: case report of paroxysmal atrial fibrillation and anticoagulation. *British Medical Journal*, **325**, 1018–1020.

Repper, J., Sayce, L., Strong, S., Willmot, J. and Haines, M. (1997) *Tall Stories from the Back Yard. A Survey of Nimby Opposition to Community Mental Health Facilities Experienced by Key Service Providers in England and Wales*. London: MIND.

Ritchie, B. (1996) Afraid to live and afraid to die. In *Speaking Our Minds: An Anthology* (ed. J. Read and J. Reynolds). London: Macmillan, Open University, pp. 9–15.

Ricouer, P. (1979) The model of the text: meaningful action considered as text. In *Interpretive Social Science: A Reader* (ed. P. Rabinow and W.M. Sullivan). Berkeley: University of California Press, pp. 73–101.

Rivers, W.H.R. (1924) *Medicine, Magic and Religion*. London, Kegan Paul, Trench and Trübner. (Reprinted by Routledge Classics, 2001).

Roberts, G. (2000) Narrative and severe mental illness: what place do stories have in an evidence-based world? *Advances in Psychiatric Treatment*, **6**, 432–441.

Roberts, G. and Wolfson, P. (2004) The rediscovery of recovery: open to all. *Advances in Psychiatric Treatment*, **10**, 37–49.

Rogers, A. and Pilgrim, D. (2001) *Mental Health Policy in Britain: A Critical Introduction*. Basingstoke: Palgrave Macmillan.

Rogers, A., Pilgrim, D. and Lacey, R. (1993) *Experiencing Psychiatry: User's Views of Services*. London: MIND/MacMillan.

Romme, M. and Escher, S. (1989) Hearing voices. *Schizophrenia Bulletin*, **15**, 209–216.

Romme, M. and Escher, S. (1993) The new approach: a Dutch experiment. In *Accepting Voices* (ed. M. Romme and S. Escher). London: Mind Publications.

Romme, M., Honig, A., Noordhoorn, E. and Escher, A. (1992) Coping with voices: an emancipatory approach. *British Journal of Psychiatry*, **161**, 99–103.

Rorty, R. (1979) *Philosophy and the Mirror of Nature*. Princeton, NJ: Princeton University Press.

Rose, D. (2001) *Users' Voices: The Perspectives of Mental Health Service Users on Community and Hospital Care*. London: The Sainsbury Centre for Mental Health.

Rose, N. (1979) The psychological complex: mental measurement and social administration. *Ideology and Consciousness*, **4**, 5–68.

Rose, N. (1985) *The Psychological Complex: Psychology, Politics and Society in England 1869–1939*. London: Routledge and Kegan Paul.

Rose, N. (1989) *Governing the Soul*. London: Routledge.

Rose, N. (1996) The death of the social? Re-figuring the territory of government. *Economy and Society*, **25**, 327–356.

Roth, M. and Kroll, J. (1986) *The Reality of Mental Illness*. Cambridge: Cambridge University Press.

Rynearson, N. (2003) Constructing and deconstructing the body in the cult of Asklepios. *Stanford Journal of Archaeology*, **2**, available on http://archaeology.stanford.edu/journal/newdraft/2003_Journal/rynearson/accessed October 7, 2004.

Sackett, D., Haynes, R., Guyatt, G. and Trigwell, P. (1991) *Clinical Epidemiology: A Basic Science for Clinical Medicine*. London: Little Brown.

Sacks, O. (1985) *The Man who Mistook his Wife for a Hat*. London: Picador.

Sadler, J.S. (2005) *Values and Psychiatric Diagnosis*. Oxford: Oxford University Press.

Said, E. (1978) *Orientalism*. New York: Pantheon.

Samson, C. (1995) The fracturing of medical dominance in British psychiatry? *Sociology of Health and Illness*, 17, 245–268.

Sayce, L. and Measey, L. (1999) Strategies to reduce social exclusion for people with mental health problems. *Psychiatric Bulletin*, **23**, 65–67.

Sayce, L. (2000) *From Psychiatric Patient to Citizen: Overcoming Discrimination and Social Exclusion*. London: Macmillan Press.

Schwartz, L. (2003) Parallel experience: how art and art theory can inform ethics in human research. *Medical Humanities*, **29**, 59–64.

Scheff, T.J. (1966) *Being Mentally Ill—A Sociological Theory*. Chicago: Aldine.

Scull, A. (1979) *Museums of Madness*. Harmondsworth: Penguin.

Seebohm, P., Thomas, P., Henderson, P. and Munn-Giddings, C. (2004) *Sharing Voices (Bradford) Participatory Action Research Evaluation: Early Findings*. London: Sainsbury Centre for Mental Health.

Seebohm, P., Henderson, P., Munn-Giddings, C., Thomas, P., Yasmeen, S. (2005) *Together we will change: community development, mental health and diversity.* London: Sainsbury Centre for Mental Health.

Shepherd, M. (1983) *The Psychosocial Matrix of Psychiatry: Collected Papers.* London: Tavistock.

Sidgwick, H., Johnson, A., Myers, F.W.H., Podmore, F. and Johnson, A. (1894) Report on the census of hallucinations. *Proceedings of the Society for Psychical Research,* **34**, 25–394.

Siegel, R.K. (1984) Hostage hallucinations: visual imagery induced by isolation and life-threatening stress. *Journal of Nervous and Mental Disease,* **72**, 264–272.

Smart, B. (1993) *Postmodernity.* London: Routledge.

Smith, M.L. and Glass, G.V. (1977) Meta-analysis of psychotherapy outcome studies. *American Psychologist,* **32**, 752–760.

Smith, N. (1992) Post-modern organisations or postmodern organisation theory? *Organizational Studies,* **13**, 1–17.

Smith, R. (2000) The failings of NICE: time to start work on version 2. *British Medical Journal,* **321**, 1363–1364.

Spiegel, D. (2004) Placebos in practice: doctors use them, they work in some conditions, but we don't know how they work. *British Medical Journal,* **329**, 927–928.

Spiegelberg, H. (1972) *Phenomenology in Psychology and Psychiatry.* Evanston: Northwestern University Press.

Spitzer, M., Uehlein, F., Schwartz, M. and Mundt, C. (1992) *Phenomenology, Language and Schizophrenia.* Springer-Verlag: New York.

Stefan, S. (1989) Whose egg is it anyway? Reproductive rights of incarcerated, institutionalised and incompetent women. *Nova Law Review,* **13**, 406–456.

Strachey, J. (1955) Editor's Introduction. In *The Standard Edition of the Complete Psychological Works of Sigmund Freud,* Volume II. London: Hogarth Press.

Szasz, T. (1976) Schizophrenia: the sacred symbol of psychiatry. *British Journal of Psychiatry,* **129**, 308–316.

Szasz, T. (1982) The psychiatric will: a new mechanism for protecting persons against 'psychosis' and psychiatry. *American Psychologist,* 37, 762–770.

Taylor, L. (1996) *ECT* is barbaric. In *Speaking Our Minds: An Anthology* (ed. J. Read and J. Reynolds). London: Macmillan, Open University, pp. 63–65.

Thomas, P. (1995) Thought disorder or communication disorder: linguistic science provides a new approach. *British Journal of Psychiatry,* **166**, 287–290.

Thomas, P. (1997) *The Dialectics of Schizophrenia.* London: Free Association Books.

Thomas, P. and Bracken, P. (2004) Critical psychiatry in practice. *Advances in Psychiatric Treatment,* 10, 361–370.

Thornhill, H., Clare, L. and May, R. (2004) Escape, enlightenment and endurance: narratives of recovery from psychosis. *Anthropology and Medicine,* **11**, 181–199.

Thornley, B. and Adams, C. (1998) Content and quality of 2000 controlled trials in schizophrenia over 50 years. *British Medical Journal,* **317**, 1181–1184.

Tien, A.Y. (1991). Distributions of hallucinations in the population. *Social Psychiatry and Psychiatric Epidemiology,* **26**, 287–292.

Timimi, S. (2002) *Pathological Child Psychiatry and the Medicalisation of Childhood.* Hove: Brunner-Routledge.

Tooth, B., Kalyanasundaram, V., Glover, H. and Momenzadah, S. (2003) Factors consumers identify as important to recovery from schizophrenia. *Australasian Psychiatry,* **11** (Supplement), 70–77.

Topor, A. (2001) *Managing the Contradictions: Recovery from Severe Mental Disorders.* Stockholm Studies of Social Work, 18. Stockholm: Stockholm University Press.

Tuori, T.I., Lehtinen, V.I., Hakkarainen, A., Jaaskelainen, J., Kokkola, A., Ojanen, M. *et al.* (1998) The Finnish National Schizophrenia Project 1981–1987: 10-year evaluation of its results. *Acta Psychiatrica Scandinavica,* **97**, 10–17.

Turner, T. (2004) Compulsory treatment can be liberating. *British Medical Journal* (rapid responses). Available on http://bmj.bmjjournals.com/cgi/eletters/329/7458/122#69003, accessed March **10**, 2005.

United States Holocaust Memorial Museum (1996) *Handicapped*. Washington, DC: United States Holocaust Memorial Museum.

Valenstein, E. (1998) *Blaming the Brain. The Truth about Drugs and Mental Health*. New York: Free Press.

van Os, J., Verdoux, H., Maurice-Tison, S., Gay, B., Liraud, F., Salamon, R. and Bourgeois, M. (1999) Self-reported psychosis-like symptoms and the continuum of psychosis. *Social Psychiatry and Psychiatric Epidemiology*, **34**, 459–463.

Vygotsky, C.S. (1978). Mind in society: the development of higher psychological processes. London: Harvard University Press.

Wahlbeck, K., Tuunaaineen, A., Gilbody, S. and Adams, C.E. (2000) Influence of methodology on outcomes of randomised clozapine trials. *Pharmacopsychiatry*, **33**, 54–59.

Walker, C. (1988) Philosophical concepts and practice: the legacy of Karl Jaspers's psychopathology. *Current Opinion in Psychiatry*, **1**, 624–629.

Walker, C. (1994*a*) Karl Jaspers and Edmund Husserl I: the perceived convergence. *Philosophy, Psychiatry and Psychology*, **1**, 117–137.

Walker, C. (1994*b*) Karl Jaspers and Edmund Husserl II: the divergence. *Philosophy, Psychiatry and Psychology*, **1**, 245–265.

Warden, J. (1998) Psychiatrists hit back at home secretary. *British Medical Journal*, **317**, 1279.

Warner, R. (1994) *Recovery from Schizophrenia: Psychiatry and Political Economy*, 2nd edn. London: Routledge.

Wertsch, J. (1991) *Voices of the Mind: A Sociocultural Approach to Mediated Action*. Harvester Wheatsheaf.

Westen, D. (1990) Physical and sexual abuse in adolescents with borderline personality disorder. *American Journal of Orthopsychiatry*, **60**, 55–66.

Whitaker, R (2004) The case against antipsychotic drugs: a 50-year record of doing more harm than good. *Medical Hypotheses*, **62**, 5–13.

Whitaker, R. (2002) *Mad in America*. Cambridge, MA: Perseus Publishing.

Wiggins, O.P. and Schwartz, M.A. (1997) Edmund Husserl's influence on Karl Jaspers's phenomenology. *Philosophy, Psychiatry, and Psychology*, **4**, 15–36.

Wigren, J. (1994) Narrative completion in the treatment of trauma. *Psychotherapy*, **31**, 415.

Williams, B., Thomas, P., Murray, I. and Lefevre, S. (1999) Exploring 'person-centredness': user perspectives on a model of social psychiatry. *Health and Social Care in the Community*, **7**, 475–482.

Williams, J. and Watson, G. (1996) Mental health services that empower women. In: *Mental Health Matters: A Reader* (ed. T. Heller, J. Reynold, R. Gomm, R. Muston and S. Pattison). London: Macmillan, Open University, pp. 242–251.

Williams, J. (1999) Social inequalities and mental health. In *This is Madness: A Critical Look at Psychiatry and the Future of Mental Health Services* (ed. C. Newnes, G. Holmes and C. Dunn). Ross-on-Wye: PCCS Books, pp. 29–50.

Winter, R. and Munn-Giddings, C. (2001) *A Handbook for Action Research in Health and Social Care*. London: Routledge.

Wittgenstein, L. (1961) *Tractatus Logicophilosophicus* (trans. D. Pears and B. McGuiness). London: Routledge & Kegan Paul.

Wittgenstein, L. (1967) *Philosophical Investigations*, 3rd edn. (trans. G.E.M. Anscombe). Oxford: Blackwell.

World Health Organization (2002) *Mental Health Global Action Plan: Close the Gap, Dare to Care*. Geneva, WHO. Downloaded at http://www.who.int/mental_health/media/en/265.pdf on 18 February, 2005.

Wurtman, J. and Suffes, S. (1996) *The Serotonin Solution: The Potent Brain Chemical That Can Help You Stop Bingeing, Lose Weight, and Feel Great.* New York: Fawcett Columbine.

Yusuf, S., Cairns, J., Camm, A., Fallen, E. and Gersh, B. (1998) *Evidence Based Cardiology.* London: BMJ Publishing Group.

Author index

Subject index